Understanding Alzheimer's

ALSO FROM NAHEED ALI

Diabetes and You: A Comprehensive, Holistic Approach

The Obesity Reality: A Comprehensive Approach to a Growing Problem

Understanding Alzheimer's

An Introduction for Patients and Caregivers

Naheed Ali

ROWMAN & LITTLEFIELD PUBLISHERS, INC.
Lanham • Boulder • New York • Toronto • Plymouth, UK

Published by Rowman & Littlefield Publishers, Inc.
A wholly owned subsidiary of The Rowman & Littlefield Publishing Group, Inc.
4501 Forbes Boulevard, Suite 200, Lanham, Maryland 20706
www.rowman.com

10 Thornbury Road, Plymouth PL6 7PP, United Kingdom

British Library Cataloguing in Publication Information Available

Library of Congress Cataloging-in-Publication Data

Ali, Naheed, 1981-
  Understanding Alzheimer's : an introduction for patients and caregivers / Naheed Ali.
    p. ; cm.
  Includes bibliographical references and index.
  ISBN 978-1-4422-1753-9 (cloth : alk. paper)—ISBN 978-1-4422-1755-3 (electronic)
  I. Title.
  [DNLM: 1. Alzheimer Disease. WT 155]
  616.8'31—dc23   2012013305

∞™ The paper used in this publication meets the minimum requirements of American National Standard for Information Sciences—Permanence of Paper for Printed Library Materials, ANSI/NISO Z39.48-1992.

Printed in the United States of America

Understanding Alzheimer's is dedicated
to my students, to Alzheimer's disease patients,
and to all who provided encouragement and
support throughout my research.

Contents

Disclaimer

This book represents reference material only. It is not intended as a medical manual, and the data presented here is meant to assist the reader in making informed choices regarding wellness. This book is not a replacement for treatment(s) that may have been suggested by the reader's personal physician. If the reader believes he or she is experiencing a medical issue, professional medical help is recommended. Mention of particular products, companies, or authorities in this book does not entail endorsement by the publisher or author.

Preface

$\mathcal{P}$eople suffering from a particular disease will have abnormal or deviated characteristics, but anyone can study the abnormalities and explore their possible cure. People want to stay in touch with friends and want to lead a happy and joyful life, and since a healthy body makes a healthy mind and keeps it sharp, it is important to learn about diseases such as Alzheimer's if one wants to keep up with life and maintain its spark.

As a person gets older, he or she faces memory and cognitive problems. It is a simple fact of nature. Forgetfulness becomes a noticeable part of everyday life with every passing minute, hour, and day. This is why it can be very difficult to recognize the early stages of Alzheimer's disease. Studying Alzheimer's disease is, in this sense, of utmost importance for aging individuals and the people who look after them. Understanding the disease in its entirety also makes it easier for patients to cope with their specific problems. Alzheimer's disease is currently the most rapidly growing neurodegenerative disease.[1] People above sixty-five years of age have a high tendency of being affected by this disease,[2] and additional statistics[3] show that almost thirty million of the world's population is suffering from Alzheimer's. Learning about other diseases is also very important because doing so provides an individual with adequate knowledge of what tests should be conducted before and after a successful diagnosis. On the other hand, one might be suffering from not Alzheimer's but rather another form of mild dementia. It is important to rule out all the possibilities of any serious illness.

It can be difficult to recognize the symptoms of Alzheimer's disease. However, it is important to recognize the early symptoms which emerge before any signs of memory loss or brain damage is actively recorded. As the complete cure for this disease is yet to be unearthed, researchers try to focus on people with a probable risk of being affected and reduce any kind of fear or other psychological factor. Alzheimer's research uses volunteers who are already affected by the disease, under the supervision of the latest technology, to determine the root cause—and possible cure—of the problem.

Elderly people want to lead a healthy and peaceful life just as much as everyone else. However, remembering the important events and tasks, such as a grandson's birthday, the last day to submit an important assignment, or the time and date of an appointment with a doctor, can be difficult with Alzheimer's disease. No one really wants to forget the important activities and tasks of life. Alzheimer's is a fatal disease that, in most severe cases, can take away one's cognitive ability to think and to remember basic events. The problem can even separate two loved ones.[4]

Alzheimer's can be categorized by three different staging systems, each explained comprehensively in part IV. The initial phase (of each of the staging systems) is usually the most difficult one to spot. It is very important for individuals who wish to provide care to their family members or to their loved ones to understand the stages of this disease. Medical studies confirm that the early phases of the disease, no matter the staging model used, can be very deceptive.[5] Physicians and scientists are trying to find a solution for detecting the first phase of the disease. They believe that, if the early phase is detected, patients can be treated easily by psychologists. The memory impairments associated with Alzheimer's can be treated but not cured, while other symptoms of the disease can be easily avoided.

The Harvard School of Public Health conducted a recent survey that focused on awareness and concern about Alzheimer's disease among participants in Europe and the United States.[6] The results of this survey were mind-boggling and showed that more than 86 percent of the participants in Europe and America are afraid of the disease and say they would be relieved to discover early on that they suffer from it, rather than finding out after the disease reaches terminal levels. The results also suggested that Alzheimer's is the second-most feared medical problem, with cancer being the first. Most of the surveyed people, especially adults, were able to identify the symptoms of the disease in themselves. They reported experiencing common symptoms such as forgetting important tasks and losing a sense of direction while on their way to college or home. Approximately thirty respondents in European countries were confident that a cure exists.[7] They believed the progression of the disease can be slowed down and that a permanent form of treatment exists.

Before moving on deeper within this book, the reader should know that the journey to treating Alzheimer's disease can be difficult because of its relation to other brain disorders. If not detected early, Alzheimer's can lead to other fatal ailments such as Parkinson's disease.[8] It would then be extremely difficult to cope with both diseases, and in most cases, the patient would have little chance of escaping death unnaturally. The root cause of brain-related illness should, therefore, be dealt with quickly to prevent any serious injury to the brain or to other vital organs. Ways of overcoming the illness should be learned as soon as possible, rather than having the patient go through otherwise avoidable challenges.

Simply put, understanding the internal (physical) and external (effects on life) characteristics of Alzheimer's disease is of utmost importance in today's society. This disease is separated into different phases or stages. These phases should be examined thoroughly in order to understand the foremost question of why this disease should be studied. Since Alzheimer's is the most rapidly growing neurodegenerative disease of the elderly population,[9] the reader should understand its progression before getting introduced to other in-depth discussions on the subject.

Patients lead normal and productive lives at the initial phases of Alzheimer's disease. The symptoms of the disease start to become apparent when it is not addressed in time. After that, there comes a point when it cannot be controlled. If the disease is not discovered in a timely manner, there is little or no chance that a patient's mental health will be restored to normal. The periodic length of any stage or phase is indeterminable. Once out of the picture, the other stages slowly continue to diminish the patient's mental health and badly affect the mental capacity to think and remember.

Stage 1 of the disease, based on the seven-stage model covered in chapter 10, does not involve any cognitive impairment as the symptoms are mild and are very difficult to spot. Individuals in the first phase do not experience any problems with remembering names and daily chores. They face no difficulty while communicating with other individuals, and they can easily recall their way home. They do not encounter any problems with carrying out their daily life activities and appear to be ordinary individuals.

Stage 2 involves a slow decline in an individual's cognitive abilities. Affected individuals will experience memory losses, forgetting the names of their loved ones, and will also have difficulty speaking to others. Furthermore, patients suffer from decision-making problems. Logical decisions will be even more difficult to execute. The patient's sleep cycle also gradually declines, causing fatigue and laziness. In addition to the said sleep issues, patients will require constant supervision since they may develop a habit of sleepwalking.[10]

An increase in the severity of the above symptoms occurs as the disease progresses. In the third or fourth stages, patients start to confuse the past with the present. Gradually, patients may find themselves confined to their beds and at the mercy of their caregivers. Such patients will slowly lose their speaking or language skills because of the disease. The last few stages of Alzheimer's disease can be fatal because sufferers cannot manage the disease alone.

Research done by Dalhousie University's Department of Medicine involving seven thousand Canadian nationals evaluated the health and aging effects on people sixty-five years of age or older.[11] At the end of the ten-year study period, more than 40 percent of the study subjects had died. The subjects developed a form of dementia and other cognitive disabilities. Of the remaining percentage, almost 20 percent of the people had developed cognitive disabilities. The investigator leading the study said that minor health problems might have had a cumulative effect on the brain, which would have caused Alzheimer's in the patients.

A healthy body makes a healthy mind and keeps it sharp. The investigators' hypothesis suggests that minor health problems are the cause of Alzheimer's because these minor issues have a cumulative effect on the brain. Experts believe that what is best for the body is best for the brain as well.[12] Minor problems in the central nervous system, if not addressed promptly, may develop into Alzheimer's disease. When the patient passes away, he or she may not be included in the statistics when measuring the magnitude of the disease because it may have gone unreported.[13]

The reader may already have a broad understanding of what Alzheimer's disease is, but some information about the disease such as the hormonal causes discussed in chapter 3, as well as unconventional treatments, are easily overlooked these days. For instance, field studies suggests that some daily activities such as drinking coffee in minor amounts might also help relieve symptoms of Alzheimer's.[14] A study on the effects of caffeine was conducted at the University of Coimbra and the University of Lisbon.[15] One experiment within the same study proved that caffeine can have a positive effect on the brain as well as on the body. Another experiment, part of the same study, proposed that moderate coffee drinkers have a probable chance of developing Alzheimer's disease.

Another reason to learn more about Alzheimer's is its sheer magnitude, both demographically and symptomatically. Clinical reports suggest that forty million people are suffering from dementia, known as a stand-alone medical condition as well as the primary symptom of Alzheimer's disease.[16] These reports also indicate major possible causes of Alzheimer's, including diabetes mellitus, hypertension, smoking, depression, obesity, physical inactivity, and low education levels. While researchers are putting forth their best efforts to find a single cause and an all-in-one solution to the disease, I encourage all to learn about this growing problem to identify people who are affected so these sufferers can be examined and treated in time.

I

GROUNDWORK

History of Alzheimer's

*W*ell into the twenty-first century, societies have had the urge to learn more about various disorders and their origins. Experts have even gone as far as finding out how each disorder affects the behavior, socialization, and growth of a person. It is crucial to also understand the origins of a disease so that progress can be made in finding a cure. It is important to keep track of a disease's origin, such as that of Alzheimer's, because people will, with time, change the perception of the disease. This altered perception will also affect the diagnosis and course of action pertaining to treatment.[1]

Mental disorders and brain-related diseases such as Alzheimer's have existed even during the time of ancient civilizations. Societies of those eras had a way of realizing that some mental behaviors were not normal. All cultures have their code of conduct, which can in turn render some behaviors boisterous or misplaced. Societies were subjected to different cultures, as some behaviors considered normal in one would be considered irregular in another.[2] Mental disorders are widespread, and globally, one in three people will, during their lifetime, display traits that can qualify as mental disorder symptoms.[3]

PREVALENCE THROUGHOUT HISTORY

Mental disorders were widespread in ancient civilizations, but even then, there was a criterion in place for telling the difference between sound mind and "mental patient." For example, ancient Egyptian and Mesopotamian cultures had a document that is now referred to as the Ebers Papyrus.[4] This document makes references to hysteria and melancholy as forms of mental disorders. The document also considered heart disease and uterine problems to be mental disorders.[5] These are not currently the phases of being in a state of mental destruction or loss of focus, but back then, it was common practice to refer to these as spells or spiritual attacks. That is why a number of treatments included the recital of magical spells even as bodily fluids were applied onto the patient.[6] Religious gatherings were hotspots for people who needed spells removed.[7]

Due to their large prevalence, mental health disorders such as Alzheimer's are not completely alienated ideas.[8] A study found that 20 percent of all Americans suffer from a mental disorder.[9] Some of these traits include schizophrenia, "shell shock," hysteria, and anxiety. Mental disorders simply lurk in the shadows and strike people unexpectedly. Because mental disorders were highly unpredictable, it was important that all who suffered had some means of getting help.[10] By the turn of the Industrial Revolution, there was a widespread creation of laws in the Western world that pushed authorities to form care programs for those suffering mental and neurological disorders. Still, very little was achieved because the people who were minding those suffering from mental disorders were merely nurses and administrational staff hired to tend to—but not clinically treat—the patients.[11]

INTRODUCTION TO HIPPOCRATES

In 400 BC, a Greek scholar named Hippocrates devised studies about mental disorders and examined a number of patients. The scholar came close to discovering that mental disorders, such as that which is known today as Alzheimer's, were caused, in a great part, from having levels of body "humors" that exceeded the normal levels. Body humors are fluids present in the body that have to be in balance for a person to be healthy. An excess or lack of them meant otherwise. In Hippocrates's time, *sanguine, melancholic, choleric,* and *phlegmatic* were the four humors examined when determining a person's psychological dispensation. In a contemporary setting, "melancholy" applies to mental or emotional states of depression. Historically, however, "melancholia" was viewed as a physical as well as mental state, and melancholic conditions were evaluated by their roots rather than how they manifest.[12] In a similar vein, melancholia was previously a reference to mental disorders that can today be diagnosed as schizophrenias or some bipolar disorders.

Hippocrates soon suggested that mental disorders came directly from the lack or excess of body humors. Back then, body humors were considered fluids that directly correlated and metaphysically expressed environmental influences in the form of pain or other physical qualities of the body. This is basically an earlier version of the contemporary view that mental instability arises from disturbances in the body's neurotransmitters.[13] Neurotransmitters are chemicals that conduct electrical signals in the nervous and musculoskeletal systems, allowing for movement and other functions. Hippocrates held the view that cases such as schizophrenia and anxiety stem from what goes on around a person. Hippocrates refuted the idea that spells, demons, or godly beings are the causes or remedies of a disease. He believed that all matter is made up of physical elements. These elements include air, water, earth, and fire. In that sense, he believed tangible things such as man's behavior and the seasons could be blamed for disease and could bring healing. Whenever the four humors were unbalanced, treatments were taken to restore stability. Common remedies included laxatives and bleeding. Primary care at the time, including for mental disorders such as memory or cognitive issues, would require rest, proper air circulation, good diet, and water. Furthermore, herbal extracts such as willow bark were used for relieving pain while a disease ran its course.[14]

Hippocrates offered a paradigm shift to traditional medicine, traversing from spiritual inclination to logic. He believed that physicians should delve into each mental symptom in a patient-to-patient basis, rather than finding conclusions and cures related to each disorder. To fulfill this, he came up with the idea of performing clinical observations. His means of observing a patient involved four stages of action. These stages of assessing a patient for what is now termed Alzheimer's included proper diagnosis, prognosis, close observation, and finally, good treatment. Hippocrates also concluded that the prevailing doctrine of the four humors would determine a person's overall health or sickness.[15]

ALZHEIMER'S DISEASE COMING TO LIGHT: ALOIS ALZHEIMER

Alois Alzheimer was a renowned scientist from Marktbreit, a municipality in southern Germany. Born in 1864, he did well in sciences at school and therefore studied medicine and did research in Germany throughout his career. He went to Tubingen and Wurzburg schools where he graduated with a medical degree in 1887. He commenced work in a country asylum in Frankfurt. It was there that he became interested in doing advanced research on the human brain. His work focused primarily on the brain cortex, and he furthered his education in subjects such as psychiatry and neuropathology. Alzheimer committed most of his years to histological and histopathological research related to the cerebral cortex, a part of the brain discussed in more detail in chapter 2. Alzheimer believed nerve cells have a lot to do with the overall pathology of a human being's nervous system. His work on the cortex was published in 1907.[16] He earned accolades afterward and was appointed the director of the asylum where he used to do his research. Motivated, he continued to investigate manic depression along with schizophrenia and other psychiatric disorders.

Alzheimer was the first to recognize Alzheimer's disease as a distinct mental disorder. It all began in 1901, when he was carefully following the case of a fifty-six-year-old woman named Auguste Deter,[17] who would pass away six years later.[18] It was around that time that similar cases were noticed. Emil Kraepelin later chose to include Alzheimer's disease as a separate type of dementia in his 1910 textbook of psychiatry since it could not be said to have a similar cause to the other cases of dementia.[19]

Looking for a post where clinical practice is possible while academic research was done, Alzheimer decided to be an apprentice of Emil Kraepelin who also worked at a medical school in Munich, Germany, in 1903. In Munich, Alzheimer created a research program that was intended only for cerebral research. He had by this time mastered theories and practices regarding the nature of the brain. By 1906, his research and discoveries had brought him to the limelight. His name grew exponentially. Alzheimer then noticed a little-known disease that affected the human brain, especially during his observation of the elderly woman mentioned earlier. This "disease" was found to be responsible for a lot of her memory loss, overall disorientation, and sporadic hallucinations. She died at the age of fifty-five.

Alzheimer joined a team of Italians who also were interested in learning the staining techniques that help identify amyloid plaques. The same research also pointed toward irregular structures in the brain known as neurofibrillary tangles. In 1906, Alzheimer convened a speech that was the first to touch on the pathology behind the symptoms manifested by dementia patients. He merged the two ideas of pathology and presenile (before old age) dementia for the first time through a string of promising experiments using microscope slides.

At any time, the original works of Alzheimer can be revisited and the specimens he worked on can be seen. Alzheimer left behind a small but important cache of reference material, including the original microscopic findings on which he based his inferences of Alzheimer's disease. This has been in Munich all along, and scientists periodically reevaluate these artifacts when needed.[20]

The examinations that Alzheimer did on postmortem specimens pointed to a number of abnormalities that were in Deter's brain. He noticed her cerebral cortex was thinner than would be a cortex with senile plaques, which are substances found normally in minimal amounts in elderly people. He also found substantial quantities of neurofibrillary tangles. With that, Alzheimer had enough reasons to delve deeper into the topic and was able to point to nerve tangles that had never before been described. As a result, Kraepelin named this newly discovered disease after Alzheimer.[21]

FRANZ NISSL AND THE HISTORY OF ALZHEIMER'S

Franz Nissl was a German-born neuropathologist who lived from 1860 to 1919.[22] He pioneered a new way of staining cells to examine them under the microscope, now called the Nissl method. This discovery was made while he was a medical student and was published ten years later. Nissl also did work in psychiatry and found a correlation between nerves and mental disease. While still a medical student, he was encouraged by his professor to submit a paper on the pathology of brain cells in the cortex. When he discovered there was a prize in neurology, he submitted the paper and won the competition.[23]

He was a friend, as well as coresearcher, of Alois Alzheimer for many years. Nissl was an excellent pianist and had a keen sense of humor. Due to his preoccupation with his work, Nissl never married. He felt keenly the weight of teaching and administration and, due in part to his kidney ailment, was unable to complete all of his work before his death. He was an administrator of a large military hospital during World War I and later died of kidney disease in 1919.[24]

PRIOR INTERPRETATIONS

Before Alois Alzheimer made his discovery in 1907, scientists, researchers, and the public community looked at dementia as if it was a natural element of the aging process, and as such, senility had to be accepted as normal whenever a person aged. According to an honors thesis regarding the progression of the now known Alzheimer's disease, that view was very common in the past.[25] Alzheimer's disease was not that different from other common types of old-age-induced dementia or even senility itself. Even after Alzheimer's findings, the disease was having difficulty getting accepted as a full-blown disease in the scientific and medical community. People would still look at the disease and its origins, symptoms, and progression and call it senility or dementia. The thesis insists that Alzheimer's was not a commonly referred term or an important issue. This was the case until neurological research gained better ground toward the late 1970s. In 1980, the Alzheimer's Association was formed; then things started to take a new turn. People started to look at Alzheimer's as a more serious disease. Alzheimer's disease was no longer considered a cause of aging exclusively, though the latter is still recognized as one of the key roles in the disease's development.[26]

ROOTS OF DIAGNOSIS

The globally accepted definition of dementia refers to a reduction in memory capacity and cognitive characteristics compared to how the patient used to function previously. As explained in further detail in chapter 5, Alzheimer's has always been diagnosed in a person when there is a constant decline in day-to-day physical and mental performance and also as a result of abnormalities stemming from clinical observation and a neuropsychological examination. Therefore, the history of Alzheimer's itself suggests that the disease cannot be diagnosed accurately simply because a patient's consciousness is blurred or when a number of other clinical abnormalities block the proper evaluation of somebody's mental state. Dementia alone is clinically tied to irregular human behavior,[27] and a brain scan cannot exclusively lead doctors to find dementia in a person. An electroencephalogram (EEG) and other common laboratory instruments will also not work, and certain causes of dementia require thorough testing. This is what the National Institute of Neurological and Communicative Disorders and Stroke/Alzheimer's Disease and Related Disorders Association (NINCDS–ADRDA) concluded after much work and research was completed by1984.[28] Thereon, scientists looked at Alzheimer's disease differently from stand-alone dementia.

ROOTS OF ALZHEIMER'S RESEARCH

Why is there is so much difficulty and anticipation in the fight to make gains with Alzheimer's research? Scientists know that Alzheimer's disease will always involve progressive brain cell malfunction, but the *reason* these cells do not work has never been too clear. Much like other persistent illnesses of the brain, health professionals are convinced that Alzheimer's is a complex consequence of various personal and social stimuli and other overriding causes.[29] Both old age and genetic traits have already been labeled as risk factors, but so many questions are yet to be answered. The emergence of more risk factors in the environment will widen the comprehension of why Alzheimer's disease develops in some patients but not in others. Although Alzheimer's disease is not considered a normal part of aging, continual aging is the most obvious risk factor associated with the disease.[30]

RESEARCH DIFFICULTY

While the current situation of Alzheimer's research in the United States will be covered extensively in chapter 15, it is important to look at why the disease has been so difficult to research throughout its history. Simply put, there are many byproducts of stand-alone dementia that can be mistaken for Alzheimer's. These include Parkinson's disease and thiamine deficiency.[31] Alzheimer's, commonly mistaken with other diseases, also took a while to be recognized as a full-blown disease because the path of development and the source of the disease varies from patient to patient.[32]

In the early stages of Alzheimer's research, scientists focused primarily on the main feature that stood out in Alzheimer's disease—notable loss of cognitive ability of a person, followed by mild forms of aggression and fluctuating mood. Using natural approaches to the disease and taking both personal and social-based approaches were not too common. Even now, it is best to have the patient taken to a care institution so treatment can be more encompassing. By the time Alzheimer's disease starts to take its toll on a patient, the families have already borne a great emotional and financial responsibility. The burden of an Alzheimer's patient is very heavy, and making matters worse, there is no 100 percent cure. Drugs are being researched with the assumption that there are insoluble deposits present in the brain of a person suffering from Alzheimer's.[33]

DRUG RESEARCH

Throughout the history of Alzheimer's disease, a substantial number of drugs have provided a decent level of relief from the symptoms. These drugs do so even though there is no cure and are therefore often welcomed as a "better than nothing" option. It is very apparent that, before a cure comes along, there needs to be adherence to the most basic of mechanisms relating to the handling of the disease. Looking back at the history of the disease and understanding its reactions to drugs of the past and present remains a priority in the interim. Nevertheless, research aimed at effective drug treatments for Alzheimer's has made great strides through history. Topics destined to provide betters solutions to Alzheimer's disease include adult stem cell research and intranasal growth factor (INF) techniques.

• 2 •

Anatomy, Pathology, and Physiology of Alzheimer's

$\mathcal{A}$natomy is defined as the science that studies the structure of the human body or of any living organism, as well as the relationships between the parts that make up either one.[1] Physiology deals with the examination of how the human body or a living organism functions.[2] For example, anatomy describes the parts that make up the nervous system such as the brain, but physiology goes into detail by giving an explanation of how the brain works in order for the entire nervous system to perform its role properly.

Pathology, on the other hand, is the medical branch that studies diseases.[3] Pathology describes and explains what a certain disease is, how the disease came to be, how it presents, its signs, and its symptoms. It focuses on the changes in the human body caused by the disease and how it affects a normal person's behavior and characteristics.[4] Since Alzheimer's disease symptoms include gradual loss of memory, intellect, skills, and the ability to learn, the disease leads to anxiety and depression. Pathological manifestations of Alzheimer's has led to psychological studies of the disease, as well as research in the area of psychotherapy aimed to help patients cope with the emotional and mental changes caused by Alzheimer's.[5] It is also important to look at Alzheimer's from the physiological point of view to fully understand how and why the brain is affected by this disease. This knowledge goes a long way in possibly preventing Alzheimer's and, maybe even one day, to find a viable cure for it.

ANATOMY OF THE BRAIN

To study anatomy related to Alzheimer's disease, one must look at the brain. The brain has nine parts, explained in the following sections.

11

Cerebrum

The cerebrum, Latin for brain, is the largest part of the brain, making up approximately 85 percent of the brain's weight.[6] The cerebrum's surface is called the cerebral cortex, thin layers of nerve cells. Under the cortex are nerve cell fibers that connect the cerebrum to other parts of the brain and to the spinal cord. This cortex is folded and convoluted into ridges called gyri and "valleys" called sulci. The sulci divide the cerebrum into four lobes.[7]

Various parts of the cortex handle the feelings and movements of the human body. The sensory cortex receives messages from the body's sensory organs. The motor cortex sends out impulses that command the skeletal muscles.[8] The largest part, the association cortex, is responsible for processing information that makes all mental capabilities such as thought, speech, and memory possible but would otherwise get hindered in Alzheimer's disease. The cerebrum is further divided into two halves: the right cerebral hemisphere and the left cerebral hemisphere. These hemispheres are joined by neuronal complexes, the largest being the corpus callosum. Normally, one hemisphere is more dominant than the other. For right-handed and most left-handed people, the left hemisphere is the dominant part of the brain.[9]

Corpus Callosum

There are more than two hundred million nerve fibers that make up the corpus callosum.[10] Its main function is to combine all activity in the left and right hemispheres of the brain. This part of the brain is functionally developed by approximately twelve years of age[11] but may improve and grow throughout a person's teenage life until he or she reaches adulthood.[12] The corpus callosum is the largest and most important connector of the two hemispheres, but there are other pathways such as the anterior commissure, the posterior commissure, and the hippocampal commissure, all of which are made up of nerve fibers.[13]

The Lobes

The right and left hemispheres of the cerebrum are both subdivided into four major lobes: frontal, parietal, temporal, and occipital. These lobes are responsible for emotions, analysis, and reasoning and how the senses function. The frontal lobes are found around the front part of the head. They deal with speech, judgment, planning and prioritizing, muscle movements, problem solving, and creativity. The parietal lobes are situated behind the frontal lobe, at the top and back part of the head. This is the part where reading, mathematics, temperature, taste, and touch are processed. The temporal lobes are located on the left and right sides, above the ears and below the frontal and parietal lobes. These lobes are involved with memory, language, hearing, meaning, learning, and sound. The occipital lobes are found in the lower back part of the brain. They take care of special recognition and vision.[14]

Cerebellum

The word "cerebellum" comes from the Latin term meaning "little brain." The cerebellum is shaped similarly to a cauliflower, found below the occipital lobe and behind the brain stem. The cerebellum deals with balance, movement coordination, and posture. It is made up of a large number of folia (leaflike nerve cells) packed together. The cerebellum consists of two hemispheres, the left and the right, connected by a structure called the vermis. The right hemisphere is joined by nerves to the left cerebral hemisphere and to the right part of the body. The left hemisphere connects to the right cerebral hemisphere and left part of the body.[15] Solid clinical research finds that Alzheimer's disease targets specific cells in the cerebellum.[16]

Hippocampus

According to medical studies, many nerve cells that are lost due to Alzheimer's disease are regenerated by the hippocampus of the brain.[17] However, clinical research has found that the hippocampus of an Alzheimer's disease patient shrinks in size.[18] The hippocampus is located on both sides of the brain, under the medial temporal lobes. It is grouped with the rest of the brain's hippocampal formation, of which the dentate gyrus, the subiculum, the presubiculum, the parasubiculum, and entorhinal cortex are parts. The hippocampus acts as a gateway for the recollection of factual events, and as discussed in chapter 4, memory loss is one of the symptoms of Alzheimer's. The hippocampus also regulates emotions and is a part of the cerebral cortex that deals with smell.[19]

Thalamus

MRI studies have found that the thalamus shrinks as a result of Alzheimer's disease.[20] The thalamus can be found in the center of the brain, below the corpus callosum. It is a gray mass that aids in the brain's sensory and motor activities. Neurons in the thalamus process sensory information, after which the information is sent to the overlying cortex and later to the cerebral cortex.[21] The thalamus has two parts: the dorsal thalamus and the ventral thalamus. The dorsal thalamus relays messages to the cortex, while the ventral thalamus acts as a shield for the dorsal thalamus.[22]

Hypothalamus

The hypothalamus is affected early on when a person gets Alzheimer's disease.[23] This gland can be found at the middle base portion of the brain, below the thalamus. It is divided by the third ventricle and is composed of cell groups or nuclei. The hypothalamus is a small region that performs many of the brain's functions. These include the control of major hormone releases, food and water ingestion, temperature regulation, sexual behavior and reproduction, the body's biological clock, stress, and emotional responses.[24]

Pituitary Gland

The pituitary gland has been found to be more active in Alzheimer's, as *growth hormone* (GH) response is higher in such patients.[25] GH is provided by the pituitary gland. This gland can be found below the hypothalamus, in an area at the base of the skull referred to as the sella turcica. The pituitary gland, also named the hypophysis, closely functions with the hypothalamus. It is shaped like a garbanzo bean and has two parts: the adenohypophysis, or anterior pituitary, and the posterior pituitary or neurohypophysis. The anterior pituitary is a gland made up of cells that release protein hormones. Meanwhile, the posterior pituitary is an annex of the hypothalamus as a group of hypothalamic neurons that drops down behind the anterior pituitary. This forms the pituitary stalk. Hormones that are secreted by the pituitary gland control neurons in the brain and affect the other endocrine glands of the body.[26]

Brainstem

The brainstem basically connects the brain to the spinal cord. It is found at the very base of the brain and is responsible for survival functions such as breathing, blood pressure, and heartbeat. It also plays a role in consciousness, basic attention, and arousal. It is composed of three parts: the midbrain or mesencephalon, the pons, and the medulla. The midbrain helps in vision and eye movement, hearing, body motion, and voluntary motor function. Slow physical movement and loss of fine motor skills are noticed regularly in Alzheimer's patients.[27] The pons region of the brain takes care of motor control and sensory analysis and is linked to sleep, consciousness, movement, and posture. The medulla, or medulla oblongata, is located between the pons and spinal cord. This is the part that deals with blood pressure, breathing, and heartbeat.[28]

PATHOLOGY OF ALZHEIMER'S

"Pathology" comes from the Greek words *pathos* meaning *suffering* and *logia* meaning "the study of." Pathology as discussed to this point is the science concerning the causes, appearances, and mechanisms of diseases. It is practiced through autopsies and examinations of tissues, organs, cells, and bodily fluids.

It includes diagnosing and monitoring diseases, as well as conducting medical research related to causes and cures of sicknesses. When considering the purpose of the field of medicine, one can say that most of medicine *is* pathology. After all, trips to the emergency room or doctor's office as a patient do not usually happen unless there is a problem.

There are different disciplines that fall under the general category of pathology, including the following:

- Anatomical pathology
- Chemical pathology
- Clinical pathology
- Forensic pathology
- General pathology
- Hematopathology
- Immunopathology
- Cytopathology
- Dermatopathology
- Neuropathology
- Pediatric pathology
- Micropathology

Each of the above disciplines focuses on a specific aspect of various diseases.

The two main divisions of pathology are clinical and anatomical pathology. All other subspecialties fall under either of these two. Anatomical pathology is when a disease, such as Alzheimer's, is studied according to visual examinations of organs and tissues. This is also when causes of death due to diseases are thoroughly studied. Gross examination is where the expert looks at visible tissues and organs, sometimes with the help of a basic magnifying glass. A more detailed process is histopathology, when haematoxylin and eosin are used on slides during microscopic examinations.[29] Immunohistochemistry is when antibodies are employed to characterize the makeup of some cancers by detecting proteins present in them. Cytopathology is simply the use of cytology to study loose cells on microscope slides. Electron microscopy, used in the diagnoses of kidney disorders and others, uses microscopes to magnify organelles in cells. In situ hybridization makes use of DNA and RNA molecules that are dyed with a fluorescent dye and can thus be studied.

Clinical Pathology

Clinical pathology is based more on the analysis of laboratory results. This involves bodily fluids, urine, blood, and tissues using chemistry, hematology, microbiology, and molecular pathology. Clinical pathology makes use of macroscopic examination, meaning an inspection with the naked eye followed by a validation using more tests. Microscopic examination is when microscopic techniques such as cytochemistry, immunocytochemistry, and also the use of fluorescent dyes allow for a magnified inspection of bacteria, parasites, yeasts, molds, or viruses. Analyzers are another process in clinical pathology. These are complex systems mainly for medical biochemistry and hematology purposes. Cell cultures are perhaps the largest part of clinical pathology. They help to identify causes of infections and diseases, including Alzheimer's.

Doctors who specialize in this field are simply called pathologists. They diagnose and distinguish diseases as well as interpret laboratory results. In fact, many cancers have been discovered by pathologists. Some of the most famous pathologists throughout time have included ancient Greek doctors such as Hippocrates, Herophilus, and Erasistratus, as well as Avenzoar of Arabia. The "father of microscopic pathology" is Rudolf Virchow.[30] Others who have contributed significantly to the field of pathology include the following:

- Edwin Klebs
- Carl Rokitansky
- Elizabeth Stern
- Julius Cohnheim
- Harry Brookes Allen
- John York
- Paul Langerhans
- Justine Johnstone.[31]

A popular forensic pathologist is Cyril Wecht, who worked on the case of former U.S. president John F. Kennedy.

PHYSIOLOGY OF ALZHEIMER'S

Physiology is the study of how the body works. The term *physiology* comes from the Greek words *physis* meaning "origin" and *logia* meaning "study of." It is also about how body parts function together and how internal and external changes affect a person, animal, or plant's movement and behavior. This is known as homeostasis. Physiological research is responsible for what people now know about the different systems of the body; life processes such as birth, puberty, and adulthood; and health-related subjects. Divisions of physiology include the following:

- Applied physiology
- Evolutionary physiology
- Defense physiology

- Cell physiology
- Comparative physiology
- Environmental physiology
- Human physiology
- Ecophysiology

Types of Physiology Explained

Applied physiology pertains to when physiology is practiced in different areas of specialization in order for stability to return to a body. Comparative physiology is the study that covers the physiology of other living things such as plants and animals, as compared to human physiology. Human physiology focuses on the human body and its normal functions, with respect to similar studies in comparative physiology. Defense physiology studies how a human body functions and reacts to life-threatening situations and the changes that happen when it prepares itself for such changes. Ecophysiology, also called environmental physiology, examines how humans and other living organisms adapt to various environmental conditions. It is closely tied to evolutionary physiology, which is the study of how organisms have functioned and changed throughout history. Cell physiology focuses more on the biological aspect and studies how a cell works and interacts with its surroundings.

People who study physiology are referred to as physiologists. Notable physiologists include the following:

- Hippocrates, "the father of medicine"
- Aristotle
- Claudius Galenus
- Persian writer Avicenna
- Andreas Vesalius, considered the founder of human anatomy
- William Harvey
- Herman Boerhaave
- Matthias Schleiden
- Theodor Schwann
- Claude Bernard
- Walter Cannon
- Knut Schmidt-Nielsen
- George Bartholomew
- Alan Lloyd Hodgkin
- Ivan Pavlov
- Albrecht von Haller[32]

Pathophysiology, alternatively called physiopathology, is a combination of pathology and physiology. Although both sciences focus on different areas, they are similar in that they both study the human body, or living things in general. Pathophysiology, then, studies the changes that take place and how a human functions as a result of a disease or an injury. This consists of physical and biological manifestations more commonly known as signs and symptoms. Pathology addresses not methods of treating a disease directly but rather primarily the disruptions in a body's condition. Thus, the pathophysiology of various diseases and injuries are commonly named after the disease or injury being studied, such as the pathophysiology of epilepsy, the pathophysiology of diabetes, or the pathophysiology of Alzheimer's disease.[33]

ALZHEIMER'S UNDER THE MICROSCOPE

Alzheimer's disease is generally caused by a continuous loss of nerve cells or neurons in the brain. It is a degenerative disease that worsens with time and affects most of the brain, particularly the hippocampus. Alzheimer's disease presents differently in each patient because its physiological and pathological evolution does not follow a set pattern. This results in complex signs and symptoms for people who have the disease. What one Alzheimer's disease patient is going through is not necessarily what another is experiencing.[34]

A brain with Alzheimer's has significant shrinkage of tissues wherein the entire brain literally becomes smaller.[35] The sulci, or grooves, widen while the gyri, or folds, shrivel, creating gaps within the brain's outer layer or cortex while losing important nerve fibers that control feelings, movements, and reasoning. The ventricles become enlarged, and as the cells in the hippocampus begin to deteriorate, a person loses his or her short-term memory and speech functions.

Moreover, Alzheimer's affects a part of the brain called the amygdala. The amygdala controls fear and anger. Therefore, damage to it results in impaired judgment and uncontrollable emotional responses, leading to outbursts of temper and possibly violent reactions. The brain stem, which manages sensory signals involving hearing, vision, and basic life functions such as blood pressure, breathing, and heart rate becomes greatly compromised as well, from as early as the onset of Alzheimer's in a patient. As Alzheimer's disease spreads throughout the cerebral cortex, the frontal lobe is damaged soon thereafter. Hence, slightly complex processes such as planning, logical thinking, cooking, driving, and learning are hampered. Alzheimer's in the frontal lobe diminishes motivation while increasing lethargy and impulsive behavior. The parietal lobes and temporal lobes suffer as well. With the parietal lobes damaged, cognitive skills such as writing, reading, mathematical abilities, and space perception deteriorate drastically. This means that a patient becomes unable to find objects and cannot estimate distances correctly. Language capabilities;

recognition of familiar things, places, and people; hallucinations; and remembering personal information are slowly lost when the temporal lobes become affected by Alzheimer's.

GENERAL PHYSIOLOGICAL AND ANATOMICAL CHANGES

The general changes of an Alzheimer's patient are in his or her inabilities to remember things and to do routine activities. Since Alzheimer's diseases works by destroying the brain gradually, more neurons eventually die, resulting in drastic physiological and anatomical changes. Therefore, a patient is constantly agitated, starts wandering, is unable to recognize anything, cannot communicate, and loses control of his or her body functions. In the most advanced stages of Alzheimer's, a patient needs complete care and constant attention. In spite of major changes in the brain, the average span of Alzheimer's is from eight to ten years, though some patients have been known to live longer than that.[36]

SIGNIFICANCE OF ANATOMY AND PHYSIOLOGY IN ALZHEIMER'S

Knowing the parts of the brain and the functions each part carries out, as well as the fundamental pathology of Alzheimer's disease, is necessary for a holistic understanding of a patient's condition. Even a basic grasp of why and how an Alzheimer's patient is acting the way he or she is helps a person to approach the situation with sensitivity and a sense of responsibility. In addition, knowing the anatomy and physiology of an Alzheimer's patient's brain will allow a person to identify signs and symptoms present in others, thus paving the way for medical assistance. This knowledge is the first step not just toward helping a patient with Alzheimer's but also to finding possible treatments for medical mysteries that have long caused great suffering and innumerable deaths. That said, the brain is responsible for all tasks essential to human survival; once a part of it has been damaged, the entire body is compromised. While recent advancements have been made in nerve cell regeneration,[37] medical research has yet to demonstrate a viable way of conducting complete brain transplants.[38] Until then, people have to learn to take good care of themselves, not just the organs such as the brain or the heart, but also the entire body in order for everything to function properly and to be free from Alzheimer's diseases well into old age.

II

CLINICAL PICTURE

• 3 •

Causes of Alzheimer's

$\mathcal{N}$eurological disorders such as cerebral palsy, progressive supranuclear palsy, idiopathic seizures (seizures of unknown cause), and Alzheimer's disease have something in common. Their physical similarities are due to the fact that, until now, their specific etiology (cause) has not been fully understood. This may be due to the complexity of brain processes and functions, as well as conflicting reports of the disease from patients and health-care professionals alike. Ongoing clinical studies such as those cited throughout this book are still conducted with the hopes of finding answers and revealing the causes of Alzheimer's disease. Thorough investigations and studies for Alzheimer's have already been made, and yet, its causation is not fully comprehended.

MAJOR RISK FACTORS

Scientists have identified familial, lifestyle-related, and environmental risk factors that predispose one to the disease. Some factors are modifiable, giving patients the chance to change unhealthy habits, but others are nonmodifiable, that is, constant and true for all. It is highly recommended to know and remember these risk factors since it can help in preventing and lessening the risk of developing the disease.

Age

Age is the primary risk factor for Alzheimer's disease.[1] The prevalence of the disease escalates with advancing age because, as people get older, the brain tends to function less effectively. This change can bring forth memory gaps and many other problems that can also progress to Alzheimer's disease.

Gender

Studies have revealed that Alzheimer's disease occurs more frequently in women than in men.[2] This is likely due to the loss of estrogen for women after menopause. Estrogen, a sex hormone found predominantly in females, possesses certain characteristics that give protection to the brain against memory loss and decline in mental functioning. With the onset of menopause, a decline in estrogen leads to a higher risk of developing Alzheimer's. Medical research proves that estrogen has direct, protective qualities against Alzheimer's disease.[3] From a broader perspective, hormonal changes are not the only reason for the increased risk of getting Alzheimer's in women. On average, women tend to live longer than men and thus have a naturally higher chance of acquiring the disease.[4]

Gene Connection

From a genetic standpoint, Alzheimer's disease has two forms of origin—the late onset sporadic and the early onset familial. Most Alzheimer's patients fall into the late onset category, accounting for 95 percent of the cases.[5] The remaining 5 percent belong to the early onset, familial type.[6] The early onset, familial type of Alzheimer's disease occurs when certain genetic mutations get passed on from one generation to another. If one of the parents suffers from the early onset, familial type, the chances are that 50 percent of the children will likewise bear the disease.[7] One defective gene passed on is enough for the development of the disease in a person. This type of Alzheimer's has been reported among individuals thirty to forty years old,[8] hence the term "early onset." The late onset, sporadic type is composed of multiple factors that result in the occurrence of the disease. It can still be brought about by genetics, lifestyle, and environmental factors. Reports state that having a parent or a sibling with Alzheimer's significantly increases the chances that a person will get the late onset type.[9]

The apolipoprotein e4 gene (APOE-4) has been implicated extensively in Alzheimer's. The presence of this risk gene can signify a late onset, sporadic type of the disease. APOE-4 is one of the APOE genes responsible for the regulation of protein production and transportation of cholesterol and fats among the cells in the body. Having at least one copy of the gene will increase the risk of getting Alzheimer's. It has been found that 40 percent of patients suffering from late onset, sporadic Alzheimer's have at least one copy of the APOE-4 gene.[10] Alzheimer's disease can still develop in those who lack the APOE-4 gene, and from the percentage above, it can be concluded that genetics do play a minor role in the development of Alzheimer's. The majority of patients with Alzheimer's disease have been found not to have genetic risk factors at all. Experts are also not recommending that parents let their children undergo genetic testing since the gene may or may not develop into Alzheimer's. One must bear in mind that Alzheimer's is irreversible, and with no cure, genetic testing is of little use until a major breakthrough occurs.[11]

DNA Mutations

Living organisms contain DNA that serves as a blueprint and a carrier of genetic information that determines the patient's characteristics. DNA provides a set of "instructions" to the cells regarding their function and purpose in an organism. DNA needs to contain all the correct genetic codes for the body to function normally and appropriately. In rare circumstances, DNA can undergo permanent changes, resulting in errors in genetic codes that can cause disorders and diseases to occur. These changes and errors are known to be DNA mutations and are irreversible and considered culprits for the development of genetic disorders. Many genetic disorders involving DNA have been discovered, including Alzheimer's disease. Of the two types of Alzheimer's disease, the early onset familial is highly genetic in nature and results in genetic mutations in one of three genes: amyloid precursor protein (APP), presenilin-1 (PSEN1), and presenilin-2 (PSEN2). These three genes are essential proteins in the body, and alterations in any of the genes result in an increased production of beta-amyloid protein.[12] Beta-amyloid protein will clump together and form highly toxic plaques in the brain, leading to neural degradation and death. The presence of beta-amyloid protein in the brain can be seen in all patients with Alzheimer's and is one of the conclusive biomarkers used for the diagnosis of the disease (see chapters 5 and 8).

Early onset, familial type is genetic in nature, which means it can be passed on easily to offspring. One copy of the mutated gene is enough to develop Alzheimer's disease later in life. There is a 50 percent chance of getting the disease when one parent is the carrier of the mutated genes PSEN1 and PSEN2, and if both parents are considered carriers, it will yield a 100 percent chance that all of the offspring will develop the disease.[13] However, APP, PSEN1, and PSEN2 genetic mutations occur very rarely, accounting for only 5 percent of all Alzheimer's disease cases.[14] Therefore, it is important for the caregiver to (1) obtain a complete family history of the patient and (2) check for the presence of early onset, familial type of Alzheimer's disease within the family to make adjustments and preparations if needed.[15]

Lifestyle

Poor lifestyle habits that could lead to high blood pressure, high cholesterol levels, atherosclerosis, and diabetes are now considered to be risk factors for Alzheimer's disease.[16] These conditions can contribute to the damage and death of brain cells by hardening the blood vessels and blocking oxygen flow to the brain. Academic research makes it clear that linkages between diabetes, which is clearly linked to lifestyle,[17] and Alzheimer's disease exist.[18] Individuals suffering from Alzheimer's concurrently with diabetes or hypertension are much more likely to die sooner as compared to those without hypertension and diabetes.[19]

Low Education Level

A study reveals that individuals with low education levels (less than six years) are more prone to suffer from Alzheimer's disease.[20] This speculation has been linked to the effects of continuous learning to the brain. Learning can stimulate the brain cells, making them stronger and healthier, and thus less likely to break down. Another study notes that individuals who achieve a higher formal education have stronger cognitive reserves that provide greater resilience against brain damage.[21] By having high levels of cognitive reserves, the risk for having Alzheimer's disease, dementia, and other neurological disorders will lessen due to protective qualities against harmful and detrimental brain changes described in the preceding chapter.[22]

There has been research to test the relationship of education and Alzheimer's disease patients, an example being a study involving patients with Alzheimer's disease where the researchers tested the patients' cognitive skills.[23] The participants of the study were grouped according to level of education. The testing specifically included patient's abilities with memory, thought, and information processing as well as their capabilities to reach for objects within their perceptual field. The test yielded results more favorable for those who have undergone formal education longer. The researchers then concluded that people who went to school longer and gained a higher degree tend to create a reserve in the brain, making the brain more capable of coping with Alzheimer's symptoms. More education also helps the brain adapt more, delaying otherwise fast degradation of the brain in patients with Alzheimer's disease. So, some people with high levels of formal education may still acquire Alzheimer's, but because of their higher education, symptoms of the disease occur with less impact and with slower progression. Based on the results of the study, researchers advise obtaining a high level of formal education. Higher education not only leads to better jobs and salaries but can be of great protection to the brain as well. The goal should be to never stop learning and thus stimulating the brain.

Exposure to Aluminum

Exposure to different toxic substances can trigger the development of different neurological disorders. Aluminum exposure is currently being considered a possible cause of Alzheimer's. Research was conducted during the 1990s where scientists injected aluminum in animals.[24] They found that aluminum produced neurofibrillary tangles in the brains of the animals that were similar to the tangles found in Alzheimer's. The advent of such neurofibrillary tangles may signify Alzheimer's disease-causing aluminum, a substance that could potentially trigger the disease. Some experts speculate that patients with Alzheimer's disease tend to be more vulnerable to aluminum, accumulating it in neurofibrillary tangles faster than others. Regardless of whether aluminum exposure will soon be widely accepted as a risk factor or not, it is best for an Alzheimer's patient to stay away from this toxic substance as much as possible.

Pollution

The identification of pollution as another relevant risk factor for Alzheimer's disease is clearly a breakthrough in the medical field. A team of researchers from the University of Southern California conducted an experiment to evaluate the effects of traffic pollution on the occurrence of Alzheimer's disease, brain damage, and inflammation.[25] Published recently, this study was also initiated to further identify other hazards of traffic, vehicular, and freeway pollution. This kind of pollution is very rampant nowadays, and Alzheimer's patients can inhale particles of air containing combinations of exhaust gas, burning fossil fuels, weathering pavements, and car parts along with the dusts from roads almost every day as they are stuck in traffic, traveling, or living near freeways. The particles from the air that people breathe in cannot be seen by the naked eye; they are so tiny yet very hazardous to one's health. The researchers created an environment resembling the vehicular traffic pollution using concrete freeway particles, with mice as the subjects. The mice were exposed to vehicular traffic pollution for five hours a day, three times a week. This lasted for ten weeks with a total of 150 hours of exposure.

The researchers then analyzed the brains of the mice after the ten-week exposure to traffic pollution and yielded significant results. Brain neurons responsible for learning and memory were largely damaged. The brain also suffered from inflammation similar to that seen in premature aging and Alzheimer's disease, as well as stunted growth of the brain neurons, impairing brain development. Particles from the traffic pollution studied were so small they bypassed filtration systems in cars. This creates a problem in finding the correct solution since patients cannot escape from these particles as long as they continue to be exposed in traffic and live in urban areas. The only thing patients can do is to stay away from traffic and the freeway as much as possible and lessen the exposure by covering the nose and mouth.

PHYSICAL BRAIN CHANGES WITH ALZHEIMER'S

As people get older, organs tend to degenerate and function less effectively, and the brain is no exception to this inevitable event.[26] Healthy elderly people may be subjected to occasional memory loss, which is normal. In patients with Alzheimer's disease, the effect of occasional memory loss is much more severe and debilitating. Certain brain changes have been found specifically for Alzheimer's disease patients that will help in the diagnosis and confirmation of the disease. Scientists are still unsure whether these changes cause Alzheimer's disease or are a result of Alzheimer's.

Senile Neuritic Plaques

Deposits of beta-amyloid protein that clump together and form plaques in the brain are found in patients diagnosed with Alzheimer's disease. Due to this finding, the plaques now serve as a cause of and an indicator that a person is suffering from Alzheimer's disease. Beta-amyloid protein is a fragment of amyloid precursor protein (APP) that is normally broken down and excreted out of the body. Due to several circumstances where the beta-amyloid protein is not excreted, it builds up in excess, forming plaques in the brain. These plaques disrupt the brain's communication pathway and repair process. Later on, the plaques destroy the brain cells, and during tissue biopsy, they are usually surrounded by dead brain cells or related debris.[27]

Neurofibrillary Tangles

Neurofibrillary tangles are recognized more as a symptom of Alzheimer's (see chapter 4) rather than a cause. However, clinical research suggests that the tangles lead to dementia,[28] of which Alzheimer's has been noted to be the leading cause.[29] These are abnormalities within a nerve cell consisting of twisted nerve fibers. The nerve fibers are called microtubules; they provide the framework and support and give structure and shape to nerve cells. Microtubules allow the transport and flow of nutrients within the cell. Within the microtubules are tau proteins that, in turn, stabilize the microtubules. When tau proteins disintegrate, microtubules disassemble, leading to the formation of neurofibrillary tangles. Under normal circumstances, neurofibrillary tangles subsequently go through neural degradation and die.[30]

CHEMICAL BRAIN CHANGES LEADING TO ALZHEIMER'S

Aside from the risk factors and abnormal brain changes that were identified by scientists, certain chemical changes also take place among patients with Alzheimer's disease. Scientists have been speculating that these changes are the causes for the disease, but until now, it remains a theory and has yet to be proved. Furthermore, discovery of these changes has led to advances in the diagnosis and treatment of Alzheimer's disease.

Acetylcholine Deficiency Leading to Alzheimer's

Nerve cells need neurotransmitters for communicating and processing different information in the brain. An example of a neurotransmitter is acetylcholine. Acetylcholine plays an essential role in the brain as it is greatly associated with processing memory, learning, cognition, and motor function. Acetylcholine in adequate amounts is beneficial for memory. This neurotransmitter makes the patient remember, learn easily, and move with strength and coordination.

Acetylcholine levels tend to be very low in patients with Alzheimer's and could later completely diminish from the brain if left untreated.[31] This phenomenon explains the reason for memory loss and learning ability amongst Alzheimer's disease victims. As the disease progresses, motor function will deteriorate as well. The reason for the loss of acetylcholine in the brain is the excess of beta-amyloid protein. As discussed to this point, beta-amyloid protein is the molecule responsible for forming neuritic plaques. It will not only form plaques but also destroy acetylcholine because it is a neurotoxic substance when in the brain. Therefore, the presence of beta-amyloid protein is the cause of acetylcholine pathology in Alzheimer's disease. Acetylcholinesterase inhibitors, explained further in chapter 6, have been added to the list of treatment options to prevent further reduction of acetylcholine. This would lead to a slower progression of memory loss, decreased learning ability, and depressed motor function of the brain.[32]

Biochemical Deficiency Explained

Research evaluating the association between the loss of growth-promoting factors in the brain and Alzheimer's disease has been taking place since the 1980s.[33] Nerve growth factor (NGF), a biochemical that promotes the proper functioning of brain cells, may be deficient in some individuals who are on the road to getting Alzheimer's disease. Experiments have also revealed that NGF in rats results in a growth of synaptic connections, especially in the hippocampus, possibly restoring memory loss.[34]

Scientists are now on the verge of investigating the possibility of safely introducing nerve growth factors in the brain among Alzheimer's patients as part of the treatment modalities used for the disease. However, a disadvantage is that NGF can be neurotoxic.[35] Increased amounts of it in the brain can also add to further nerve cell destruction and the development and progression of Alzheimer's disease.

Amyloid Changes Leading to Alzheimer's

Some studies find that amyloid changes in the brain are brought on by Alzheimer's itself,[36] while other clinical reports maintain that such changes are both the cause and the result of the disease.[37] The exact relationship remains unclear.[38] The role of amyloid in Alzheimer's disease will be discussed in further detail later, but first, it is important to understand that amyloid is an abnormal protein made by the cells from the bone marrow that can be deposited anywhere in the body—not just the brain. High accumulation of amyloid protein in a specific organ or tissues is toxic if it does not get excreted and will lead to the development of amyloidosis. Amyloidosis may affect only a part of the body known as local amyloidosis or it may spread throughout the body affecting multiple organs known as systemic amyloidosis. It affects vital organs such as the heart, kidneys, liver, spleen, lungs, and brain. Amyloidosis alters the structure and function of the organs and may lead to multiple organ failure up to the death of the patient. It is a serious and life-threatening disease that occurs in rare occasions. The amyloid light (AL) version of amyloidosis affects 1,200 to 3,200 new patients annually in the United States.[39]

Early detection of the disease is needed as prompt treatment is necessary to reduce mortality rates caused by the disease. Though one study found that Congo red testing should not be a preferred means to diagnose amyloidosis,[40] others suggest differently.[41] Congo red testing is nonetheless widely accepted as a diagnostic test for amyloidosis and involves a biopsy of the affected tissue. After the biopsy, the tissue is coated and stained with a special dye (Congo red). The test is positive if the amyloid protein gives off an apple-green glow when viewed under polarized light. Once amyloid protein is seen and detected, medication therapy is soon initiated to stop the former's progression and reduce any resultant complications, but it is important to remember that there is no complete cure for amyloidosis.[42] Treatment therapy is geared toward relieving the symptoms, stopping their otherwise speedy progression, and preventing organ failure and includes many other interventions to prolong the life of the patient.

Inflammation

Inflammation is a physiological process that occurs whenever the body is in contact with a harmful stimuli and an unknown, potentially threatening organism. Inflammation can surface in any part of the body, depending on the area of invasion by the pathological stimuli or organism. In the brain, neuroinflammation can occur and go undetected due to the absence of pain receptors in the brain. Neuroinflammation yields more harmful effects as compared to the inflammatory processes in the periphery. Researchers note that inflammatory response plays a role in exacerbating the pathological processes of the disease, thus contributing to the development and progression of Alzheimer's disease.[43] Inflammation in this regard comes about from the presence of microglias and astrocytes in the brain. A microglia is a cell that provides support and protection to the neurons. It is a type of macrophage (a strong immune system cell) in the brain that acts to defend the central nervous system. If there are harmful lesions and organisms that contact the brain, the microglias initiate an inflammatory response to fight back. Although the microglia can render protective effects on the brain, they can also be neurotoxic at the same time. As beta-amyloid proteins deposit in the brain and form senile plaques, microglias are activated, forming clusters around the senile plaques. This gives off reactive oxygen species and releases the chemokines and cytokines named interleukines 1 and 6 that have toxic and detrimental effects on the brain, harming otherwise healthy neurons along the way.[44]

The continued release of cytokines in increased amounts by the microglias as the microglias try to remove the senile plaques will only add to the inflammatory burden, destroying and degrading neurons. Interleukin-6, a type of cytokine, is seen in high concentrations among patients with Alzheimer's disease. This leads to a conclusion that inflammatory responses occurring in the brain greatly contributes to the disease process by worsening and giving further damage to the neurons. These findings are highly significant as they add to the full understanding of the disease process. Still, there are unanswered queries to the full relationship of neuroinflammation and Alzheimer's disease. Scientists are still not sure if neuroinflammation contributes to the development of the disease or occurs secondary to the disease process. Its actual timing of activation and occurrence is still not fully understood. Further probes into the topic are currently undergoing.[45]

Free Radicals as Possible Causes of Alzheimer's

Free radicals are molecules that possess an unpaired electron and are highly unstable. Due to the instability of free radicals, they tend to latch on to other molecules and steal their electrons to render themselves stable. The unpaired electrons can bind to large molecules such as proteins and fatty acids, and alter DNA's structure and function. These alterations result in cell damage, cell degradation, and consequently—cell death. The central nervous system (CNS), which primarily constitutes the brain and spinal cord, is highly sensitive and reactive to free radical damage that results in more serious injuries as compared to other systems of the body. The brain accounts for 20 percent of oxygen usage in the body,[46] and a high metabolic rate can increase the amount of free radicals that the CNS carries.[47] The CNS is also rich in fatty acids, which are readily oxidized and contain low amounts of enzymes and antioxidants that fight free radicals. These identified properties of the central nervous system, specifically in the brain, will lead to more free radical attacks that can cause brain damage. Such free radicals and oxidative stress on the brain increase the likelihood of Alzheimer's, as the two are closely associated with neuronal death, a typical characteristic of the said disease.

Studies have also discovered that beta-amyloid proteins are capable of producing free radicals in the brain.[48] Free radicals are released as soon as the beta-amyloid protein forms plaques and surround a brain cell. These plaques were found to have toxic effects on the cells of the hippocampus, the part of the brain that is responsible for memory. The findings of the scientists indicate that beta-amyloid protein destroys brain cells in many ways that may lead to a faster progression of the disease.

ANALYSIS

Knowing the possible etiologies (causes) is a major step in finding out other significant details concerning any given case of Alzheimer's disease. The possible causes serve as the backbone that bridges other approaches to the disease. The importance of trying to identify the causes and risk factors are threefold. First, the entire disease process and its complications will be known, which is crucial in formulating the overall action plan to prevent things from getting worse. The key to promote health and prevent the occurrence of just about any disease is having patients and caregivers that know and understand its causes. Second, appropriate clinical testing will be laid out for the patient so that correct diagnoses can be made. Correct diagnosis is also crucial in treating a patient suffering from Alzheimer's, or any other disease. Third, the appropriate treatment and preventive measures can be given if the causes of a disease are known.

This chapter explored a few studies of unusual causative factors of Alzheimer's, such as the role of aluminum in increasing the chances of Alzheimer's.[49] Some of these studies have deemed that ingestion of certain aluminum compounds can actually lead to Alzheimer's, although these studies are still inconclusive and tend to be contradictory at best. Nevertheless, scientists are hoping that, once the surefire cause of Alzheimer's has been clearly defined, the medication that could put a stop to it would be found.

Since medical research has yet to uncover a specific cause of Alzheimer's, patients have difficulty understanding the disease. Several risk factors and different changes, when identified, are enough for people to understand the nature and course of the disease. Alzheimer's disease affects not only the physical aspect of a person but the emotional and social aspects as well. That is why obtaining knowledge on the risk factors and associated changes leading to Alzheimer's disease will help the patients and their families to cope better and understand its complexities. Knowing the risk factors leading to Alzheimer's helps caregivers handle and approach patients appropriately, feel the patients' burdens, and realize specific needs. In broader terms, there will be a significant improvement on all aspects of care for patients suffering from Alzheimer's disease once the causes, risk factors, and symptoms are well understood.

· 4 ·

Symptoms of Alzheimer's

*E*veryone is susceptible to disease, but some might not take notice until the situation has finally developed into something potentially fatal. The likelihood of any disease can be hindered, and one can always avoid further development of a disease by knowing its symptoms. Having a keen understanding of the symptoms is the key to detecting any disease, whether Alzheimer's or another, while still at an early stage. An Alzheimer's patient can experience immediate medical relief from symptoms, though only with a slight possibility of being cured. One must also be aware that some diseases can only be treated to alleviate symptoms but are incurable in nature. In the following sections, the symptoms of Alzheimer's will be discussed thoroughly to help the reader understand the results of such a disease.

First, a symptom is different from a medical sign. As defined in medicine, symptoms are the characteristics of a disease that are felt internally by the patient.[1] These characteristics include experiences from injury, illness, or ailments such as chills and shivering during a fever, or vertigo and nausea during a hypertensive crisis. On the other hand, a medical sign is a definite hint of a disease that a doctor can visualize or quantify. A sign entails the physical manifestation of the injury, illness, or disease including high temperature associated with fever, rapid pulse, and high blood pressure during hypertension. Simply put, a symptom is more subjective compared to a medical sign, which is more objective and verifiable by individuals other than the patient. Both are important, but the latter helps the doctor more when it comes to identifying the symptoms of Alzheimer's.

MENTAL SYMPTOMS

Research shows that people with Alzheimer's disease experience extreme memory loss.[2] This is characteristic of a specific Alzheimer's stage known as mild cognitive impairment (MCI), believed to be the most fundamental sign for elderly people who suffer from preliminary Alzheimer's. The forgetfulness of a patient suffering from Alzheimer's disease can be organized into two different categories: retrograde and anterograde amnesia.[3] Retrograde amnesia involves the loss of recent memory possibly connected to a traumatic incident that occurred before the start of the disease. The second, anterograde amnesia, involves loss of memory of incidents happening after acquiring the disease itself. A patient with Alzheimer's disease usually starts with retrograde amnesia. After a few months, the disease slowly progresses and shows signs of anterograde amnesia, making the patient suffer from severe and permanent memory loss.

Retrograde Amnesia

According to research, Alzheimer's disease starts with retrograde amnesia.[4] Academic sources state that retrograde amnesia is memory loss of events that happened prior to an incident.[5] Studies suggest that a patient experiences forgetfulness of episodic and declarative memories at the start of the disease due to damage in parts of the brain responsible for storage of such memories.[6] These parts include (1) the hippocampus, which deals with memory consolidation, (2) the diencephalon, which is in the front part of the brain and consists of other important structures, and (3) the temporal lobes, essential for processing facts. Damage in these areas of the brain can cause problems in a patient. Such problems can include impaired thought organization, categorization of verbal material, disturbance of language comprehension, and impaired long-term memory. In this case, Alzheimer's patients completely forget their own personal information such as their name, phone number, and address.[7]

Retrograde amnesia patients have been clinically found to have higher levels of irritability.[8] At the start of the disease, patients may not be able to recall where they live or were born. Patients also forget all the events that occurred since birth—information that could probably define their entire existence. From the damage caused to the rightward region of the temporal lobes, patients can also suffer from nonrecognition of nonverbal materials such as music and drawings, and can have difficulty naming objects such as a clock, a ball, or other objects typically seen around the home. In addition, retrograde amnesia patients experience minor language problems, including forgetting what they have recently heard and having a tough time understanding what is being said by another person or even themselves.[9] For example, when a patient with retrograde amnesia listens to a relative who is talking about a birthday, the patient may ask for the story to be repeated. The patient may ask, "What are you talking about?" or, "What was that again?" Another manifestation of anterograde amnesia is trouble with following basic directions for an already familiar task. This may involve forgetting how to ride a bike, how to cook, or how to prepare breakfast. The patient also experiences difficulty in planning, organizing, and concentrating, and this most often leads to specific personality changes.

Anterograde Amnesia

According to a peer-reviewed website, anterograde amnesia is the inability to create new memories after the onset of the disease, which leads to a short-term memory loss or difficulty in recalling the past.[10] A textbook on the subject of clinical neurology mentions that anterograde amnesia is really the loss of memory pertaining to what occurred before a specific event, rather than after.[11] This type of amnesia can happen together with retrograde amnesia, and when it does, the phenomenon is clinically referred to as global amnesia.[12]

An Alzheimer's disease victim who is suffering from global amnesia has varying degrees of forgetfulness and experiences declarative memory loss. The person still retains nondeclarative memory, also known as procedural memory. For instance, a patient with anterograde amnesia might still remember how to ride a bike, use the phone, cook a recipe, or prepare a breakfast but might forget the actions taken after completing the tasks. This can be well portrayed in a scenario where, after eating breakfast, a female patient makes a telephone call. After hanging up the phone, the patient forgets she had breakfast and might ask others what she did before calling, what was for breakfast, or even whether it was breakfast or lunch. The patient may also question the identity of the person on the phone, why the person was calling, or why she was on the phone with them. When Alzheimer's patients have loss of procedural memory that is not considered global amnesia, they simply suffer from procedural transient amnesia.[13]

DEMENTIA AS A SYMPTOM

According to reports, a person who suffers from Alzheimer's disease also experiences some form of dementia.[14] Dementia is mostly experienced by older people from age 85 onward and is manifested by loss of mental skills affecting the patient's daily life. A study involving more than two thousand participants found that the rate of dementia is very high in elderly patients of low socioeconomic status.[15] Via another report, dementia can also be explained as a progressive set of symptoms that targets and damages some parts of the brain responsible for memory, language, problem solving, and attention.[16] As the patient gets older, dementia also gets worse. A person who is suffering from this disease experiences general symptoms such as memory loss, moodiness, and communicative difficulties. For instance, patients may forget their home address after going to the store. They can become more aggressive and impatient, losing their temper easily, or experiencing too much anxiety about what is happening in the surrounding environment. The patient may also develop difficulty speaking and writing in a later stage or during severe dementia.

As demonstrated by other research, dementia can also be a result of alcoholism, drug ingestion, hormonal and vitamin imbalance, and depression.[17] Dementia caused by such factors is reversible, while dementia caused by various diseases such as Alzheimer's is irreversible. According to data, dementia is divided into two major categories: cortical and subcortical.[18]

Dementia, while technically not a disease, is really an outcome of other diseases that affect the anatomy and physiology of the brain. Alzheimer's is one such disease that causes dementia, but there are many others. Since there are a lot of possible sources of dementia, the types of dementia have been classified according to the part of the brain most involved. Other categorizations of dementia are based on whether it can be treated. In effect, Alzheimer's is a combination of four subcategories: progressive, primary, secondary, and cortical dementia.

Only around 10 percent of dementia cases can be treated.[19] Treatment in this case would mean the dementia is reversible or has been stopped completely. Normal-pressure hydrocephalus, brain tumors or brain cancer, hypothyroidism, neurosyphilis, poisoning, vitamin B_{12} deficiency, and dementia due to medications are some of the treatable cases. Nontreatable dementia are those that come with severe brain disorders such as Alzheimer's, Lewy body disorder, Binswanger's, Pick's or frontotemporal dementia, Huntington's, Creutzfeldt-Jakob disease, Parkinson's, HIV-related dementia, and head trauma.[20]

Progressive, Primary, and Secondary Dementia

Progressive dementia is when patients lose more of their abilities to function physically, emotionally, and mentally over a period of time. It can happen very rapidly in some diseases, but in Alzheimer's, progressive dementia occurs slowly. Primary dementia is inherent to a disease and is not a result of anything else. Secondary dementia comes from other injuries or physical disorders, as a resulting symptom.

Cortical Dementia

Cortical dementia is caused by damage in the cerebral cortex and outer layers of the brain responsible for thinking abilities, memory skills, and language. When the cerebral cortex is damaged, the Alzheimer's sufferer experiences impaired initiation and sequence of physical tasks. In this case, the patient goes through severe memory loss as well as aphasia, the inability to recognize and understand certain words. Cortical dementia can lead to negative changes in social behavior.

Subcortical Dementia

Subcortical dementia results from damage in some parts of the brain beneath the cortex.[21] This type of dementia is very different from cortical dementia because a person with such problems experiences severe motor abnormalities such as a slow rate of thinking and an inability to initiate activities. These abnormalities can occur conjointly with emotional disturbances and problems with physical movement and pain sensation. An example of this is Binswanger's disease (see chapter 12), Parkinson's disease, Huntington's disease, HIV–AIDS, and Steele-Richardson-Olszewski syndrome (progressive supranuclear palsy or PSP). Such abnormalities can be exemplified in a scenario where a patient is pinched yet only feels the pain seconds afterward. This is due to a slowed reaction time and malfunction of motor skills because of damage in the subcortical parts of the brain.[22] Additionally, there are various types of dementia that are named according to the condition that caused the disease.[23] These types are explained in the following sections.

Vascular Dementia

Vascular dementia refers to symptoms that are caused by a disease, such as Alzheimer's disease.[24] A patient who suffers from this condition goes through short-term memory loss, difficulty in solving problems, and trouble with concentrating; these symptoms are due to the death of brain cells when the supply of blood in the brain is hindered. Factors that hinder the supply of blood include hypertension, heart problems, high cholesterol, and diabetes. Other factors, such as a lack of physical activity, alcohol addiction, and heredity, can also worsen an Alzheimer's-related case of vascular dementia.[25] The most noticeable symptoms of this state include depression, epileptic seizures, acute confusions, hallucinations, delusions, physical and verbal aggression, and restlessness. For an example, a woman suffering from vascular dementia might be found walking and chatting with an imaginary friend but then forget where she is going. In this case, the patient is not only imagining or hallucinating but also forgetting her destination. One may also suffer from vascular dementia and exhibit some symptoms of Parkinson's disease such as trembling movements.

There are two types of vascular dementia. The first is called stroke-related dementia, which is described as a permanent damage in the brain due to a hindrance of blood supply in the brain. The other is known as small vessel disease–related dementia, described as direct damage to small blood vessels in the brain. The effects of stroke-related dementia on a person depend on which part of the brain is damaged. When the damaged area of the brain is responsible for movement of limbs, the person is paralyzed, but when the area is responsible for speech, the person will have difficulty communicating clearly. Stroke-related dementia is also the reason an Alzheimer's patient, after experiencing a severe stroke, tends to be more forgetful than usual, possibly causing a family member to simply think it is senility. Stroke-related dementia can be categorized in two ways. Dementia that is caused by a single stroke is known as single-infarct dementia, while dementia that is caused by a series of small strokes is called multi-infarct dementia. A person under this condition might experience slurred speech, weakness on one side of the body, and blurred vision. Research confirms that, even in the absence of preexisting dementia, a stroke leads to Alzheimer's disease.[26]

Small vessel disease–related dementia is also known as subcortical vascular dementia. When the problem turns severe, it turns into Binswanger's disease. A person who is suffering under such a condition experiences walking problems,[27] but brain lesions, found in many Alzheimer's patients, are a critical process in diagnosing Binswanger's.[28]

Dementia with Lewy Bodies (DLB)

Lewy body dementia happens when abnormal protein outgrowths called Lewy bodies infiltrate the brain. Symptoms are different from Alzheimer's and other diseases that manifest dementia. A Lewy body dementia patient suffers from hallucinations and paranoia and demonstrates signs similar to Parkinson's, such as shuffling movements and rigid muscles. Records show that DLB accounts for 10 percent of dementia in aged people.[29] The condition is a combination of the effects from Alzheimer's disease and Parkinson's disease, and causes 15 percent of all dementia found in elderly patients.[30] A person suffering from DLB experiences problems in body movement. When DLB is present in the brain, the disease can disrupt its normal function and hinder the work of important hormones, turning the problem into a progressive neurological disease. The person with DLB experiences the same symptoms of Alzheimer's disease and Parkinson's disease, continuously worsening. For instance, a person under such conditions has trembling limbs, muscle stiffness, and loss of facial expression combined with attention and alertness issues. Other significant symptoms include hallucinations and sleeping problems. When an Alzheimer's patient with DLB experiences such symptoms, he or she will fall asleep easily but will awaken to tell everyone about an undesirable nightmare. Even if this nightmare is repetitive, the patient tends to hallucinate and think the nightmare is in fact reality. The patient might say they saw a killer, although it is quite obvious the killer only exists in his or her dreams. This scenario would also be true for a traumatic event the patient is reminded of exclusively through nightmares. The patient may not realize it is just a dream, but as the event keeps repeating in his or her mind, paranoia can sometimes take place.[31]

Lewy body dementia occurs when round, atypical structures referred to as Lewy bodies develop in areas of the brain that control thinking and movement functions. Lewy body dementia is the second-most prevalent form of progressive dementia after Alzheimer's disease.[32] It causes the patient to lose the various aspects of mental abilities requiring both rationalization and motor functioning. A person with this condition may also show extreme and varied degrees of inattentiveness, exhibited by daytime drowsiness[33] and aimless gazes into space. Symptoms of muscle rigidity, tremors, and slow movements commonly seen in patients with Parkinson's disease may also be present in patients with Lewy body dementia. Other symptoms may also include cognitive problems, memory loss, and confusion.[34]

The cause of Lewy body dementia is not known, but it is closely tied to both Alzheimer's and Parkinson's diseases. Several factors could increase the risk of DLB. Unlike Alzheimer's disease, people with Lewy body dementia develop impairments late into the progression of the disease. In addition, Lewy body dementia patients suffer from Parkinson's-like symptoms such as shaking, which is not typical of Alzheimer's.

Dementia Pugilistica

Dementia pugilistica is a condition that many outside of the boxing profession are unaware of and can get misinterpreted as basic dementia or Alzheimer's. This type of dementia can also be referred to as boxer's syndrome, punch-drunk syndrome, or chronic traumatic encephalopathy. Dementia pugilistica is caused by the trauma that boxers receive to their brain during a boxing match. Other athletes can suffer from this condition as well. Dementia pugilistica can appear many years after the boxer has retired from the ring. The signs and symptoms of this condition include poor coordination, slurred speech, loss of memory, and impaired cognitive functions. Although this condition is caused by repeated trauma, it is similar to other dementias in how it progresses and is treated.[35]

Frontotemporal Dementia

Frontotemporal dementia is a rare type of dementia that is a result of damage in areas of the brain responsible for a person's behavior, emotional responses, and language, such as the frontal and temporal lobes.[36] This type of dementia is also called Pick's disease, frontal lobe degeneration, and motor neuron disease. In this case, the patient experiences change in both personality and behavior even though the memory remains unaffected. Research indicates that patients become egocentric when suffering from a specific type of frontotemporal dementia known as semantic dementia.[37] Their behavior changes, causing them to lose their ability to understand others and thereby distressing the caregiver.[38] They become the opposite of themselves. For instance, a sociable person becomes introverted, going from being assertive to becoming the silent type. A patient might be very friendly and vocal in the first place but suddenly turn very self-serving as the disease progresses. Also of note is the inappropriate behavior wherein the patient makes rude comments and jokes at the wrong moment.[39] The patient become very aggressive and gets easily distracted by other people's actions. As the disease worsens, the patient may already experience change in eating habits such that they eat either excessively or less, and prefer certain flavors such as sweet, sour, or salty over and over again. During the later stages of frontotemporal dementia, the patient becomes forgetful, similar to Alzheimer's disease. The patient forgets families, relatives, and loved ones.

Braak's Dementia

Also known as Braak's disease or argyrophilic grain disease, this type of dementia is an emotional disorder involving behavior change, aggression, and delusions.[40] The symptoms of this disease are very similar to Alzheimer's. The characteristics of Braak's disease observed in the patient include the following: memory loss (short term at primary stage), emotional disturbance, hallucinations, stubborn or violent behavior, and personality changes. Persons suffering from argyrophilic grain disease have difficulty in formulating sentences, writing and reading, and finding words while speaking. Since Braak's dementia is really a disease of old age, the signs are only visible when the patient reaches around seventy, with memory failure reaching four to eight years into the past. Persons also suffer from mild amnesia and irritation. As many experts state, argyrophilic grain disease is a form of dementia that worsens with advancing age.[41]

Dementia/Senile Dementia of the Alzheimer's Type

Dementia of the Alzheimer's type hinders the patient's ability to recall things that happened quite recently because the brain cells that deal with learning are affected. Changes in that section of the brain's cellular matter hamper the victim's ability to think and behave properly. Each alteration diminishes the patient's capacity to feel oriented. By the same token, he or she undergoes a marked change in mood, along with noticeable confusion. In addition, the patient may develop a baseless suspicion regarding some event or may have trouble speaking.

Older adults fall victim to senile dementia of the Alzheimer's type. It is also important to note that dementia of the Alzheimer's type (DAT) and senile dementia of the Alzheimer's type (SDAT) are collectively known as Alzheimer's disease. When referring to each of them individually, these two forms of dementia are respectively known as early onset Alzheimer's disease and late onset Alzheimer's disease.

OTHER PHYSICAL AND VERBAL SYMPTOMS

Alzheimer's disease also manifests physical symptoms.[42] Most of the physical symptoms caused by the disease occur in the later stages of life and usually target a person's motor skills. Motor functions develop in the motor cortex in the region of the cerebral cortex and are responsible for a series of movements combined to produce the proper actions to master a particular task. When motor skills are altered due to the disease, various disorders can be felt through both the gross and fine motor skills, which then become the physical symptoms of Alzheimer's disease. Gross motor skills are responsible for activities oriented for larger muscles, such as walking and running, while fine motor skills engage smaller muscles to perform simple activities such as buttoning shirts and feeding with a spoon.

Gross and Fine Motor Skills

Patients suffering from Alzheimer's disease experience physical symptoms of both gross motor skills and fine motor skills, detected by using different methods. First, the patient experiences a breakdown in mobility and movement. For gross motor skills, patients experience tremors that can result in walking difficulties. Most patients under this condition either tremble before standing or exhibit shaky limbs while performing simple steps. Alzheimer's disease causes stiffness to limbs, which can make muscles contract at irregular intervals. If that is the case, patients may need the aid of a cane or wheelchair. Soon afterward, related shortcomings take place in the fine motor skills of the patient. Many Alzheimer's patients that experience defective gross motor skills also experience problems in fine motor skills such that they even have difficulty with grasping a cane, and thus can fall. Patients may also lose the ability to smile, causing them to look grumpy or emotionless, and they might lose their ability to move on their own while sleeping.

Urinary Symptoms

Strong clinical evidence proves that Alzheimer's disease patients suffer from urinary symptoms such as incontinence, or the incapacity to control urine and bowel functions.[43] When it comes to gross motor symptoms, patients with Alzheimer's disease, aside from forgetting where the bathroom is located, also experience difficulty in controlling their bladder and bowel movements. In some instances, the patient does not realize what he or she has done. As far as fine motor skills are concerned, patients can reach their bathroom but experience difficulty in opening the door, unbuttoning a shirt, or reaching for the bathroom tissue. This is why Alzheimer's patients suffering from such problems get enrolled in physical therapy—to orient and maintain conscience of such issues. Caregivers still need to assist patients all the time, even accompanying them to the bathroom or bedroom, as well as helping with these tasks.

Apraxia

Another physical symptom is apraxia, which targets both the gross motor skills and fine motor skills of a patient with Alzheimer's disease. In this case, patients lose the ability to perform daily basic activities such as bathing, brushing teeth, or feeding themselves. When not well taken care of, patients might seldom eat due to forgetting the right activities for the day or the non-recognition of the activity that is supposed to be done at the moment. That is why most patients with severe Alzheimer's disease need caregivers to aid them with almost all of the daily basic activities to survive. On the other hand, the symptom can be felt in the gross motor skills due to the loss of physical instincts. This includes a loss of the most basic function of the body such as chewing, swallowing, and speaking. When apraxia affects the patient's ability to talk, it is called apraxia of speech.[44] The change is a result of the brain not performing basic functions of swallowing or breathing. In such a later stage, Alzheimer's disease can cause various illnesses; for instance, pneumonia can be caused by aspirating food into the lungs as a result of neuronal inactivity. Pneumonia and its relation to Alzheimer's are discussed further in chapter 17.

Atrophy

Atrophy is defined as a decrease in tissue size and is a significant characteristic of Alzheimer's disease. The size of the brain is diminished in Alzheimer's patients.[45] A study done by the University of Kansas School of Medicine showed that increased cardiorespiratory (heart and lung) fitness resulted in reduced brain atrophy in patients with Alzheimer's.[46] The patients who were studied had early stage Alzheimer's, with the other group lacking any dementia. All were subjected to a chain of treadmill exercises as well as an MRI scan (a diagnostic process described in the next chapter). The O_2 (oxygen) levels were measured before, during, and after the treadmill tests. The patients then had another MRI following the exercises. Alzheimer's disease victims who lacked dementia had results showing better overall cognitive abilities. There were marked results indicating that cardiorespiratory fitness did reduce brain atrophy. More recent studies indicate that physical fitness could possibly delay the onset of the disease in many individuals,[47] and this study seems to confirm that. It should be noted that the test was performed on patients in early stages of Alzheimer's who were evaluated for signs of brain atrophy even before the official study began.[48]

Difficulty with Speech

Verbal symptoms experienced by a patient suffering from Alzheimer's disease include impaired speech and linguistic skills. Alzheimer's disease damages the language center of the brain. When this happens, the patient may undergo occasional mispronunciation of words. For instance, a patient might utter "wharf" instead of *what*. When the Alzheimer's disease gets worse, the patient gradually experiences speaking difficulties and slurred speech, and presents with incoherent communication. This is why, at times, patients are difficult to converse with. An Alzheimer's sufferer at a later stage could have difficulty pronouncing the *r* in *wharf*, verbally transforming the word into "whalf." A person listening might not immediately comprehend the sentences.

Another example is when a patient seems to be chewing something inside his or her mouth while talking. Although the patient might not notice it, a medical professional could assert that the patient is mumbling due to stiffness of tongue muscles. In this case, the symptoms affect the gross motor skills wherein the tongue is kept from working the right way. As an Alzheimer's patient grows older, the verbal symptoms also get worse such that the slurred vocalization is reduced to grunts and moans. In this case, words are very rarely spoken. The caregiver seldom hears the patient speak, and when the patient does make an attempt, the speech is entirely mispronounced. This inability in communicating clearly can lead to the patient's state of low self-esteem and low rate of socialization.

One of the functions of the brain is to control speech. When someone suffers from Alzheimer's, speech is often affected. More specifically, the patient struggles with meaningfulness of language as opposed to the mechanical aspects of speech production. It is not articulating the word but rather generating the word appropriate for meaningful communication that becomes increasingly difficult. As Alzheimer's disease spreads through the nervous system, the patient progressively loses the ability to communicate effectively with others and therefore becomes increasingly isolated from society. It certainly makes sense to encourage senior citizens to develop a habit of regular aerobic exercise before signs of mental deterioration are seen. Participating in a class where others are present also provides the opportunity to socialize and interact with other elderly people, thus reducing depression and the inevitable sense of isolation that plagues the Alzheimer's patient.

In later stages of Alzheimer's, the patient becomes almost mute and is unable to communicate verbally. This makes it very difficult for the caretaker as they cannot always ascertain what is making the patient upset. It is almost similar to working with a baby who cannot communicate its needs. This can be distressing and unnerving if the caregiver is an adult offspring of the patient. An Alzheimer's patient may become distressed when disorientated, when too hot or cold, when needing the bathroom, and when hungry or thirsty. A sensitive caregiver will learn to pick up signs of approaching distress and circumvent an increase in agitation in the patient. Oftentimes, a walk outside in the garden distracts and soothes the patient and provides fresh air and exercise. Talking is not necessary in order to walk together—a hand around the shoulder gently guiding the patient communicates in a reassuring nonverbal way and can bring positive results.

ANALYSIS

According to one report, Alzheimer's disease is becoming such a critical health issue in America that scientists have had to accelerate efforts to find its cure.[49] As with any disorder or disease, the symptoms are the focus. A person suffering from the disease can only undergo medical treatment that prevents symptoms from getting worse, but the treatment does not heal the person. Alzheimer's patients are occasionally treated by using devices to compensate for impaired cognitive functions and to maintain general health.[50] For depression and other mental outcomes (see chapter 11), patients may be treated with antidepressants, but long-term use of such medications can bring on anticholinergic effects (see chapters 5 and 6). Before complicated medications or treatments are prescribed for an Alzheimer's patient, the caregiver and patient must understand which symptoms are being targeted. Presently, there are approximately five million Americans suffering from Alzheimer's disease, while as many as sixteen million will have it by 2050.[51] A sadder fact of such an epidemic is that the symptoms worsen at the fastest pace when the patient reaches very old age. If the symptoms are recognized early, people with Alzheimer's are more likely to receive an early, accurate diagnosis and proper medical treatment before it is too late.

UNCOVERING THE SYMPTOMS EARLY

While the victim of Alzheimer's might not realize what is happening to them, a member of the family should have the capability and the knowledge to detect early symptoms of Alzheimer's disease, especially when the family has an elderly person living with them. This helps the family prepare for the painful fact that a loved one who could be suffering from Alzheimer's disease might lose happy memories and fail to recognize close family members. Preparing for Alzheimer's is not simply a matter of educating the rest of the relatives.

Early detection of Alzheimer's symptoms also reduces hospitalization and impairment. Patients at an early stage of Alzheimer's do not necessarily have to live in hospitals. Conditions such as depression can be addressed with urgent care before the situation worsens. Through early detection of Alzheimer's disease, the family can also prepare to make critical life decisions such as financial planning and living wills that help to avoid further problems and complications within the family. Financial planning involves setting a budget for the treatment of and medication for the symptoms, while living wills place legal frameworks into place to protect the family members as well as the sick person. One way would be to have powers of attorney or dividing wealth. Another advantage of early detection of Alzheimer's disease is protection and safety for the patient and family. When the symptoms are discovered by caregivers accurately, certain activities will need to be supervised, limited, or stopped. These activities include driving, use of firearms for hunting, certain sports activities, and using machineries. In the absence of early detection of symptoms, it is not impossible for a sick person to cause harm to the family. The patient who is suffering from dementia might pull a trigger on a family member instead of a bird due to some memory loss and confusion. Even worse, patients might shoot themselves, causing immediate unexpected death. Some severely ill Alzheimer's patients may have to give up their jobs in case they harm someone at work.

Furthermore, knowing the early signs and symptoms of Alzheimer's disease allows prompt treatment for the reversible problems associated with the disease.[52] Examples of these reversible problems include pseudodementia, thyroid problems, dehydration, malnutrition, infections, and medication problems. The first symptom is important. Pseudodementia is a psychological issue that manifests much like dementia and includes difficulty in thinking clearly, problems in concentrating, and trouble with making decisions. When a family member is unaware of this, the Alzheimer's disease victim might be subjected to wrong treatment, which can cause severe complication and hazard to both parties.

Caregivers should also know the conditions behind the symptoms. For example, they should understand the possibility of hypothyroidism when the patient has thyroid problems or malnutrition due to forgetfulness, as well as difficulty in concentrating due to some infections. These symptoms can simply be used as indications that the person might be suffering from Alzheimer's disease.

Knowledge of the early signs and symptoms of Alzheimer's disease makes possible the various treatments that can slow its progression. When patients are diagnosed, hopes for a cure are more conceivable. In addition, early detection allows family members to prepare themselves with knowledge of the different types of dementia and other deceptive symptoms that could lead to further danger in the absence of any standalone treatment. In the end, knowledge is power, and although science and medicine cannot yet provide exact and precise solutions to Alzheimer's disease, awareness of the symptoms is beneficial for both patients and caregivers.

• *5* •

Diagnosing Alzheimer's

*R*esearch has shown that true Alzheimer's disease begins decades before severe cognitive decline starts to occur.[1] New guidelines stress that the disease should be detected and diagnosed early, long before the client or patient develops dementia,[2] which is characterized by the deterioration and breakdown of a person's mental functions.[3] This is more so because, in spite of its high incidence, Alzheimer's is commonly misdiagnosed or unrecognized in the early stages.[4]

RECENT ALZHEIMER'S DIAGNOSTIC GUIDELINES

The National Institutes of Health, along with the Alzheimer's Association, led in the development of the diagnostic guidelines for Alzheimer's disease released in April 2011. A distinguishing feature of the new guidelines for research on the early stages of the condition is reflecting on a deeper understanding of the disease. The National Institute on Aging/Alzheimer's Association diagnostic guidelines for Alzheimer's disease lays out some fresh approaches for clinicians and gives scientists more advanced guidelines for research on diagnosis. It is believed that updating the diagnostic guidelines will bring the guidelines up to speed with research on the disease.

The original clinical criteria from 1984 constituted the first set of diagnostic guidelines for Alzheimer's disease but only described the later stages, when manifestations of dementia are already obvious.[5] With limited knowledge of the disease circulating at the time, Alzheimer's was defined as having only one stage—dementia—and the diagnosis of dementia was based only on its clinical symptoms. Those without symptoms of dementia were simply assumed to be disease-free.

47

NEW CRITERION FOR DIFFERENTIATING
ALZHEIMER'S FROM OTHER DISEASES

Because Alzheimer's causes damage to the brain before one finally notices symptoms, a string of major changes were implemented, relating to how the disease is diagnosed and how patients are cared for. There were new documents published that described a new criteria for differentiating and diagnosing the disease alongside other forms of dementia.[6]

Key contrasts stand between the way Alzheimer's disease was officially diagnosed in 1984 and how Alzheimer's will continue to be diagnosed from now on. Some patients can possess many variations of amyloid plaques in the brain cells without having any symptoms or hints of illness. Furthermore, the idea that the population can portray mixed forms of dementias, (e.g., vascular dementia and Lewy body dementia) can only begin to gain further approval rather than dispute.

Diagnosing Alzheimer's is not a waltz in the park, as even some of the current methods, such as the usage of biomarkers, have their own downsides and should be used for basic research purposes only. Consistent roadblocks in the quest to find a cure could prevent experts from discovering a one-step diagnosis. As pioneers of stipulated guidelines for Alzheimer's, the National Institute on Aging (NIA) and Alzheimer's Disease Centers (ADCs) program note that the newer criteria they support look at Alzheimer's disease from a different light.[7] Such criteria help people to identify and start dealing with the disease from a much earlier stage, rather than simply waiting to be sure the issue at hand is in fact Alzheimer's.

What warranted this shift in the proposed criteria? Because information regarding the non-Alzheimer's dementias used to be considered rudimentary up until 1984, the old criteria appears vague when it is time to define the distinctions between Alzheimer's and similar medical issues. Some pathological and neuropsychological properties of the disease would be uncovered by experts decades after Alois Alzheimer made his discoveries, but the fact that the symptoms of neuropsychiatry disorders can be tied to Alzheimer's disease was still not enough to woo people before the early 1980s.

The common correlation with cerebrovascular disorder, Lewy body disease, and Alzheimer's disease seen in elderly people does not get the recognition it deserves. Therefore, only in the last ten or so years has there been better understanding of the differences. Certain overlaps of the non-Alzheimer's types of dementias with true Alzheimer's have started to surface. Issues such as these have been factored into the new criteria. The main clinical criteria have been covered in the recommendations for Alzheimer's dementia or mild cognitive impairment (MCI). Because of the severity of the later stages of Alzheimer's disease (covered in chapters 8 and 9), something needed to be done to confirm diagnosis in a purely clinical setting. Many of the recommendations that arise from preclinical Alzheimer's research groups are simply intended for research and academic purposes, with the overall effect being the lack of clinical backing.

BIOMARKERS IN THE DIAGNOSIS OF ALZHEIMER'S

There have been widely researched biomarkers that point to Alzheimer's disease.[8] These biomarkers are formally incorporated today in the criteria for diagnosing the disease. There is agreement between related work groups that more work is needed to validate the use of biomarkers. For example, elaborate biomarker comparison tests need to be done, as well as a more elaborate validation of the disease using postmortem exams. Further work on the standardization of biomarkers is required before people can confidently adopt the recommendations put forward in a widespread manner, irrespective of what stage the disease has reached.

Purpose

Biomarkers continue to stand as diagnostic traits of Alzheimer's. In that sense, biomarker standardization should be not a "luxury" but *essential*. Biomarkers are gaining acceptance and will in fact make research results more credible and easier to interpret. To obtain standardized, reliable, and credible diagnostic caliber readings, biomarker tests should be used more often with harmless research conducted via clinical trials and clinical care.[9]

Usage

Clinical diagnosis of Alzheimer's can only be confirmed upon autopsy of the brain, when plaques made of amyloid proteins and tangles of tau proteins are found. These plaques and tangles, often regarded as a form of biomarkers, are definitive proofs of incidence of Alzheimer's disease. Updated diagnostic guidelines encompass the whole spectrum of the disease as it slowly changes over many years—even decades. The guidelines now include symptoms found in the earliest preclinical stages, such as mild impairment of cognition and dementia due to the physiological causes of Alzheimer's disease. They also include refinements to present guidelines for diagnosing incidence of MCI. These guideline updates address the usage of diagnostic imaging procedures and biomarkers found in a person's blood and spinal fluid that (1) may aid in establishing diagnosis and (2) is indicative of certain changes in the blood and body fluids that are effects of Alzheimer's disease. Biomarkers are being used increasingly in research for detecting an early onset of the disease and to track disease progression but cannot be routinely employed in clinical diagnosis in the absence of extensive testing and evaluation.[10] The more popular biomarkers are low levels of the beta-amyloid protein and high levels of tau proteins. That these biomarkers may be found in people with no cognitive challenges underlines the possibility that Alzheimer's disease begins long before symptoms become evident.[11]

EARLY "DIAGNOSIS"

By observing early the symptoms covered in chapter 4, an informal caregiver can detect, but not legally diagnose, a case of Alzheimer's disease. Medicine alone cannot stop or completely reverse the onset of Alzheimer's disease, but early detection and diagnosis gives patients better chances of benefiting from treatment and lessening anxieties about unknown and unexplained conditions.[12] Early detection and treatment commenced in the early stages may help preserve brain function for a longer period of time, even years. This may be so even if the underlying disease cannot be cured.[13] It also gives patients more time to plan and provide for the future, and more opportunities to be involved in decision making about current and future living arrangements, personal care, and financial and legal matters. Early diagnosis also gives the patients or doctors and other caregivers more time to develop and establish a therapeutic approach.[14] Prompt detection gives patients more chances to get maximum benefits from treatments available and to maintain longer a certain level of independence,[15] more so because some medication for Alzheimer's disease can only work in the earlier stages.[16] Early detection might also give Alzheimer's victims better chances of being involved with and benefitting from clinical drug trials.[17]

Clinical Drug Trials and Early Diagnosis

Clinical drug trials improve the overall process of early detection and prompt diagnosis of Alzheimer's. An Alzheimer's disease clinical trial is essentially a research study where scientists test and determine the safety, efficacy, and side effects of a drug or other treatment.[18] These trials also enable a client to take advantage of support and care services, thus making it easier for the person and the family to handle and cope with the situation. Considering the importance of early diagnosis, a physician should be consulted if you or someone you know manifests any of the warning signs and symptoms. The early signs and symptoms are usually obvious more to family members, caregivers, and friends than to sufferers because sufferers might find it difficult to figure out what is wrong.[19]

FINDING THE RIGHT SOLUTIONS

A medical test or procedure alone cannot show whether a client has Alzheimer's disease.[20] Diagnosing Alzheimer's disease necessitates a careful and complete medical assessment. It is thus important for a client manifesting symptoms of Alzheimer's to be evaluated by a doctor. A doctor or physician can usually determine if a patient has dementia. However, it may be difficult to ascertain whether Alzheimer's disease is the cause.[21] The entire ordeal could be confusing to the elderly, and it is easy to mistakenly assume their memory problems are just ordinary forms of "forgetfulness" that some people undergo as they age. Presently, doctors can diagnose probable incidence of Alzheimer's with about 90 percent accuracy by ruling out other health problems, using simple processes of elimination.[22]

Family Doctors

From a patient's standpoint, the first step in diagnoses is choosing a physician with whom the former is comfortable. Many clients with concerns regarding memory loss and other symptoms of dementia often go to their primary care doctor,[23] but such a physician may not be a specialist in cognition problems or dementia. A family practice doctor could perform brief screening tests that can help to detect cognitive deficiencies. A good reason to start with one's primary care doctor is familiarity with the patient's medical history. This provides for more physician-patient comfort as well as important data needed for a diagnosis. Moreover, he or she knows the patient better, which may enable the patient to talk more about sensitive matters and better enable the family doctor to spot changes in the patient's mental functioning.[24]

Specialists

Although a primary care doctor usually oversees the diagnostic process, he or she will refer the client to a specialist for the official diagnosis and treatment of Alzheimer's disease. These specialists include neurologists, psychiatrists, psychologists,[25] geriatricians, geriatric psychiatrists, neuropsychologists, and other specialists.[26] A neurologist is a doctor who specializes in diseases of the nervous system,[27] which includes the brain.[28] A psychiatrist specializes in mental disorders—their diagnosis, prevention, and treatment.[29] A psychologist has been trained to provide testing of a person's memory and other mental functions.[30] A geriatrician is a physician who has had targeted education and experience in the medical care of the elderly.[31] He or she understands how the human body changes as a person ages and whether symptoms are indicative of a serious issue.

A geriatric psychiatrist specializes in the mental and emotional challenges of the elderly and can evaluate cognitive problems. A neuropsychologist administers memory and thinking evaluations for the patient.

Support Groups

The local chapter of a national Alzheimer's support group can be of help in identifying the proper specialists.[32] Moreover, ADCs all over the United States also offer services helpful for the overall diagnostic process.[33] It is very important to find a doctor experienced in diagnosing Alzheimer's disease. Obtaining a second opinion would be advised, especially if the doctor diagnosed the disease by way of hurried assessments. A doctor who is experienced in determining Alzheimer's disease would conduct a complete assessment and examination to rule out other conditions with similar symptoms. It would be prudent to inquire about the diagnostic procedures to be used before booking an appointment and to look for another doctor if the evaluation does not seem comprehensive enough. Even so, the doctor who eventually makes the Alzheimer's diagnosis may not be the doctor who will manage the subsequent long-term care. Once Alzheimer's disease is determined, it may be necessary to find another physician experienced in giving ongoing care to meet the various needs of such a patient. The family or family member of the client thus needs to choose a knowledgeable doctor and one who communicates well with them.

EVALUATION AND ASSESSMENT PROCESS

Sometimes, Alzheimer's disease victims refuse to see a doctor for assessment. They are often in denial about having cognitive challenges. In such cases, the family member or friend may have to pretend the doctor's visit is a regular physical exam or is for a preknown, accepted condition such as hypertension or a specific complaint such as a headache. This might give the doctor a chance to start the evaluation for Alzheimer's and has to be prearranged with the doctor as being the real purpose of the visit. The patient may feel stressed about visiting the doctor for evaluation. To help minimize this, a feasible level of preparation would benefit the client. Whoever accompanies the client should be someone familiar to the client and who knows the client's current symptoms, medical history, and concerns.[34] The patient as well as any accompanying person should be prepared for the doctor to ask about noticeable symptoms, when the symptoms began, how often they occur, and whether they are getting worse.[35] It always helps to write down in advance any questions about issues and concerns one may want to mention during the visit.[36]

Outpatient Assessment

A thorough evaluation of an Alzheimer's patient is usually done on an outpatient setting.[37] A patient's family member, friend, or caregiver may be asked to accompany the patient so useful information can be provided about the patient's mental status.[38] In certain areas, the process can take more than one visit. The diagnostic tests can be done over the course of several days to avoid "tiring out" the patient. Other than the treating doctor, the full diagnosis of Alzheimer's can involve nurses, technicians, social workers, psychiatrists, and other specialists.

It takes several days for results of the doctor's review. An equivocal or unconfirmed diagnosis is sometimes given because doctors are often hesitant about diagnosing Alzheimer's disease in the outpatient setting without enough time to observe the progression of the cognitive failures.[39] A doctor might only give a diagnosis of "possible Alzheimer's disease," "probable Alzheimer's disease," or some other condition characteristic of a patient with memory difficulties. A "possible" case of Alzheimer's means the cognitive problems may be due to another condition. A "probable" case of Alzheimer's disease means no other cause for the problems can be pinpointed.[40] Such equivocal evaluations usually entail a repeat assessment in six to twelve months. A more firm diagnosis is sometimes possible at these later evaluations, but when the cognitive impairment is gradual, repeated testing at annual intervals may be recommended.[41] An absolute confirmation of Alzheimer's disease is only possible upon examination of brain tissue if and when the hallmark signs of the disease are there.[42] These hallmark signs include decisive amounts of tau tangles, made of the tau proteins mentioned earlier, and plaques made of beta-amyloid proteins.[43]

Presently, new outpatient diagnostic tools and updated criteria enable doctors, both primary care physicians and specialists, to make a diagnosis of probable Alzheimer's disease with a reasonable level of accuracy. Cognition impairment should be evaluated in people not only with cognition concerns but also who, though not showing any obvious symptoms, have risk factors for the disease such as age and family history.[44]

The diagnostic criteria used in diagnosing Alzheimer's disease in the outpatient setting include a failure by the patient in at least three functions of cognition. These three functions can be any of the following: memory, use of language, personality, the ability to understand what is seen, spatial orientation, or calculative skills.[45] Diagnosing Alzheimer's disease beyond hospital grounds (outpatient setting) necessitates careful medical evaluation, which would include a thorough personal medical history of the patient, a physical examination,[46] a neuropsychological evaluation, laboratory tests,[47] neurological testing,[48] and various other diagnostic tests that help to rule out conditions with dementia-like symptoms other than those suggestive of Alzheimer's disease.[49]

PATIENT'S HISTORY

A detailed history of the patient is obtained to identify changes in the patient's cognition and behavior. The patient's history may necessarily have to be corroborated by the patient's caregiver or an informed source in view of the client's possibly altered mental status.[50] This helps the evaluating physician to assess the client's past and present health status. It also assists the doctor in assessing where there are any other medical problems, developing a treatment plan, and managing the client's health in the future.

Constituents

For a thorough patient history, the doctor asks questions geared to obtain identifying information of the Alzheimer's victim, such as the following:

- Name
- Age
- Concerns with daily activities of living
- Data about other symptoms
- History of past and current injuries
- Past illnesses and surgeries
- Present health status

The patient history also includes a psychosocial history, with marital status, the patient's employment and living situation, sexual history, and important events of the patient's life. The process also involves an evaluation of the patient's mental state, which may be obtained through a series of questions asked to assess whether the patient is having symptoms of depression or other psychiatric illness. The family history usually contains data of key medical problems that appear to run in the patient's family,[51] including whether family members may have had Alzheimer's disease or other forms of dementia.[52] The doctor will inquire about any medications the patient is taking, including herbal supplements and nonprescription drugs.

Additional Information

The Alzheimer's disease patient's personal and medical history serves as the basis for the physician's diagnostic workup. It may appear to be overwhelming for all parties involved, but a thorough medical history enables the doctor to determine possible diagnoses upon which to base the ensuing medical evaluation. For example, a doctor might immediately subject a patient with acute mental changes and difficulty in walking to a computed tomography (CT) scan of the brain from the start, rather than in the later part of diagnostic testing as a final test. This is because the aforementioned symptoms may indicate an accumulation of cerebrospinal fluid in the brain—normal-pressure hydrocephalus—for which an early and prompt detection and treatment could preclude permanent damage to the brain.[53]

WHEN DIAGNOSIS GETS PHYSICAL

A physical examination (PE) is integral to an Alzheimer's disease victim's totalized care. The PE enables the assessing physician to evaluate the overall physical status of the client. It provides the doctor with more information and data about a medical complaint of the patient and assists both parties in formulating a fitting treatment plan. Assessment of the following is usually included in a complete, annual PE for an Alzheimer's patient,[54] irrespective of any prevailing neurological symptoms:

- Vital signs, including body temperature
- Condition of the skin
- Blood pressure and pulse
- Eyes and nose
- Breasts
- Genital and rectal area
- Neck and throat
- Chest, including heart and lung sounds
- Abdomen
- Bones and muscles
- Height and weight
- Head and ears
- Neurological functioning

As described in chapter 3, many medical conditions can cause dementia-like changes. To refresh the reader's memory in the context of Alzheimer's disease diagnosis, these medical conditions are listed as follows:

- Heart failure
- Kidney failure
- Thyroid problems
- Liver disease[55]
- Depression
- Excessive alcohol use
- Drug interactions
- Certain vitamin deficiencies[56]

Moreover, older people do not always have or manifest the typical symptoms of a disease. The general sensation of pain is often dulled in the elderly, so much so that, for example, it is not rare for confusion instead of chest pain (angina), to be the main symptom manifested in some cases of a heart attack.[57]

Neurophysical Examinations

By conducting a neurophysical exam, a physician can learn about the condition of particular areas of the brain by testing and assessing a patient's muscle tone, muscle strength, reflexes, coordination, senses, eye movement, and pupillary response to light. A weakness on either the left or right side of the body or unequal reflexes may indicate localized damage in the brain that may be due to a tumor or a stroke. Involuntary movements or tremors may suggest a degenerative condition such as Parkinson's disease.[58]

Lumbar Puncture

A lumbar puncture (LP) is the insertion of a spinal needle usually between the third and fourth lumbar bones for the purpose of, among others, obtaining cerebrospinal fluid (CSF) for analysis and measuring CSF pressure.[59] It is important to note that LP also establishes the absence or presence of blood in the spinal fluid, as well as other central nervous system abnormalities. The LP aids in the diagnosis of tumors and brain abscesses. It is also used to determine levels of beta-amyloid and tau proteins in the cerebrospinal fluid, which are biomarkers for diagnosing Alzheimer's disease.[60] While LP may have had a limited role in the diagnosis of the disease a long time ago, the technique may be more widely used now that diagnostic markers for the disease are getting to be more specific.[61] CSF screening via LP is a great diagnostic process, and there has been plenty of recent medical research about CSF and its relation to Alzheimer's. (CSF will be discussed further in chapter 15).[62]

Neuropsychological Exams

A neuropsychological evaluation that includes an assessment of the patient's mental status is conducted to determine specific areas of impaired mental functioning as compared to areas of unimpaired functioning.[63] A neuropsychological test analyzes the relationship between the state of the brain and behavior. It is employed especially when the client is having serious difficulties with memory, understanding language, remembering words and names, concentration, visual-spatial issues, and various other symptoms of cognitive difficulties. This test aids in the diagnosis of a disease such as Alzheimer's that affects thinking, emotion, and behavior. The test is employed in tandem with a comprehensive interview and may include screenings to evaluate memory, language, the ability to change behavior, planning and reasoning abilities, and personality and emotional stability. The effects of Alzheimer's disease on a patient's daily functions are also better understood by doctors and families through neuropsychological testing.[64]

While performing a neurological examination, the physician will carefully assess the patient for problems that may indicate disorders of the brain outside of Alzheimer's disease and will be on the lookout for tumors, fluid accumulation, and signs indicative of small or large strokes and Parkinson's disease. A mental status test, included in a full neuro-psychological examination, assesses a person's memory, ability to solve simple problems,[65] orientation, language skills, and comprehension. Here, the doctor may ask the patient to perform basic mental exercises such as duplicating creative designs, counting backward, memorizing words, and following written instructions.[66]

Other Areas Examined

A doctor conducting a full neurological exam on an Alzheimer's patient may choose to assess the cardiovascular system, the lungs, the kidneys, the liver, and other organs for possible signs of abnormalities. The doctor will also examine the client's eyes and vision and ears and hearing because sensory problems can significantly add to a patient's cognitive challenges. The nervous system,[67] which includes the brain, the spinal cord, and the nerves,[68] is thoroughly assessed because any abnormalities can signify a brain disorder other than Alzheimer's disease.

DIAGNOSTIC TESTING

Laboratory tests are conducted to rule out infectious diseases or metabolic disorders that can cause altered mental functioning in patients. These tests include the following:

- Complete blood count (CBC)
- Chemistry panel
- Thyroid-stimulating hormone (TSH)
- Folate level
- Serum B12
- Acetylcholinesterase
- Syphilis
- Human immunodeficiency virus (HIV)[69]

CBC

A CBC is a laboratory test that determines the quantity of red and white blood cells as well as other blood elements per cubic millimeter of blood.[70] An increased white blood cell count is indicative of possible infections and inflammatory diseases. An inflammation in the brain may cause cognitive problems, while a deficiency in hematocrit and hemoglobin levels in the blood can indicate anemia,[71] which can cause confusion and disorientation.[72] The presence of a specific gene identified as a risk factor for Alzheimer's disease may be found through a blood test.[73]

Chemistry Panel

A chemistry panel tests for various substances in the body, comparing the results to normal values. For instance, above-normal levels of lead in the body can cause anemia[74] and disorientation.[75] A chemistry panel tests for various substances in the body, comparing the results to normal values. The sedimentation rate is the speed that red blood cells settle in a vertical column of plasma and is a measure used to monitor inflammation or malignant diseases.

TSH

A TSH test measures TSH concentration. A TSH deficiency can cause mental lethargy or memory problems that might otherwise be misinterpreted as Alzheimer's symptoms. The TSH testing process requires a blood sample from a patient. The doctors want to see if the patient's levels of TSH are within the normal ranges. Under otherwise normal circumstances, the Alzheimer's patient should have around 0.4 milliunits per liter (mU/L) of TSH in their blood.[76] Children and newborns will have slightly higher levels of the hormone in their blood stream. If the level is too low or too high in the patient, the attending physician will decide on a course of treatment in conjunction with the treatment for Alzheimer's disease if necessary.[77]

Folate and Vitamin B12 Test

A folate-level test is a blood test used to detect anemia caused by a lack of folic acid. Vitamin B12 is needed to convert inactive folate to active folate, which is necessary for the function and generation of red blood cells (RBCs). A deficiency in RBCs causes anemia. Anemia might cause the confusion or disorientation found in Alzheimer's patients.[78] Doctors perform folate and B12 tests when they suspect a person might suffer from several different Vitamin B deficiencies. The test, like many other medical tests, starts by drawing blood. Phlebotomists measure the amount of the blood available in the patient's red blood cells. By adding a simple chemical that reacts to folic acids, a doctor can determine the patient's vitamin B level. Vitamin B deficiencies can lead to depression if left untreated, but increasing the Alzheimer's disease sufferer's folic acid intake restores the levels of this vitamin to normal. Liver, dark green vegetables, citric acid, and supplements help return a person's folic acid level to normal also.

Acetylcholinesterase Test

This blood test is used to detect acetylcholine levels which are sometimes,[79] but not always,[80] found to be irregular in Alzheimer's patients. Acetylcholinesterase is the enzyme responsible for breaking down acetylcholine, an important neurotransmitter. It is used to help the doctor rule out any conditions that may be mistaken as being caused by Alzheimer's disease.[81] The acetylcholinesterase test is used to gain a measure of how much acetylcholinesterase enzyme exists in the Alzheimer's patient's red blood cells. This test can also be used to evaluate the toxicity levels of organophosphates, a certain kind of pesticide. For this test, a health-care practitioner will draw blood from an arm vein: after the practitioner has tightly fastened a tourniquet (rubber strap) above the vein, he or she will cleanse the area and insert a needle into the vein, collecting one to two tubes of blood. The tubes are sent to the lab, where chemicals are added to the sample to test its acetylcholinesterase levels.[82]

Syphilis Testing

Syphilis is associated with dementia, a claim strongly supported by medical research.[83] This is especially true for neurosyphilis in aging patients, so testing for syphilis may be part of the diagnostic process for Alzheimer's. Neurosyphilis may also cause anemia and changes in fluids within the brain that can result in altered mental functioning.[84] Diagnosis of neurosyphilis in an Alzheimer's patient involves the use of two major testing techniques. A technique called dark field microscopy is the most accurate way to diagnose syphilis in the case where an active condyloma latum or chancre is present. The results and outcome of this procedure is, however, limited to the operators' experience, to the number of treponeme-related lesions, and on whether treponemes that are nonpathologic are present in body lesions. As for nontreponemal detection techniques, the infection normally produces antibodies that are not specific and will react to the application of a substance known as cardiolipin. This is used as a base for several conventional tests that are nontreponemal, such as plasma reagin and venereal disease evaluations.[85]

HIV Testing

An HIV infection can affect cognitive function, demonstrated by mental slowing and impaired memory and concentration.[86] Because these symptoms are closely associated to those of Alzheimer's, it may be a good idea to get tested for HIV as part of the process of verifying an Alzheimer's patient's symptoms. An Alzheimer's patient can test for HIV at home,[87] but it is best performed by a health care professional. The main objective is to search for an infectious organism, and testing for HIV reflects a scientific understanding of how the human system responds to a foreign body. That infected man or woman has a particular protein in his or her bloodstream. An enzyme-linked immunoabsorbent assay (ELISA) screens for the presence of that specific antibody. That ELISA can alert a doctor to the presence of that marker about six to twelve weeks after the virus first invades the body. Only in two rare situations can it prove ineffective. One of those is for an infant born of an HIV-infected mother. The other concerns the person who has taken part in a trial for a possible vaccine.[88]

X-RAYS AND ELECTROCARDIOGRAMS (EKGS)

A chest X-ray produces images on a photographic film, of bones and cavities filled with a contrast medium, to show anatomical changes of targeted aspects of the chest area.[89] It can be used to rule out disorders that cause dementia-like symptoms.[90] An electrocardiogram gives a record of the electrical activity of the heart and can show cardiac abnormalities such as an enlargement or decrease in blood flow. Cardiac disorders may cause cognitive problems such as those characteristic of Alzheimer's.[91] X-rays are also used in the diagnostic processes for pneumonia, a respiratory condition from which Alzheimer's disease patients suffer.[92]

COMPUTER-GENERATED IMAGERY (CGI)

A host of other diagnostic procedures are also done to rule out other conditions that cause similar symptoms as Alzheimer's disease. As well as chest X-rays and EKGs,[93] neurologic diagnostic procedures such as the following can be conducted:[94]

- Computed tomography (CT)
- Positron emission tomography (PET)
- Single-photon emission computed tomography (SPECT)

- Electroencephalogram (EEG)
- Magnetic resonance imaging (MRI)
- Magnetic resonance spectroscopy (MRS)[95]

CT Scans

A CT scan is a noninvasive and painless procedure, a type of brain scanning used to detect the following:

- Tumors
- Lesions
- Intracranial bleeding
- Fluid accumulation
- Cerebral atrophy
- Infarctions
- Shifts in brain structure[96]
- Hemorrhages
- Stroke
- Infractions

When taking place within the brain, the above irregularities may cause alterations in mental functioning.[97] Computed tomography scans show changes in the brain, both functional and structural, such as a size reduction that could be attributed to Alzheimer's disease. A size reduction of the brain, or atrophy, is a sign of Alzheimer's in its later stages.[98]

PET and SPECT

A PET scan is another imaging technique that allows study of the chemical functions and metabolism of the brain. It has many other uses, including early detection of dementia.[99] A SPECT is a variation of a CT scan that is used to reduce the imaging time and purveys three-dimensional, very clear pictures of the brain.[100] It is used to assess specific functions of the brain and to see how blood flows in certain cerebral areas. This test can also show abnormalities critical in the diagnosis of Alzheimer's disease.[101]

EEG

An EEG produces a record of brain wave activity to diagnose impaired consciousness, brainstem and seizure disorders, and brain lesions.[102] EEGs are carried out on the brain to detect any electrical abnormality. In order to conduct the test, the person performing the electroencephalogram sets electrodes on the scalp of the patient. The electrodes then detect the electrical movement of the brain and relay that message to a computer, from where the expert can interpret. The movement in a normal brain follows a certain pattern. When this pattern is irregular, the interpreter can detect the problem immediately.

Although the EEG is commonly used for checking for seizure disorders,[103] it is very helpful in the diagnosis of Alzheimer's.[104] In order to get a good diagnosis of the dementia, patients going through EEGs are required to lie or sit still to avoid affecting the brain activity. This test determines the extent of Alzheimer's. There is a difference in the signals recorded from a patient suffering from Alzheimer's and going through normal aging and the signals from a patient with dementia. Therefore, the doctor can determine if the patient is having permanent or temporary dementia. EEG tests also help rule out other brain irregularities caused by aging itself.[105]

MRI and MRS

An MRI is another painless, noninvasive test that provides more detailed images than a CT scan.[106] It is used for imaging the abnormalities of the brain, brainstem, and spinal cord.[107] An MRS scan allows observance of certain substances in the brain without using radioactive materials. It is used to observe changes due to Alzheimer's disease, strokes, brain tumors, seizure disorders, and other conditions affecting brain function.[108] All these procedures can aid in narrowing down a diagnosis but could not definitively show the microscopic abnormalities in brain tissue that define Alzheimer's disease and, therefore, cannot confirm the disease with certainty.

GENETIC TESTING

As discussed to this point, research has shown that having a sibling or a parent afflicted with Alzheimer's disease does increase one's risk of developing the disease. Thus, Alzheimer's disease has been a subject of intense genetic studies. Research has shown four mutations of genes linked with the disease. Three of these genes located on chromosomes 1, 14, and 21 respectively are associated with early onset Alzheimer's, wherein symptoms start to appear between the early forties and midfifties. A fourth gene located on chromosome 19, identified as the apolipoprotein E4 (APOE-4), increases the risk of susceptibility to the late onset form of the disease—the more common form—which manifests after age 55. Genetic testing for this gene is controversial. Before undertaking the test, one should discuss it properly with a genetic counselor or one's doctor. Having the APOE-4 gene increases the risk of eventually developing Alzheimer's, but many people without the gene develop Alzheimer's and not everyone who has the APOE-4 gene gets Alzheimer's disease.[109]

DISCLOSURE OF DIAGNOSIS

A person has a legal and moral right to know about his or her full medical status. With the exception of special circumstances, doctors have to disclose the diagnosis to the client who has Alzheimer's disease. It may even be necessary to firstly advise the family in cases where the patient may not fully understand it. Disclosure in the early stages of the disease would be more beneficial to the patient as it would give the person better chances to maximize quality of life and be involved in making future plans compared to a disclosure given at the advanced dementia stage, where it would no longer be so meaningful. Plans may include long-term care options, end-of-life decisions, advanced directives such as living wills, and agreeing to be part of Alzheimer research. However, telling a patient and the family about an Alzheimer's diagnosis may be difficult if the prognosis (outlook) of the disease is not the best. The disclosure process might thus necessitate a joint meeting with the client and the family. The disclosure process goes smoother if doctors consider the cultural values and family dynamics before revealing the diagnosis. The presence of the whole evaluating team to answer questions would help, and the possible progression of the disease has to be discussed at the time of disclosure. The doctor and the client or family have to agree on a particular care plan that matches the client's values and beliefs.

As part of the disclosure process, one issue that has to be understood is that the disease is a degenerative disease of the brain leading to cognitive and behavioral changes—not a normal consequence of aging. Another is that Alzheimer's disease does not have the same effect on everyone, so there is no sure way to know how it will progress in a particular patient. It has to be understood that, while the disease cannot be cured or reversed, some of the symptoms can be treated or alleviated through the right diagnosis. Caregivers also have to understand that communicating the diagnosis allows the patient a chance to maximize the quality of his or her ensuing life. They should also keep in mind that any assistance in the diagnostic process from the patient, even if ancillary, is helpful.

ANALYSIS

Alzheimer's patients and caregivers need to understand that progress is continually made in diagnostics for Alzheimer's disease, and one way to support the progress is through involvement in clinical drug studies. These studies are crucial in the diagnostic advancements. Moreover, the family and patient's caregiver has to be involved throughout the diagnostic process, treatment, and care planning. The diagnosis and pertinent information for care of the patient has to be disclosed to them. For Alzheimer's patients who are not diagnosed early, as they become increasingly dependent on caregivers, the latter will ultimately become the primary engine for data gathering and, thus, be the key element in diagnosing the disease.[110]

III

TREATMENT OPTIONS

· 6 ·

Pharmacological Treatment
of Alzheimer's

$\mathcal{G}$enerally considered the most prevalent form of dementia, Alzheimer's disease is one of the few medical issues that currently have no cure; some of the others are diabetes, leukemia, and AIDS. In the United States alone, Alzheimer's is the seventh-most common cause of death.[1] A report suggests that, in 1987, Alzheimer's occurred in at least 45 percent of the population aged 85 and above.[2] Although this disease is mostly prevalent in adults, especially in those who are already in their geriatric years, it is worth noting when considering treatment options that the earliest signs may manifest at a younger age, especially if it is the early onset Alzheimer type. A number of factors such as age, gender, general health status, and predisposition can lengthen or shorten the life expectancy of a patient. Efforts are being made to find both medicinal and natural ways to cure Alzheimer's, and other research faculties examine ways to at least ease the symptoms that come with the disease.

There is currently no direct cure for Alzheimer's because scientists have not completely unraveled the mystery of what causes it in the first place. Although may people associate the disease with aging, scientists are still at a loss on what causes the formation of amyloid plaque in the brain tissue.[3] Early diagnosis of the symptoms, as described in the preceding chapter, can actually be beneficial to the patient from a treatment standpoint. Early diagnosis can not only lead to timely treatment of reversible symptoms such as memory loss but also ensure correct determination of whether the patient is actually suffering from Alzheimer's or is simply having pseudodementia.[4] It would also provide a way for health-care professionals and family members to make a plan for how they are going to approach the situation in the long term.

Doctors and other health care professionals whose specialties lie in the treatment of Alzheimer's make use of various pharmacological options in order to ease their clients' problems. Pharmacological interventions necessitate a careful examination of how the medication biologically affects the patient's disease. Specialists are looking forward to new findings and developments that they can derive from prescription treatments, since that may be where the cure for Alzheimer's remains hidden. Drugs that are being used to treat Alzheimer's disease can be divided into two general classifications: those that deal with the symptoms related to memory and learning and those that deal with the behavioral symptoms that are unresponsive to nonmedicinal methods. Current medications can also be grouped into either medications that deal with N-methyl D-aspartate (NMDA) receptor antagonization or medications that deal with cholinesterase inhibition.

MEDICATIONS AT A GLANCE

Currently, the U.S. Food and Drug Administration (FDA) has approved five medications for treating Alzheimer's. This includes donepezil (considered the topmost medication when it comes to this dreaded disease), galantamine, memantine, rivastigmine, and tacrine. Of these five, donepezil is the one being used for all stages of Alzheimer's. On the other hand, memantine is more suited for patients with moderate to severe cases, while the rest on the list are more suited for mild to moderate cases, according to an article from the Alzheimer's Association.[5]

N-METHYL D-ASPARTATE
RECEPTOR ANTAGONISTS

One of the most common classifications of medication that doctors prescribe to their Alzheimer's patients is the NMDA receptor antagonist. Typically, NMDA receptors allow the transfer of brain signals from the brain to the spinal cord and to the rest of the body. NMDA receptors play an important role in learning, memory, and cognition—the same areas that usually suffer the most once a person succumbs to Alzheimer's disease. An increase or decrease in the chemical compounds present in the NMDA receptors can impair brain functions. This is where NMDA receptor antagonists come in handy. NMDA receptor antagonists are a class of drugs that typically inhibits abnormal brain actions by binding the NMDA receptors with the brain cells and blocking *neurotransmitter glutamate* activity. NMDA receptor hyperactivity causes memory deficits as the brain ages and can also cause agitation, hallucination, paranoia, confusion, mood swings and learning deficits,[6] all of which are part of the symptoms of Alzheimer's (see chapter 4).

Memantine

Memantine (brand name Namenda) is one kind of medication being prescribed by a number of doctors to their patients in order to deal with the NMDA receptor antagonists. This prescription drug was first synthesized in 1968 by Eli Lilly and Company. From then on, it became recognized as the first novel class medication in treating Alzheimer's disease. It is a renowned treatment for moderate to severe Alzheimer's, but its effect on mild to moderate conditions is still unknown. This drug has been shown to be successful in gradually slowing down the deterioration of a patient's mental condition. Researchers believe that memantine really controls glutamate, a brain chemical whose overproduction has been known to kill brain cells.[7] It is normally taken orally, with or without food. During the initial stages of the medication, the patient has to take the medicine once a day, with the doctor gradually increasing its dosage over time. Some of the common side effects the patient may experience include tiredness, body aches, constipation, dizziness, and headaches. Although very rare, there are some patients who show severe allergic reaction to this drug. These reactions range from swelling of the face, tongue, or mouth area to severe dizziness and breathing problems.[8]

Memantine is a derivative of amantadine, a drug used in treating Parkinson's disease. However, memantine is more potent for Alzheimer's, as studies have reported that amantadine is a weak NMDA receptor antagonist.[9] Memantine is also prescribed to patients who are intolerant or have contraindications to acetylcholinesterase (AChE) inhibitors.[10] Namenda is one of the top brands of memantine medications today that comes in either tablet or liquid form. Once the patient has successfully tolerated lower dosages, he or she would be given a daily dosage of twenty milligrams. Memantine medications are not commonly advised by specialists because it can be expensive. One should also avoid mistaking it for other NMDA receptor antagonists as the combination could increase the risk of side effects. Alzheimer's patients who suspect that they might be pregnant or are currently breastfeeding their baby should not take this medication as it has shown to be quite harmful to the unborn child. The lowest dosage of Namenda is five milligrams although a higher dosage, seven milligrams, is also marketed as Namenda XR.[11]

Blurred vision, tightening of the chest, difficulty in breathing, and a fast heart rate are just some of the side effects of Namenda that warrant an immediate visit to the doctor. Conversely, amantadine is typically used for the treatment of flu in children as young as one year old and in patients suffering from Parkinson's disease. Its other off-label uses include treatment for attention-deficit hyperactivity disorder (ADHD) and chronic hepatitis C. In patients with Alzheimer's disease, amantadine has been proven to reverse immobility and help with word formation.[12] Researchers have found that amantadine stimulates the production of nerve cells.[13] Patients taking amantadine may suffer from such side effects as nausea, lightheadedness and dizziness, and insomnia. There are very few reported cases of severe allergic reaction to amantadine. Of those few cases, reactions include:

- Depression
- Anxiety
- Hallucination
- Confusion
- Hypotension
- Agitation
- Fast, irregular heartbeat
- Swelling of the extremities

Such cases warrant an immediate trip to the doctor's office or emergency room. Amantadine is also rarely prescribed to patients that are also taking atropine, atropa belladona, diphenhydramine, antipsychotic medications, quinine, stimulants, and intranasal flu vaccine. When combined with amantadine, these medications can increase the possibility of severe side effects.[14]

CHOLISTERASE INHIBITORS

A cholinesterase inhibitor is a medication that restores the function of the muscles and the nerves by breaking down acetylcholine, thus allowing for a better transmission of signals from the brain. Cholinesterase inhibitors are prescribed by specialists to patients with early to moderate cases of Alzheimer's. This class of drugs works by either increasing the levels of acetylcholine in the brain or strengthening nerve cells' response to it. Acetylcholine is a neurotransmitter found within a person's peripheral and central nervous system. This assists in the brain's memory and thought and judgment functions, which is why it can aggravate the Alzheimer's symptoms if there is a decrease in the amount of acetylcholine present. This class of drug works best if taken continuously. Not doing so can cause the disease to deteriorate further in as soon as a month.[15]

Galantamine

Galantamine is one of the top prescription cholinesterase inhibitors today. One of its most popular brand names is Razadyne, or what used to be known as Reminyl. Razadyne is a drug prevents the breakdown of the acetylcholine neurotransmitter and creates a balance among the neurotransmitters present in the brain. As with other Alzheimer's disease medications, Razadyne does not cure the said disease but merely improves qualities such as memory, awareness, and the ability to execute daily activities. Razadyne is typically taken orally with food twice a day. As with other medications, the patient starts with a lower dose in order to prevent drastic side effects until the target dosage has been met. It usually takes four weeks of continuous use before significant effects can be felt.[16] A patient taking this medication may suffer from a few side effects such as diarrhea, headache, lack of appetite, and vomiting, among others. Severe allergic reactions, on the other hand, may include decreased urination, breathing problems, tremors, and irregular heartbeat.[17] Razadyne should not be combined with medications for depression as this could lead to severe complications. The lowest dosage available for this medication is four milligrams. Razadyne has shown some promising results in the treatment of patients with moderate to severe Alzheimer's.[18]

Other popular galantamine brands include Nivalin and Lycoremine. Like any other medications, galantamine may interact with other medications. If the Alzheimer's patient is already taking aspirin, anticholinergics, or atropine, among others, taking galantamine might increase the possibility of a severe side effect. Oftentimes, doctors will remove patients from a medication for forty-eight hours before introducing galantamine.[19]

Rivastigmine

Rivastigmine is another type of cholinesterase inhibitors prescription. It is used to deal with patients suffering from mild to moderate dementia associated with Alzheimer's disease as well as Parkinson's disease. However, it is the only medication approved for use in cases of dementia related to Parkinson's disease.[20] There have been very few cases of side effects to rivastigmine, although there are still a number of patients undergoing treatment using the said medication who have diarrhea, dizziness and headache, increased sweating, and weight loss. Severe side effects to the medication include chest pain, confusion, tremors, and bloodlike vomit.[21] Rivastigmine is also not recommended for patients currently taking anticholinergic medications or nonsteroidal anti-inflammatory drugs (NSAIDs). A patient planning to take rivastigmine needs to inform his or her doctor about any heart condition, stomach and bladder problems, asthma, instances of epilepsy or seizure, and allergies.[22]

One of the more popular brands of rivastigmine is Exelon. Exelon comes in a capsule form and as a skin patch, but both require a prescription. The skin patch has a once-daily dosing and is usually popular for its continuous administration, much like how a nicotine patch works. Exelon works in a similar way to that of Razadyne and Aricept, which is why it is important for the patient to discuss any existing medication or condition before taking this drug.[23] It has been known to address behavioral problems, especially agitation, being experienced by patients with Alzheimer's disease. Overdosing on Exelon has led to life-threatening muscle weakness as well as seizures and slowing down of heart rate. The lowest available dosage of Exelon is generally around one and half milligrams.[24]

Donepezil

More popularly known in the market as Aricept, this drug is considered the most popular of all the medications for Alzheimer's disease. It was approved by the FDA in the early nineties after having proven it does not pose any undue health risks, although as with most medications for Alzheimer's disease, it merely improves the patient's condition and slows the disease's progress but does not completely stop the disease. Donepezil is particularly effective in addressing mild to moderate dementia associated with Alzheimer's. Typically, it is taken orally once a day, commonly at night, with or without food. Patients taking anticholinergic medication as well as those taking ketoconazole are advised to avoid taking it for around forty-eight hours before using donepezil. Anticholinergics in general have a tendency to counteract donepezil, while ketoconazole blocks the metabolism of donepezil in the liver. An increased amount of donepezil that has not been metabolized can increase side effects.[25] Some of the most common side effects of this medication include diarrhea, vomiting, and nausea. These can be avoided, however, if the medication is slowly introduced to the patient over a period of time. If the patient shows signs of unexplained weight loss, severe diarrhea, seizures, stomach or intestinal ulcers, or swelling of the mouth and throat, he or she needs immediate medical attention.[26]

Tacrine

Tacrine is another medication used for dealing with mild to moderate dementia associated with Alzheimer's. However, it is not recommended for patients who have an above-average level of bilirubin in the blood as well as those that have previously taken the medication and have developed jaundice. There is also a risk of liver damage with continued use of this medication. Other medications such as NSAIDs and cholinergic medications may also increase the risk of side effects. Though one research study found that NSAIDs protect a person from Alzheimer's disease,[27] these medications are also known to increase the possibility of stomach or bowel bleeding when combined with Cognex,[28] the brand name for tacrine hydrochloride. In contrast, a clinical report says that gastrointestinal symptoms arising from tacrine use can be alleviated by simply lowering the dosage.[29]

Tacrine is taken orally between meals on a regular schedule. It may be taken with or without food, although if the patient develops an upset stomach, he or she should take the medication with food. As a precaution, this medication should not be taken with alcohol.[30] Patients may also have a difficult time finding this drug as the manufacturers of Cognex are no longer actively marketing the medication.

MORE ON PRESCRIPTION DRUGS

Regardless of the brand of medication, the doctor would normally start with a low dosage and move on to the next one until the Alzheimer's patient's tolerance has been set. This gradual introduction of higher dosages is done to prevent severe side effects.[31]

Generally speaking, both NMDA receptor antagonists and cholinesterase inhibitor groups can provide positive effects for patients after six to twelve months. Since each of the groups typically addresses the same, probable cause of Alzheimer's, there is very little difference if a patient shifts from one medication to another as long as it is within the same group. Because NMDA receptor antagonists deal with a different cause of Alzheimer's than do cholinesterase inhibitors, there are times when doctors prescribe a combination of both in order to achieve better results for the patient.

OTHER DRUGS BEING CONSIDERED FOR ALZHEIMER'S

Aside from NMDA receptor antagonists and cholinesterase inhibitors, there are other drug classifications today that are being developed and are aimed at curing Alzheimer's disease.

Bapineuzumab

One of these is bapineuzumab,[32] a medication to address the buildup of beta-amyloid plaques, brain deposits that are a possible cause of Alzheimer's (see chapter 3). Currently, bapineuzumab is being assessed for treating mild to moderate dementia associated with Alzheimer's. The trial program for this drug is already on its third phase and continues today. Results of the second phase of the study have indicated that the side effects of the medication are minor and temporary except for the occurrence of vascular edema. Lowering the dosage seems to have addressed this side effect to a certain extent.[33]

Dimebon

Today, there are many clinical trials being undertaken to find more medications that can help treat dementia and Alzheimer's disease. Dimebon (iatrepirdine) and PBT2 (Prana Biotechnology 2) are two drugs that are being studied today for their possible therapeutic benefits to Alzheimer's. Dimebon is an over-the-counter (OTC) drug and has the same components as the Russian antihistamine drug Dimebolin, used to treat hay fever.[34] The drug is in its final phases of development as a treatment for Alzheimer's, with results so far showing stabilization of the disease in patients with mild to moderate symptoms.[35] The third phase involved patients who were being treated with donepezil. What set Dimebon apart from other treatments for Alzheimer's is its ability to protect the brain cells from further damage and promote survival. Mitochondrial function is relatively more stable when Dimebon is used (see chapter 5).[36]

Dimebon is not without a downside. Although well tolerated by participants in the clinical trial mentioned above, some of the observed side effects include dry mouth and depression. Some of the participants have also experienced drowsiness, possibly due to the drug's antihistaminergic properties.[37] A major 2008 experiment confirms the benefits of Dimebon for Alzheimer's disease,[38] but the drug failed a more recent, much larger clinical study and is unavailable for use in the United States.[39] It is also no longer available in Russia, its country of origin, as an OTC medication.[40]

PBT2

PBT2 is showing some potential as a treatment for Alzheimer's. Having already passed its initial phase of trials, PBT2 has shown it can be well tolerated by Alzheimer's patients over a twelve-week period of administration. It has also been said to directly restore the neurons in the brain, allowing an Alzheimer's patient to gain back his or her cognitive skills or memory. The PBT2 is a metal-protein-attenuating compound that has been shown to lower the concentration of amyloid-ß in the cerebrospinal fluid (CSF), the same compound that causes toxicity when interacting with copper and zinc. It is also the same compound that can be found in the plaques of the brain tissue of people with Alzheimer's disease. This toxicity plays a major role in the development of Alzheimer's disease.[41] PBT2, however, has its own share of side effects. Some of the participants in the clinical trials for this medication have shown signs of headache, dizziness, and fatigue. There were also some participants who developed hypertension during the course of the treatment. PBT2 continues to undergo testing and research on patients with proven mild to moderate Alzheimer's disease.[42]

HDAC Inhibitors

Another drug currently being studied was originally intended to treat cancer, the histone deacetylase (HDAC) inhibitor.[43] HDAC is an enzyme that takes out acetyl attachments from molecules. This class of medication comes from HDAC blockers that, although do not directly treat Alzheimer's, can help in improving the memory performance of patients with Alzheimer's. HDAC inhibitors are able to increase the gene transcription of the subject's DNA as well as the spool acetylation. According to a website intended for senior citizens,[44] the drug has had success in mice in which Alzheimer's disease, in a form similar to that found in humans, was induced.[45]

Statins

Another class of drugs that might be used to treat Alzheimer's in the future is statins. These drugs actually comprise a class of drugs currently being used by doctors for lowering cholesterol. In one study, it was observed that patients who took the medication had fewer plaques as well as other visible signs of Alzheimer's,[46] but larger-scale clinical research studies (similar to those presented in chapter 15) have not yet been organized to really figure out whether statins are able to produce significant long-term effects. Patients who have taken statins as part of medication for cholesterol have reported side effects such as the following:

- Headache
- Nausea
- Flushing of the skin
- Diarrhea or constipation
- Sleep problems
- Abdominal cramping
- Bloating
- Inflammation of the muscles

Should statins prove to actually help slow down the progression of Alzheimer's, the above symptoms are just some of the many that an Alzheimer's patient might need to deal with. The patient would also need to keep away from such foods as grapefruit and bitter oranges, since these prevent statins from being metabolized. As with any pharmacological treatment, increased levels of the drug in the body can also increase the risk of side effects.[47]

Carbamezepine

There is also a current study being conducted to test the possibility of carbamazepine, a medication used in dealing with epilepsy, as a treatment method for Alzheimer's disease.[48] Initial findings from the study have shown that about three-quarters of the participants had marked improvement in their cognitive functioning. Although not yet officially conclusive, such findings definitely shine a light for people who have long waited for a really effective medication, as patients seems to tolerate the drug quite well.[49] However, some of the more serious side effects that patients who are willing to take carbamazepine may suffer from the following:

- Anemia
- Suicidal thoughts
- Irregular heartbeat
- Unexplained bruising
- Yellowing of the white of the eyes
- Worsening of seizures
- Difficulty urinating

Patients who exhibit these symptoms need immediate medical attention.

Axona

There are also a number of prescription medications derived from food products that are being marketed as a solution to some of the symptoms of Alzheimer's disease. One such item is known commercially as Axona. Considered a "medical food,"[50] Axona is said to have no contraindications and may be successfully combined with NMDA receptor antagonist medications as well as cholinesterase inhibitor medications. However, it also has its share of side effects. Patients have been known to suffer from diarrhea, flatulence, and dyspepsia after prolonged intake of Axona. This medication is available only with prescription and is quite effective in dealing with symptoms brought about by mild to moderate Alzheimer's disease. Care should be given when ingesting this medication as there have been no recent studies done that have replicated the initial results of the second phase of Axona's major clinical trial.[51]

SUMMARY

Although there are a number of FDA-approved medications that can help in dealing with the symptoms of an Alzheimer's disease patient, no specific drug can really put an end to this degenerative disease. Even FDA-approved medications might prove to be harmful to an Alzheimer's patient if not taken properly or if not enough disclosure is made by the physician before prescribing a drug. When it comes to drugs yet to be FDA approved or those still undergoing clinical trials with both positive and negative effects, it is important to know that all existing medical conditions should be taken into consideration before asking for a prescription. As with any pharmacological approach, it is important to get second opinions from other doctors to get a better understanding of what would work versus what would prove fatal for a person. For obvious reasons, people do not like to see themselves suffering from the effects of Alzheimer's and should therefore take care of their health beginning at a young age. A major step in pharmacological treatment is determining a person's risk factors for developing this debilitating disease. Once determined, he or she should make the appropriate lifestyle changes and research the pharmacological options.

· 7 ·

Natural Treatment of Alzheimer's

There is no known cure for Alzheimer's disease,[1] and while pharmaceuticals currently in market may slow progression of the disease and improve the general quality of life for both the Alzheimer's patient and the caregiver, Alzheimer's medications do not work for everyone.[2] For people who are either genetically predisposed or going through behavioral symptoms of Alzheimer's, it is important to know how to approach the disorder naturally. In choosing the natural approach to treating Alzheimer's, a patient benefits from the therapeutic and restorative properties offered by conventional medication without the side effects, which often prove more debilitating than the disease itself.[3] A natural approach is also recommended for Alzheimer's patients who have failed to respond to traditional prescription medication.

Several alternative treatments and natural approaches in the treatment of Alzheimer's disease flood the medical industry today. To narrow down the topic, herbal and animal-based supplements are the natural remedies outlined in this chapter. Some well-sourced and recommended modifications of the Alzheimer patient's living and social environments are also discussed at length.

HERBAL REMEDIES

Caprylic Acid

Caprylic acid, the fatty acid produced when processing coconut or palm kernel oil, has been touted as a leading remedy to combat the early stages of Alzheimer's disease. Following ingestion, caprylic acid breaks down into a substance called ketone bodies. These ketone bodies provide the brain with an alternative energy source. The assumption of caprylic acid's curative powers lies heavily on the proven fact that patients suffering from Alzheimer's tend to have a metabolic deficiency, rendering the brain cells unable to utilize glucose vital for the brain's energy.[4] However, some researchers caution against a dependency on caprylic acid, explaining that as a medium chain fatty acid, caprylic acid tends to be easily absorbed and digested by the body and may result in mild to severe indigestion, heartburn, bloating, abdominal pain, vomiting, constipation, or diarrhea.[5]

Ginkgo Biloba

Ginkgo biloba is one of the oldest living tree species and a staple in traditional Chinese medicine. Due to its reported encouraging effects on diverse ailments such as circulatory disorders, tinnitus, multiple sclerosis, and vitiligo, ginkgo biloba has become a very popular herb in the United States. It has also claimed results in enhancing and sharpening memory. The dried green leaves of ginkgo biloba contain the chemicals flavonoids and terpenoids, and are thought to have resilient antioxidant properties that help in eradicating harmful substances called free radicals in the body. Ginkgo biloba also contributes to an increase of blood flow to the brain and has been widely used in Europe and the United States to combat Alzheimer's and to delay the onset of dementia.[6] Comparative studies indicate that ginkgo biloba extract yields the same benefits as some existing pharmaceuticals aimed at Alzheimer's patients.[7] As with most prescription drugs and supplements, ginkgo biloba is not without its potential side effects. Generalized weakness, nausea, dizziness, restlessness, heart palpitations, and diarrhea or constipation are just some of the milder side effects of ginkgo biloba documented so far. Ginkgo biloba may be particularly harmful for patients with blood circulation disorders, as well as patients who are taking certain types of antidepressant drugs. More serious side effects such as seizures, hemorrhagic stroke, and gastrointestinal bleeding have also been reported.[8]

Huperzine A

Huperzine A is a natural cholinesterase inhibitor derived from the Chinese herb huperzia serrata. Solid medical research concludes that huperzine protects a person's nervous system.[9] Its antioxidant and neuroprotective properties means that it may be constructive for patients suffering from Alzheimer's disease and the early stages of dementia. Long-term studies show a marked improvement in patients' cognitive and noncognitive functions after taking huperzine.[10] Studies also show that Huperzine A shares some chemical properties with some FDA-approved Alzheimer's medications and that it not only cures but also prevents further damage of nerve cells caused by Alzheimer's disease and improves memory.[11] In spite of this, rivals of Huperzine A are quick to draw attention to some of its common side effects, namely, seizures, changes in heart rhythm, blurred vision, nausea, dizziness, muscle cramps, and a considerable increase of sweat and saliva. Patients are cautioned to consult a medical professional before taking Huperzine A with certain conventional prescription drugs because certain combinations can cause adverse reactions.[12]

Tramiprosate

Tramiprosate is an amyloid-beta antagonist used to avert the buildup of the toxic amyloid plaques, which trigger a brain abnormality now largely recognized for the development of Alzheimer's disease.[13] Originally known as the medical drug homotaurine, it has since been renamed tramiprosate and marketed as a natural health product, possibly owing to the discovery of its presence in certain species of seaweed.[14] Some of the frequent side effects reported by Alzheimer's patients taking tramiprosate are intermittent and gastrointestinal in nature, namely, mild to moderate nausea, vomiting, and diarrhea.[15]

ANIMAL-BASED SUPPLEMENTS

Omega-3 Fish Oil

Many blame modern dietary habits as the primary cause of today's lifestyle-associated diseases, which often result in minor inflammation in the body.[16] A diet high in omega-3 fish oil comes highly recommended by researchers because of its anti-inflammatory properties and as an affordable and easily available defense against Alzheimer's disease. Omega-3 fish oil is present in fatty fish such as salmon, halibut, and sardines. It is also found in certain plant oils such as flaxseed oil, rapeseed oil, walnuts, and tofu. Studies show that the omega-3 fatty acid docosahexaenoic acid—originating from fish oil—spurs the production of LR11, the protein responsible for annihilating plaque deposits of the beta amyloid protein believed to have a harmful effect on brain neurons.[17] Some side effects reported from patients taking omega-3 fish oil consist of the following:

- Initial abdominal discomfort
- Easy bruising or bleeding
- Gastrointestinal bleeding
- Impaired vision
- Hemorrhagic stroke

- Hives
- Rashes
- Itching
- Wheezing
- Breathing difficulties[18]

Hyperglycemia, or high blood sugar, was also noted in Alzheimer's patients suffering from diabetes.

Phosphatidylserine

Phosphatidylserine (PS) is an indispensable molecule produced naturally by the human body that plays an important role in keeping cells undamaged and whole. It also moves nutrients into cells and drives out waste. Clinical evidence substantiates the fact that PS aids in alleviating memory loss and depression among the elderly, resulting in sharpened memory and an improved, focused thinking ability.[19] PS was initially sourced from the brains of cows, but this method was abandoned after concerns about mad cow disease were brought to light. Other sources come from chicken heart, chicken liver, and pigs' innards (spleen, kidneys, and liver), but the majority of supplementary PS today is derived from soybeans, white beans, and other plants.[20] Documented side effects of PS are rare and consist mostly of mild gastrointestinal discomfort. Still, studies indicate that PS may disrupt the effects of a number of conventional prescription drugs, and a word of caution is advised when mixing PS with other drugs without the endorsement of a physician.[21]

Coenzyme Q10

Coenzyme Q10, or CoQ10, is a substance inside the cell located specifically in an area that is largely credited as the energy-producing center, called mitochondria. CoQ10 is a producer of the molecule called adenosine triphosphate (ATP), which, aside from getting heralded as an antioxidant, serves as the cell's primary source of energy for protein production.[22] CoQ10 is also available in supplementary form and is said to be beneficial to the general improvement of Alzheimer's patients diagnosed with low levels of CoQ10. Further benefits of CoQ10 include an improvement in immune functions, a delayed aging process, and longevity of health.[23] Some of the possible side effects reported by patients taking CoQ10 are minor and include the following.

- Loss of appetite
- Heartburn
- Nausea
- Vomiting

- Rashes
- Headaches
- Insomnia
- Irritability
- Fatigue
- Flu-like symptoms

Since CoQ10 is known to lower blood pressure, it is advised to constantly monitor the Alzheimer's patient's blood pressure before, during, and after taking CoQ10.[24]

Vitamin E

Vitamin E is an antioxidant celebrated for its defense of body tissue, cells, and organs from free radicals.[25] This vitamin is even more popular as an effective beauty product and is credited to having a profound antiaging effect on skin. Anecdotal evidence blames vitamin E deficiency as one of the key causes for neurological diseases such as anemia, eye disorders, and cognitive difficulties.[26] Owing to anti-inflammatory characteristics, vitamin E is considered a potential treatment for diabetes and high blood pressure. Vitamin E is also given special credit for boosting the mental and physical capabilities of Alzheimer's patients.[27] Recent clinical evidence also points out that a diet rich in vitamin E can considerably reduce a person's risk of getting Alzheimer's.[28] Excellent sources of vitamin E include the following:

- Nuts and seeds (peanuts, almonds, sunflower seeds, and hazelnuts)
- Leafy green vegetables (spinach, watercress, broccoli, and mustard greens)
- Fruits (avocado and kiwi)
- Vegetable oil (wheat germ, corn, and soybean oil)
- Fortified breakfast cereals
- Eggs
- Fruit juices
- Margarine and spreads[29]

On a contentious note, a considerable number of deaths from intravenous vitamin E overdose have been reported for which there have been no concrete answers.[30] Vitamin E is also known to promote and increase the risk of bleeding. In some cases, vitamin E has been found to cause a slew of side effects including the following:

- Nausea
- Diarrhea

- Intestinal cramps
- Fatigue
- Headaches
- Blurred vision
- Gastrointestinal bleeding
- Hemorrhagic stroke[31]

CHANGING THE LIVING ENVIRONMENT

According to a home-care website, nearly six million people in North America struggle with Alzheimer's disease today.[32] This number is expected to reach fifty million in the next five decades. The grandness of these numbers indirectly implies the future burden that might surface on the shoulders of caregivers and family members. Since the living environment plays a crucial role in increasing or lessening such a burden, it is important to understand how minor changes at home can help treat Alzheimer's.

Diet and Exercise

Proper diet combined with consistent exercise still holds true when it comes to preventing and treating Alzheimer's disease. Changing the living environment by way of diet and exercise can help improve the symptoms of Alzheimer's. In fact, studies have shown that a diet high in saturated fat and cholesterol increases the possibility of getting Alzheimer's disease and related ailments.[33] A calorie-restricted diet that includes foods high in omega-3 fatty acids (such as fish) can reduce this risk by 30 to 50 percent. Combined with an exercise regimen of at least thirty minutes a day, three times a week, diet and exercise improves heart rate and blood circulation, bringing down the risk of getting Alzheimer's by 50 percent.[34] (Diet and its role in Alzheimer's disease are covered more extensively in chapter 16.)

Family Time

Having a daily routine gives a semblance of consistency and regularity, which are mutually beneficial to Alzheimer's patients and their caregivers. Maintaining a sense of structure and familiarity within the patient's living surroundings is also of vital importance.[35] Further examination into the topic shows that family caregivers of patients suffering from Alzheimer's disease tend to suffer from psychological distress, which can result in depression, thereby compromising their caregiving functions.[36] Short and concentrated counseling sessions, together with continuous support, have proven to yield a positive and long-lasting effect in counteracting the inevitable depression. This can reduce the overall stress levels of everyone concerned with the situation at hand, including the patient, professional caregivers, and the family members.

Moving in with a family member afflicted with Alzheimer's disease can be tough and stressful. Some difficult decisions and overwhelming changes are bound to take place. This is why researchers are quick to point out how family members can help pave the way to better understanding of and interaction with a loved one suffering from Alzheimer's disease.[37] First and foremost, they advise how family members must not allow themselves to feel stigmatized by the disease. Children are especially prone to stigmatization converging from their peers, so it is imperative that these children be made to learn about the circumstances of Alzheimer's disease, aside from the expectations and inevitable changes that might unfold.[38]

In the attempt to keep the structure and familiarity constant in the living environment of an Alzheimer's patient, experts recommend getting family members involved in the patient's daily or weekly activities. Children or grandchildren must not be kept in the dark from the realities of Alzheimer's disease. Instead, they must be taught about the challenges their grandparent is struggling with, and how they can help their loved one cope. In this way, children learn to empathize with the challenges their loved one is going through. Involving the grandchildren in a routine that is set by the caregiver is a novel method of helping them cope with the patient's struggles while benefiting the Alzheimer's patient. Grandchildren are encouraged to spend time with a grandparent who is suffering from Alzheimer's disease. This should not exceed twenty minutes, as the patient can be prone to mood changes and short attention spans.[39] Nevertheless, much can be accomplished within this short time frame. Young children are inquisitive by nature, and a genuine curiosity for the past can be harnessed by letting them look over photo albums and watch old home movies together with an Alzheimer's-afflicted grandparent. The children can also be encouraged to engage the patient in memory games and help them with simple tasks such as recording important dates on a calendar. Uncomplicated chores such as folding newly washed laundry together are also quantifiable in the sense that it makes the patient feel useful and indispensable. These moments of routine interaction and activity between grandparent and grandchildren may even aid in reminiscing about forgotten memories.[40]

Traveling

While most people do not associate it with healing, traveling can be therapeutic. Aside from the obvious change in living environment, traveling gets the Alzheimer's patient to go outdoors, as he or she moves about between destinations, and perhaps boosts the body's level of vitamin D along the way. Travel also breaks the tedium of monotony and adds variety to life, which is something everyone, not just people undergoing an illness, can appreciate. Travel leaves the patient feeling rejuvenated, refreshed, and chock-full of memorable events.[41]

CHANGING THE SOCIAL ENVIRONMENT

Research shows that, for patients struggling with Alzheimer's, social interaction and recreation can be therapeutic.[42] These are undoubtedly natural approaches to Alzheimer's and are recommended options for treating the disease. Further studies also prove that Alzheimer's patients who get involved in structured activity exhibit cognitive benefits and are less prone to the more disturbing behavioral symptoms of Alzheimer's disease, such as aggression.[43] They are also less likely to get frustrated and wander. In order to be effective however, it is essential that this therapeutic recreation be developed into a routine. When an Alzheimer's patient is active, a habit is developed along with a sense of expectation. This contributes to the patient's feeling of stability and self-worth.[44] Depending on the capabilities, skills, interests, and hobbies of the Alzheimer's patient, suggested home activities include the following:

- Walking
- Gardening
- Cooking
- Painting
- Watching videos
- Singing
- Playing an instrument
- Listening to music

Home movies are likely to spark recognition and ignite memories.

Reducing Social Stress Naturally

As social creatures, people crave companionship and require regular interaction with peers. Scientific research shows that socially isolated people are at a higher risk for Alzheimer's disease.[45] Therefore, when faced with a loved one suffering from Alzheimer's disease, it is important for family members to nurture that kinship and for close friends to stay supportive. Moreover, while interaction and communication are encouraged, psychologists and self-styled new age gurus agree on one thing: the power of positive thinking can greatly contribute to an improved physical state and less social stress. Clinical psychologists who are into the study of the mind-body connection have noted how high stress levels can produce abnormal alterations in the body's immune system, resulting in higher levels of stress hormones and inflammation—always a red flag as far as the immune system is concerned. The same study further claims how psychological and chronic stress can hinder the healing of wounds and even weaken the efficiency of vaccines and medication.[46]

As discussed throughout this writing, long-standing evidence also points to social stress as a mitigating factor in building up frustration and aggression in Alzheimer's patients. Because of its regenerative, relaxing results, massage therapy is one of the suggested programs not only for Alzheimer's disease victims but also for patients suffering from various health conditions.[47]

To take advantage of this suggested link between a positive state of mind and a sound body, it is practical to apply treatments that reduce social stress to people undergoing life-altering illnesses. Alzheimer's patients, since they are prone to bouts of depression and mood swings, can greatly benefit from this. One way to accomplish this is to surround the Alzheimer's patient with positive, upbeat, and emotionally supportive people—they can be family members, neighbors, friends, or colleagues. What is important is that the patient develops a continuous and positive emotional connection with them.[48]

Another way of diffusing and relieving social stress in the Alzheimer's patient's immediate surroundings is to keep a pet that can be taken to gatherings, provided the patient is not allergic to it. Anyone who has raised and nurtured a pet knows the tremendous bond and comfort, not to mention the love and security, these animals can provide. Strong research shows the significance of the human-animal bond in physical impairment, mental illness, dementia and trauma recovery, and even child development.[49] Pet therapy further shows the strengthening of a patient's resilience against emotional, mental, and physical crises. Additionally, most pet owners who are grappling with an illness tend to be aware of how their pets have enhanced their health and overall quality of life.[50]

Human beings seek recreation to satisfy themselves against boredom and to relieve social stress. As discussed previously, Alzheimer's patients are prone to boredom and stress, which can lead to depression. It is crucial that they are provided recreational stimulation that allows them to cope with their illness by experiencing pleasure and recapturing their dignity. While the need for recreational stimulation is still there, Alzheimer's patients, especially those in an advanced state of the disease, can no longer create this themselves and require assistance.[51] Choosing the right recreational activities, therefore, must be approached with care. If the activity is too complicated for the patient to comprehend, the patient may end up getting frustrated. Recent research suggests that leisurely activities, including those known to reduce stress, may lower the chances of getting Alzheimer's.[52] The research indicates that activities should not be aimed at keeping Alzheimer's patients busy; rather, activities should provide a way to create significance in their daily lives. Some important factors to be assessed when choosing an activity for the Alzheimer's patient include attention span, language level, cognitive ability, and mobility. It should also aim to promote social interaction and normalize the patients' lifestyle, maximize functional performance, promote pleasure and enjoyment, and increase self-esteem. Taking all these into consideration, some recreational activities for Alzheimer's patients are discussed below.

Music and Dancing

Music is generally rewarding for everyone, more so with Alzheimer's patients. Studies affirm that Alzheimer's patients become more alert and display better memory skills when exposed to music. Dancing to the music is also a fun and excellent way to get the Alzheimer's patient to exercise and encourage physical wellness.[53]

Arts and Crafts

The list is endless when it comes to arts and crafts projects, and the benefits are just as numerous. Getting Alzheimer's patients involved in an arts and crafts project encourages them to utilize and focus on their fine motor skills. It also enhances and maintains their communication skills, thereby improving personal relationships. An arts and crafts project also stimulates their creativity and expression and elicits a general sense of accomplishment, pride, and enjoyment from their work. Most Alzheimer's patients are prone to changes in mood, skill, and behavior, so the caregiver needs to be flexible and must be sure the project adapts to the patient's abilities and interests.[54]

Games

Integrating games into the daily program of Alzheimer's patients brings about a certain level of excitement for them. While behavioral researchers do not suggest children's board games (this may offend some patients), a simple game such as bingo has actually been pinpointed as a reliable source of therapeutic mental stimulation, with a reported increase in alertness and awareness. Puzzle games with large, brightly colored pieces also aid in boosting cognitive functions in the patient. While picture dominoes and counting games are some of the other popular and easily available games, recent studies have added computer and electronic games conceptualized mainly for Alzheimer's patients. Depending on the patients' needs, these games are programmed to work on different levels and to provide and enhance stimulation to attention and memory, often with promising results.[55]

Sports

Activities that expose Alzheimer's patients to the outdoors and physical exertion are also recommended, be it gardening, raking the leaves, a walk to the park, or a simple game of catch using balloons or large, soft balls. These physical activities help in strengthening and maintaining muscle coordination, increasing flexibility, reducing muscle and joint pain, and enhancing and promoting the patients' general health. Additional benefits include the release of nervous tension and anxiety and decreased restlessness and agitated behavior.

Comedy

Very recently, some researchers have come up with the novel idea of using improvisational comedy as a tool in helping Alzheimer's patients in the early to middle stages of the disease to cope. This natural approach to the disease intends to free patients from the worries and stress of losing their cohesive grasp on words, thoughts, and actions, with humor and laughter as primary instruments. Furthermore, this type of program "fools" the patient's brain chemistry into forging new barriers against the onslaught of memory loss brought about by Alzheimer's disease. Patients who have tried this improvisational approach ("improv" comedy) have declared positive results, describing it as freeing, imaginative, creative, playful, and funny.[56]

Medical practitioners engaged in the treatment and care of Alzheimer's patients note that, before beginning any activity for the patient, it is imperative that the caregiver (1) properly assess the patient's skills beforehand, (2) keep the activity simple and safe, (3) provide both verbal and visual instructions, and (4) play up on the patient's past interests.[57] Patients in the early stages should never hesitate to try something new or, if necessary, to repeat the patient's favorite activities, which may establish a routine in the long run. These reminders can go a long way in creating activities that are meaningful, engaging, and helpful to the patient.

Experts also encourage Alzheimer's patients to socialize with their peers and to get them involved and aware of what is going on in their immediate community.[58] A simple, uneventful trip to the movies, the mall, or the beauty salon can give patients a sense of "staying connected" to the world and provides them with confidence, a sense of pride, and a strong identity.

ANALYSIS

With the advent of easily accessible alternative medicines and numerous natural therapies, it is very easy for an Alzheimer's patient to get drawn into various treatments and programs, often without a doctor's sanctions or prescriptions. These give way to questions that warrant objective responses—questions such as the following: What are the benefits of using natural supplements vis-à-vis prescription drugs in the treatment of Alzheimer's disease? What are the drawbacks? Countless natural supplements, herbal remedies, and other forms of alternative therapies are available in the market today, and most of these claim to defeat almost every disease and illness known. Of particular interests here are illnesses that usually come with advanced age, such as Alzheimer's disease, rheumatism, and osteoporosis. Natural supplements and herbal remedies are not a cure-all for lifestyle diseases such as cancer, cirrhosis, asthma, heart disease, diabetes, gout, obesity, and stroke. However, proponents of herbal medicine and natural supplements are quick to point out that the safest way for humans to supplement their diet would be the natural way, courtesy of readily available, natural food supplements.[59] They have several convincing arguments to support this. One argument is that natural supplements and remedies are just as effective as prescription medicine but with fewer side effects, making these safer to use over time. Another advantage is pricing. Since all prescription drugs undergo a very extensive research, testing, and marketing process, natural supplements generally turn out to be less expensive than prescription drugs. Moreover, unlike prescription drugs, natural supplements do not require a physician's prescription, thus making them easier to obtain. Natural supplements can readily be purchased over the counter or even through the Internet.

As a warning, supporters of pharmacological approaches such as those covered in the preceding chapter, maintain that natural supplements are not without its disadvantages. This is evidenced by the fact that the term *natural* does not have the same meaning as *harmless*. For instance, certain natural supplements are known to induce a trance such as that which is drug-related in some patients, while specific key elements in the supplements may prove incompatible with the body's system, especially when taken simultaneously with specialized forms of conventional medication. This can prove particularly harmful in cases where an early onset Alzheimer's patient is pregnant, breastfeeding, or about to undergo surgery, or where complications such as blood thinning and resistance to anesthesia have been known to occur from mixing natural supplements with conventional prescription drugs.[60] Because government regulation of natural supplements is not as stringent as it is with prescription drugs, there is a considerable risk of acquiring supplements of inferior quality. This variance in quality among supplement brands and manufacturers makes it difficult to arrive at the proper dosage for the patient. Natural supplements should be stored with care. This is especially important when the Alzheimer's disease victim lives with children (see chapter 19).

Believing that natural remedies do not harbor any side effects would expose a giant misconception. Whether these remedies are combined with doctor-prescribed medications or not, gastrointestinal disorders such as nausea, vomiting, and diarrhea have been documented in some patients taking natural supplements for Alzheimer's disease, as well as blood thinning, vertigo, and dizziness.[61] Then there is the alarming possibility of overdosing.

Some natural supplements do not come with instructions, which can lead to self-medication.[62]

If there is anything that most advocates from both ends of the healing spectrum agree on, it is the necessity of consulting a licensed physician or herbalist before starting on any medication, whether pharmacological (traditional) or natural (supplementary). This warning holds true when getting on a regimen comprised of both traditional and supplementary medication. When it comes to the short- and long-term drawbacks of supplementary medicine, the risks involved remain high.

IV

SETTING THE STAGE

· 8 ·

Three-Stage Model of Alzheimer's

$\mathcal{A}$lois Alzheimer first identified a set of brain cell abnormalities as a disease in 1906 but did not propose any staging system to describe this disease.[1] Almost a century later in the 1990s, another German researcher, Heiko Braak, described six stages of Alzheimer's disease, termed the Braak stages 1 through 6.[2] The latter staging system helped to systematically clarify the pathological processes of Alzheimer's.[3] Between these two discoveries, a staging scale called the Global Deterioration Scale for Assessment of Primary Degenerative Dementia (GDS–APDD) was established in 1982. The disease process of dementia was classified into seven stages, based on the extent of the patient's cognitive decline. Although the GDS is a general staging system for dementia, it is most applicable to persons with Alzheimer's. This is because some other dementia types do not always comprise memory loss, such as frontotemporal dementia.[4]

In July 1984, a report on the criteria for diagnosing Alzheimer's disease was published for the first time. This report was a joint effort of the National Institute of Neurological Disorders and Stroke (NINDS) and the Alzheimer's Disease and Related Disorders Association (ADRDA). The report was based on the history of patients with Alzheimer's as well as their clinical examinations, which included neuropsychological and other laboratory assessments. The criteria was thus commonly connoted as the "NINDS–ADRDA criteria" but is hereinafter referred to for clarity as the 1984 criteria.[5] These criteria were adopted by the global medical community.[6] Their reliability and validity as diagnostic evaluators of probable Alzheimer's were generally accepted and utilized. In terms of the sensitivity and specificity of these criteria, several pathological studies have yielded high values for these two parameters (81 percent and 70 percent, respectively).[7] If the success of a set of diagnostic criteria for neurological disorders was measured by its longevity of use, then the nearly thirty-year survival of the 1984 criteria says plenty. No one can deny that advances in genetics and pathological assessment techniques, among others, have been made since 1984. Consequently, the National Institute on Aging (NIA) and the Alzheimer's Association (AA) tasked three expert international workgroups in 2009 to revise, modify, and update the 1984 criteria. This new set of criteria and guidelines is the result of about two years' worth of studies. More than forty international Alzheimer's researchers and medical practitioners performed in-depth reviews of the 1984 criteria to enable improvements via the integration of accumulated research from the last thirty years.[8]

PURPOSE AND BENEFITS

Staging systems in general are very useful for understanding the progress of a disease and can be the basis for selecting the proper interventions.[9] Staging systems are especially important for neurological disorders. The early detection of these disorders enables therapeutic strategies to be developed and applied. An efficient staging method benefits not only the patient but also the study of the neurodegenerative disorder itself in the clinical setting. Advances in the fields of epigenetics, biomarkers, and imaging techniques have contributed to the staging of brain disorders.[10] The three-stage model of Alzheimer's comprises a preclinical stage, a mild cognitive impairment (MCI) stage, and a dementia stage.[11] These stages are discussed in the following sections.

STAGE 1: PRECLINICAL

The first stage of Alzheimer's in the three-stage model is officially known as the preclinical stage but is also called the mild, early,[12] or presymptomatic stage.[13] Stage 1 lasts from two to four years. A distinction should be made between this stage and what are called "early onset" and "familial" Alzheimer's. These latter two are not synonymous with the first stage of Alzheimer's. In fact, they are not stages of Alzheimer's at all. Early onset Alzheimer's is often seen in patients with ascendants (parents or grandparents) who developed Alzheimer's when they were young.[14] Familial Alzheimer's is another Alzheimer's classification in terms of genetic risk factors. Familial Alzheimer's runs in families, compared with "sporadic" Alzheimer's, where no obvious inheritance pattern is seen. Less than 5 percent of Alzheimer's cases are true familial Alzheimer's, whereas sporadic Alzheimer's is much more common. All familial Alzheimer's types thus far known have an early onset.[15]

Presentation

In the preclinical stage, no sign or symptom may exist. The person may not have any sort of memory problem, and even a medical professional interviewing the patient may not see any dementia symptoms.[16] This may be confusing for some. How can this be an Alzheimer's stage? Actually, the concept of a preclinical disease stage is not new. Symptoms are not always necessary for predicting a human disease. Cancer can be detected at a "carcinoma in situ" stage, and a myocardial infarction (heart attack) can be predicted by the narrowing of coronary arteries. Type II diabetes, hypertension, renal insufficiency, and osteoporosis are all frequently detected via laboratory tests or biomarkers. Hence, the possibility that Alzheimer's could one day be preclinically diagnosed exclusively by the presence of biomarker evidence does exist.[17]

There may also be very mild to moderate cognitive decline or neurodegenerative changes in the preclinical stage. These include frequent memory loss of recent events (such as recent conversations and actions), repeating of questions, and some difficulties in expressing and understanding language. There may also be mild coordination problems with writing and using common objects. The occurrence of apathy, indifference, depression, or mood swings is also possible.[18]

Biomarkers for the First Stage

Amyloid beta (Aß, or beta-amyloid) protein accumulation is a major biomarker for the preclinical stage of Alzheimer's.[19] A biomarker is a substance in the body that can be measured to reliably indicate the presence (or absence) of a disease, or even just the risk for developing a disease. An example is the blood glucose level as a biomarker of diabetes. Another example is the cholesterol level as a biomarker of the risk for heart disease.[20] Clinical data from normal older persons suggest that Aß is associated with changes in brain functions and structure. On this basis, the earliest detectable pathological change was hypothesized to be in the form of Aß accumulation. However, Aß accumulation may not solely produce the clinical manifestations of Alzheimer's. Cognitive decline may occur with Aß accumulation but only if accompanied by synaptic dysfunction or neurodegeneration. In recognition of these hypotheses and individuals who may never progress beyond the stage of Aß accumulation, the following staging schema for the preclinical stage was established: (1) asymptomatic cerebral amyloidosis; (2) amyloid positivity with evidence of synaptic dysfunction or early neurodegeneration; and (3) amyloid positivity with evidence of neurodegeneration and subtle cognitive decline.[21]

When an Alzheimer's patient in the first stage has cerebral amyloidosis without noticeable symptoms, he or she has biomarker evidence of Aß accumulation together with a high tracer retention on a positron emission tomography (PET) amyloid image or a low Aß42 in the cerebrospinal fluid (CSF). However, additional brain changes that suggest neurodegeneration or subtle cognitive or behavioral symptoms may not be detected. A study has suggested a CSF Aß42 cutoff value that may predict the development of cognitive impairment—seen in the late phases of stage 1 or early on in stage 2—to

Alzheimer's dementia.[22] Nevertheless, the possible use of a similar threshold value for predicting the decline of individuals with normal or almost normal cognition remains unconfirmed. Moreover, it remains unknown whether a threshold from the cortical region or another anatomic region provides the most reliable predictive value.[23]

Recent data suggest a strongly inverse correlation between CSF Aß42 and quantitative PET amyloid imaging. However, some patients going through the first stage may demonstrate decreased CSF Aß42 but would not be considered amyloid positive on the PET scans (described in chapter 5).[24] These findings reflect that either different thresholds are needed for different techniques or a decreased CSF Aß42 value indicates earlier accumulation. There may also be genetic implications specific to CSF or PET markers of Aß.[25]

In amyloid positivity with evidence of synaptic dysfunction or early neurodegeneration (i.e., the first stage), a patient is positive for amyloid and has one or more markers of "downstream" neuronal injury related to the preclinical stage. The current, most highly validated neuronal injury markers are as follows: (1) elevated CSF tau or phosphorylated tau, or p-tau; (2) Alzheimer's-pattern-like hypometabolism; and (3) cortical thinning or gray matter loss with a specific anatomic distribution. Another future marker may be default network connectivity measured by functional magnetic resonance imaging (fMRI). Although some studies have revealed that amyloid-positive patients have significantly greater abnormalities on these markers on the average (compared with those who are amyloid negative), there are significant variations among patients. People who are amyloid positive and have evidence of early neurodegeneration may be in the later stages of preclinical Alzheimer's. The feasibility of detecting differences among these other biomarkers of preclinical Alzheimer's remains unclear. However, some evidence has implied the possible detection of early synaptic dysfunction before volumetric loss using functional imaging techniques such as PET and fMRI.[26]

In amyloid positivity with evidence of neurodegeneration and subtle cognitive decline, a patient has biomarker evidence of amyloid accumulation and early neurodegeneration, as well as subtle signs of cognitive decline. This patient is in the last part of preclinical Alzheimer's (the first stage) and is nearing the border of the clinical criteria for MCI (mild cognitive impairment). This patient may demonstrate decline from his or her own baseline, even if he or she is still able to perform within "normal" standard cognitive measures. More sensitive cognitive measures, particularly the evaluation of episodic memory, may be able to reveal very subtle cognitive impairment in an amyloid-positive Alzheimer's patient. Self-complaint of memory decline or other subtle neurobehavioral changes may be acceptable as useful predictors of preclinical Alzheimer's progression. However, the combination of biomarkers and a patient's subjective assessment of "self" is still more reliable and verifiable.[27]

Medications for preclinical Alzheimer's are mostly the cholinesterase inhibitors. They slow the breakdown of acetylcholine, a neurotransmitter that is decreased in the brains of Alzheimer's patients. Acetylcholine functions in memory and is used by the hippocampus and cerebral cortex. As discussed to this point, these two brain regions are major areas affected by Alzheimer's disease. However, cholinesterase inhibitors do not cure the disease or reverse the damage that has been done to the brain. They merely improve the patient's symptoms and slow down the disease's progress. To date, five cholinesterase inhibitors have been given the green light for use in the United States for patients in the preclinical stages of Alzheimer's: tacrine (Cognex), donepezil (Aricept), rivastigmine (Exelon), and galantamine (Razadyne). (See chapter 6 for the characteristics of these drugs.) These medications mainly work to improve or stabilize memory and thinking skills. Research has shown that cholinesterase inhibitors help slow the decline of mental functions and behavioral problems.[28] Consequently, the ability to perform everyday tasks is also improved.[29]

Caregiving in the First Stage

A person caring for someone with preclinical Alzheimer's first needs to learn as much as possible about Alzheimer's. Understanding what to expect about the disease will help with care planning and transitions. A caregiver should also avoid thinking that he or she is alone on this journey. Even with an utmost dedication, help in caregiving during the first stage of Alzheimer's will be needed at some point. It is very important to have support in caring for an Alzheimer's patient. A patient with preclinical Alzheimer's mostly needs reminders from the caregiver about daily activities and help with driving.[30]

STAGE 2: MILD COGNITIVE IMPAIRMENT

The second stage of Alzheimer's is officially known as the MCI stage and lasts from two to five years. This stage is also called the moderate or middle stage.[31] The symptoms may be moderate or moderately severe. The patient can no longer hide some problems. There is persistent and pervasive memory loss, such as forgetting about personal history and not recognizing family and friends. Speech tends to be rambling, reasoning is unusual, and current events, time, and place are confused. The patient is more likely to become lost, even in familiar settings; to have a disturbed sleep pattern; and to experience mood and behavior changes that may be aggravated by stress. Delusions as well as aggressive and uninhibited behavior may also be exhibited. There is slowness, rigidity, and tremors in mobility and coordination.[32]

Presentation of Symptoms

Generally, persons with MCI have mild problems performing complex tasks that they could easily perform previously. Such tasks include preparing a meal, shopping, or paying bills. They may take more time in doing rather simple things, become less efficient, and commit more errors than in the past. Nonetheless, they can still maintain their functional independence with activities of daily living (ADLs) with minimal help. These cognitive changes should be sufficiently mild such that no significant social or occupational functioning impairment is apparent. Intraindividual change must be evident before MCI can be diagnosed. If only one evaluation has been performed, change will need to be inferred from other sources. Such sources include the patient history or evidence of cognitive impairment beyond what is expected for that patient.[33]

A person with MCI has an impaired episodic memory or an impaired ability to learn and retain new information. This condition is very common in MCI patients who inevitably progress to a diagnosis of Alzheimer's dementia. Because there might also be other cognitive domain impairment among persons with MCI, domains other than memory need to be examined as well. These domains include executive functions (e.g., reasoning, planning, and problem solving), language (e.g., comprehension, naming, expressive speech, and fluency), attention control (e.g., simple and divided attention), and visuospatial skills. Moreover, atypical clinical presentations of Alzheimer's may manifest, including the visual and language variants of Alzheimer's. The former variant involves posterior cortical atrophy, and the latter is sometimes called logopenic progressive aphasia (LPA).[34]

Genes

There are autosomal genetic mutations involved in Alzheimer's and genes that increase the risk for this disease and that might be meaningful in the MCI stage. The development of MCI is most likely to progress to Alzheimer's dementia when an autosomal dominant form of Alzheimer's is known to be present, such as the amyloid precursor protein (APP) and the phosphatidylserine 1 and 2 (PS1 and PS2) mutations. Notably, early onset Alzheimer's develops in almost all of these mutation occurrences. The duration within which MCI progresses to Alzheimer's dementia (the third stage) varies among different individuals.[35]

The genetic influences on the development of late onset Alzheimer's dementia are also significant to the MCI stage. The only genetic variant currently widely accepted as a mark of increased risk for late onset Alzheimer's dementia is the presence of one or two ε4 alleles in the apolipoprotein E (APOE) gene. In contrast, the ε2 allele marks decreased risk. A person who meets the clinical, cognitive, and etiologic criteria for MCI and is also APOE ε4 positive is more likely than a person without APOE to progress to severe Alzheimer's disease within only a few years. A number of other genes play important, though smaller, roles than APOE. These genes also confer changes that may heighten the risk of MCI progression to Alzheimer's.[36]

Treatment

The treatment for the MCI stage may include a structured-group cognitive development program, multisensory stimulation, behavior management, meaningful activities and engagement, and early psychological therapy. A structured cognitive group development program involves exercises that enhance memory and thinking, as well as those that stimulate multisensory and reminiscence functions. This program usually runs for several weeks and aims to improve memory and day-to-day activities, as well as to orient the patient with reality. Multisensory stimulation helps improve the quality of life via music and pet therapies, as well as massage and aromatherapy.

Behavior management treats problems seen in a stage 2 Alzheimer's patient, such as depression and aggressiveness. Behavior management may be provided by a nonclinical caregiver with instructions from a doctor and support from a nurse. Meaningful activities and engagement include having conversations, cooking and playing games, and painting and drawing. All of these can help the patient express and induce a sense of well-being. Early psychological therapy or counseling helps patients deal with feelings of despair, loss of control, and insecurity. Group therapy, which sometimes involves family members and friends, is practical support to help a patient feel less isolated and happier.[37] All these can improve the patient's quality of life, make the work of caregivers easier, and postpone confinement to a nursing home.[38]

Caregiver's Role

Alzheimer's disease patients in the MCI stage are often aware of their disabilities and their risk of developing dementia. Therefore, they need to make decisions together with their primary caregivers about participating in daily activities that are routine but meaningful; tackling more serious issues (e.g., financial and legal, such as executing a durable power of attorney or a living will); and designing a suitable care plan. Caregivers need to be educated about interventions and must have early training to prepare for possible future behavioral disturbances.[39] Caregivers need to provide structure, reminders, and assistance with ADLs to persons with MCI. Last, medications for the MCI stage include cholinesterase inhibitors (see chapter 6).[40]

STAGE 3: DEMENTIA DUE TO ALZHEIMER'S

The third stage of Alzheimer's is officially known as the dementia due to Alzheimer's stage and lasts from one to three years. This stage is also called the severe or late stage of the three-stage model of Alzheimer's disease.[41] Given that this is the final stage of the disease, the symptoms are already severe. A person loses the ability to respond to the environment and to speak. Ultimately, the person can no longer control movement.[42] There is confusion about the past and present. In addition to the loss of the ability to remember, the abilities to communicate or process information are also absent to a certain extent. Incapacitation occurs accompanied with a severe to total loss of verbal skills. Proper self-care is simply out of the question. Falls and immobility are very likely to happen if the patient lives alone. More importantly, problems with swallowing, incontinence, and illness also arise. There are extreme alterations in mood and behavior that lead to hallucinations and delirium.[43]

Probable versus Possible

Dementia in this stage is classified as (1) probable Alzheimer's dementia, (2) possible Alzheimer's dementia, or (3) probable or possible Alzheimer's with evidence of severe pathophysiological processes of the disease. The first two classes are established for use in clinical settings. The third is currently intended only for use in research. In probable Alzheimer's dementia, the documented cognitive decline of a patient increases the certainty that the condition is an active and evolving pathological process. However, the certainty that the problem is of Alzheimer's pathophysiology is not necessarily increased. The definition of probable Alzheimer's dementia with documented decline is twofold: (1) evidence of progressive cognitive decline on subsequent evaluations based on information from informants and (2) cognitive testing in the context of either clinical evaluation or standardized mental status examinations. There is also evidence of a causative genetic mutation in the APP, presenilin-1 (PSEN1), or presenilin-2 (PSEN2) genes. This evidence increases the certainty that the condition is caused by Alzheimer's pathology. Interestingly, the presence of the ε4 allele of the apolipoprotein E gene is not sufficiently specific to be considered in this category.[44]

In Alzheimer's dementia, there is an atypical course and an etiologically mixed presentation. An atypical course meets the core clinical criteria in terms of the nature of the cognitive deficits.[45] However, there is either a sudden onset of cognitive impairment or insufficient historical detail or objective cognitive documentation of progressive decline. An etiologically mixed presentation meets all core clinical criteria for Alzheimer's dementia.[46] There is evidence of (1) a concomitant cerebrovascular disease characterized by a history of stroke associated with the initiation or worsening of cognitive impairment or by the presence of many, extensive infarcts or severe white-matter hyperintensity burden;[47] (2) features of dementia with Lewy bodies besides the dementia itself; or (3) evidence of another neurological or nonneurological medical comorbidity or medication use that could substantially affect cognition.[48]

In probable Alzheimer's dementia with evidence of the Alzheimer's pathophysiological process, the major Alzheimer's biomarkers may be broken down into two classes based on the biology they measure. The biomarkers of brain Aß protein deposition are (1) low CSF Aß42 and (2) positive PET amyloid imaging. There are also biomarkers of neuronal degeneration or injury. The three major biomarkers in this category are (1) elevated CSF tau (both total tau and phosphorylated tau, or p-tau); (2) decreased 18fluorodeoxyglucose uptake in the temporoparietal cortex as observed on PET; and (3) disproportionate atrophy in the medial, basal, and lateral temporal lobes, as well as in the medial parietal cortex, as seen on a structural MRI. Although total tau and p-tau are treated equivalently, p-tau may be more specific for Alzheimer's than for other dementia types.[49]

Treatment

In addition to cholinesterase inhibitors, memantine (Namenda) is also approved in the United States for the treatment of the dementia from this (third) stage of Alzheimer's. Namenda regulates the activity of glutamate, a neurotransmitter that is important in learning and memory. This is different from other drugs for Alzheimer's that affects acetylcholine levels. The activity of glutamate is often disrupted in Alzheimer's. Namenda functions differently from cholinesterase inhibitors. Studies have shown that its combination with other Alzheimer's drugs may purvey a synergistic effect, compared with any single-drug therapy.[50] A previous controlled clinical trial studied patients receiving Aricept (donepezil) and Namenda (memantine).[51] The results of the study revealed better cognition and other functions than in patients receiving only Aricept. Health care providers might also prescribe medications for treating the other medical conditions that people with stage 3 of Alzheimer's can experience. Anticonvulsants, sedatives, and antidepressants are prescribed to treat seizures, agitation, sleep disorders, depression, and other problems related to dementia. Research from 2005 showed that using Zyprexa (olanzapine) and Rispedal (risperdone) for treating elderly people with Alzheimer's dementia leads to an increased risk of death for the patients.[52] These two are "atypical" antipsychotic drugs that target behavioral problems. Heart problems or infections were the causes found for the mortality. The Food and Drug Administration (FDA) has issued a public health warning to alert patients and caregivers alike regarding these drugs.[53]

Home Environment

Home environment safety is very important in planning the care of persons with Alzheimer's dementia. A research team from Thomas Jefferson University reported that people with dementia, including those who may be going through the third stage of Alzheimer's, particularly those who live alone or with a family caregiver, face several fundamental safety concerns.[54] These concerns are injuries (from falls, ingesting dangerous substances, sharp objects, fire, or burns), leaving the home and getting lost, and an inability to rapidly respond to a crisis situation. Maximizing home safety is not difficult. An extensive range of environmental strategies can be used to make a home safe for a third-stage Alzheimer's patient. As expected, everyday competencies will decline with memory loss. People with Alzheimer's dementia will have an increased difficulty in navigating spaces as well as deciphering and processing cues and stimuli from the environment. Consequently, caregivers need to periodically reevaluate the physical safety of the home and plan new approaches for maintaining all-around safety. Caregivers of people with Alzheimer's need to provide round-the-clock intensive support and care.[55]

THE THREE-STAGE VERSUS THE
SEVEN-STAGE MODEL

The first four stages of the seven-stage model correspond to the preclinical stage of the three-stage model. The fifth and sixth stages correspond with the MCI stage, and the seventh stage corresponds with the dementia stage.[56]

Advantages

The seven-stage model of Alzheimer's is covered in more detail in chapter 10, but it is important to now compare this model to the three-stage model discussed in this chapter. The three-stage model is more advantageous because of its two main approaches: (1) it incorporates biomarkers of the underlying disease state, and (2) it formalizes the different stages of disease in a set of diagnostic criteria. Incorporating biomarker tests, tests that measure Alzheimer-related biological changes in the brain, is important because these tests are very objective. The 1984 criteria were ultimately based on the clinical judgment of a doctor about the etiology of the symptoms of a patient. The doctor gathers medical history from the patient or from family members and friends. The results of cognitive and general neurological assessments are also taken into consideration. The three-stage model proposes the addition of biomarker tests, which delve into the biological processes underlying the symptoms. Moreover, the formalized set of diagnostic criteria is very appropriate because it encompasses a stage (the preclinical stage) wherein symptoms such as memory loss have not yet occurred and one's ability to carry out ADLs (activities of daily living) has not yet been affected. The 1984 criteria required severe memory loss and cognitive decline that affected daily life before making an Alzheimer's diagnosis and taking action.[57]

Given that the three-stage model is relatively new, the seven-stage GDS model is probably still more widely used. Moreover, the new criteria and guidelines do not actually call for an immediate preclinical Alzheimer's diagnosis. The guidelines for the MCI stage are established to distinguish it from mild cognitive decline from other causes. Due to its brevity, the three-stage model is still very convenient and easily applicable in a clinical setting. This model is similar to the available criteria and guidelines in facilities specializing in memory and research. For criteria for the Alzheimer's dementia stage, experts are still working to clarify existing guidelines that can also be used in doctors' offices.[58]

ANALYSIS

The three-stage model of Alzheimer's needs to be updated periodically, especially when intended for use in trials with the main goal of discovering prevention strategies. The updates should focus on three main improvements. The first one: fully incorporating the temporal lag between the first ever pathological event and the initial appearance of signs. The second: establishing or providing complete or better explanations for the biological mechanism underlying the key clinical features of Alzheimer's, such as memory loss and overall cognitive deterioration. Third and last: identifying new or different therapeutic targets.[59]

Doctors, scientists, and experts need to know the most recent staging methods for any neurological disorder, not just Alzheimer's. There is a currently growing recognition that neurobiological processes may start many years before any measurable clinical sign and functional impairment appear. The importance of the preclinical identification of asymptomatic people who have an increased risk for a neurological disease is gaining momentum. Health care providers need to understand the functional relationships (or stages) among the key components of a disease so they can identify the most optimal preventive and therapeutic approaches, which are of course the ultimate goals of any staging system.[60]

· 9 ·

Six-Stage Model of Alzheimer's

$\mathcal{W}$hen Professor Heiko Braak found out about the correlation between a disorder in biochemical processes in the brain and the increasing intensity of Alzheimer's more than twenty years ago, little did he guess that his six stages of Alzheimer's (the Braak stages) would mold into one of the standards for diagnosing and classifying the disease for decades to come.

A NEW CONCEPT

Both Braak and his wife Professor Eva Braak (1939–2000) were teaching at Frankfurt's Anatomical Institute of the Johann Wolfgang Goethe-University and working on the leading edge of research.[1] They searched for new techniques to investigate the course of Alzheimer's. The research was carried out by a team of scientists under the guidance of the Braaks using detailed anatomical analyses. In 1991, the study group released a landmark article regarding the neuropathological staging of Alzheimer's disease that was published in the journal *Acta Neuropathologica*.[2]

A RESEARCHER'S LIFE

Born in the city of Kiel in northern Germany in 1937 as the younger son of Drs. Phil and Elisabeth Braak, the young Heiko Braak was raised in an academic environment. His inclinations toward mathematics and natural science began to manifest early on, and so it was only natural that he chose to study medicine, enrolling himself in studies at the universities of Kiel, Hamburg, and Berlin. In 1963, he graduated from medical school and received his PhD at the Anatomical Institute of the Christian Albrecht University of Kiel. In an interview he gave in 2008, Braak stated he had been interested in researching the human nervous system from the very start.[3] He is said to have been very disappointed when he found out that psychiatrists at the time were not primarily interested in the human nervous system and that, if they considered it from any angle besides anatomical, they considered their patients' sexual lives a more valid point of interest. This situation made him change from psychiatry to anatomy, where physical, not mental, clinical research was valued. Even in the anatomy department, Braak was the only one working with tissues from autopsy, as the investigation method at that time included working with the electron microscope, which did not work well on dead organic material.

Braak's early research papers feature the form and structure of the central nervous system of cartilaginous (bony) fish, in particular, a species called Chimaera monstrosa (ratfish), and on spinax niger (black shark).[4] In 1970, he completed his studies in anatomy at the University of Kiel and climbed the professional ladder within the university from instructor of anatomy to assistant professor, and finally, to associate professor.[5]

From 1979 until 2002, Braak held the directorial position at the Institute for Clinical Neuroanatomy of the Johann Wolfgang Goethe University in Frankfurt.[6] He followed his passion for science after his official retirement in October 2002 and was appointed to the position of guest researcher at the Dr. Senckenberg Anatomical Institute at the University of Frankfurt, where his work was supported by the German Federal Research Council. Braak's main research focus still remains with the investigation into age-associated brain changes versus age-associated degenerative diseases of the human brain. He has made major discoveries on dementia-related problems such as those described in chapters 2 and 4, including Parkinson's, argyrophilic grain disease (AGD), multiple system atrophy, Pick's disease, and progressive supranuclear palsy, in addition to cortical basal degeneration.[7] As one of the most honored contributors of scientific research in the field of neuropathology and neuroanatomy, Braak is recognized among several societies and institutions,[8] including the American Association of Neuropathologists (AANP). In 1998, Braak was a guest of honor at the Sixth International Alzheimer's Congress in Amsterdam. Together with his wife Eva Braak, he won major prizes for his contributions to the field of Alzheimer's research. In 2003, he was a guest of honor to the Third German Parkinson's Congress in Dresden, Germany. He was awarded the Lundbeck Prize for Parkinson's Disease Research jointly with Kurt Jellinger.[9]

New research by Braak and his team of experts at the University of Ulm has revealed that Alzheimer's is really a systematically progressing disease very much like an infection that starts spreading from a specific section of the brain.[10] The damaging process seems to start at a very early age.

THE METHOD

Determining the six stages of Alzheimer's involved examining the brains of deceased people using staining techniques to enhance visualization of the problems in question. At the time, it was very uncommon to work that way; researchers were either using the electron microscope or the brains of rats and mice for scientific comparison. As Alzheimer's disease was gradually categorized into six stages, it became obvious that the process of deterioration of brain activity was due to a deformation of tau protein. Scientists also believe that a different protein called the amyloid beta protein was the cause of the process of deterioration.

Anatomical evaluation eventually led to the visualization of the tau protein. The six-stage model of Alzheimer's really represents a scientifically proven scale of intensity and progression of the accumulation of tau tangles in the brain, including information about the location of the "tangling" process in the cerebrum's various regions. The tau protein is the body's own substance that is used by the brain cells of every healthy individual as a kind of scaffolding material, but when it gets out of control, problems occur. In all cells of the human body, the so-called microtubuli (small tunnels) formed by tau proteins and others serve as a stabilization element giving form and structure to the cell, ensuring the processes of communication and transport of chemical messages between cells. In the case of the six-stage model of Alzheimer's, the tau proteins are found to be subject to an ongoing process of mutation, causing the microtubule to destabilize. The reasons for this progressive malfunctioning of the tau protein are still rather unclear.

As the Alzheimer's patient gets older and goes deeper into the phases of the six-stage model, the tau proteins get shaped into filaments inside the neuron.[11] The tau filaments lose their rigidity and form tangles—clinically referred to as neurofibrillary tangles (NFTs). The NFTs form clusters that overcrowd the neuron and eventually lead to its bursting. This inevitably leads to the death of the nerve cell. The decay of the neuron then starts off a major pathological chain reaction, which gradually spreads to involve more and more brain cells. So far, scientific research has found the complete destruction of brain cells to be an irreversible process. The traces of destruction in the brain of affected individuals can be likened to the destructiveness of a tsunami wave. With relentless insinuation, neurofibrillary tangles spread and damage more and more neurons, literally invading one region of the brain after another, starting from the hippocampus on to the temporal lobe and the neocortex. This development affects the brain signals and impulses that are carried from lower regions of the brain to higher regions.

ADDITIONAL ATTEMPTS TOWARD CATEGORIZATION

As symptoms can fluctuate quite a bit and seem to vary daily or even hourly, it appears that the individual manifestation of the illness has to be considered from a particularly personal point of view for each and every patient, especially when it comes to practical experience.[12] This fact speaks against the method of staging in Alzheimer's disease altogether, especially where the categorization of outwardly detectable symptoms into stages is concerned. For the same reason, it is quite difficult to place an Alzheimer's disease victim in a specific stage of the six-stage model. In the past, there have been several attempts to classify the stages of Alzheimer's disease. Stage qualifications such as the three- or seven-stage model focus on the symptoms of the disease, for example, how Alzheimer's affects the quality of life as the disease progresses. When speaking of a staging system that is directly related to symptoms, it is important to re- member that symptoms are never uniform in every patient and that stages never really follow a straight pattern. Individual phases can overlap.

OTHER STAGING MODELS IN COMPARISON

The three-stage model is the one model that has enjoyed major recogni- tion so far. In that model, the stages are subdivided into early, middle, and late phases of progression.[13] The subdivisions of the three-stage model were found to be insufficient and too broad by many researchers, leading to the formation of newer ways to categorize Alzheimer's. There was a call for a new system that would offer a more hierarchical structure.

Theorizers of the most recent staging system, the seven-stage model, suggest that Alzheimer's disease is a gradually progressing disease. They also suppose that other illnesses, concurrently with dementia, would be clearly dis- tinguishable at all levels. The third principle involved in their consideration was that certain social functions and behaviors of humans are common to society and that they can be used for general reference. The variety of pos- sible functional loss was categorized in the Functional Assessment Staging (FAST).[14] (The seven-stage model of Alzheimer's will be discussed in more detail in the next chapter.)

The major difference between the traditional three-stage model and the six-stage model is that the latter uses different parameters. The three- and seven-stage versions focus on categorizing symptoms, whereas the six-stage model of Braak concentrates on the degenerative neurological process of tau- protein malfunctioning and on how it gradually affects the various parts of the brain. In the six-stage model, the gradual decay of neurons is categorized based on direct anatomical observation. These observations include the intelligence of the patient, behavior, and the existent or nonexistent ability to cope with everyday situations, considered marginally as a point of reference. This establishes the work of Braak as truly scientific since it is based on empirical research, not on assumptions.

A LOOK INTO THE BRAIN

The scheme of stages established by Braak in 1991 is divided into six categories that are subdivided further when considering the regions of the brain gradually affected by neuronal death.[15] The reason for various areas of the cortex being affected prior to others is that they are much more sensitive and tend to be subject to lesions more easily. By way of a lecture, Braak distinguishes exactly six stages giving evidence of the propagation of the disease.[16] The various phases are subdivided with respect to the location of the changes within the neurons (nerve cells) and the severity of the destructive process. The first two stages are summarized as being related to the transentorhinal region of the brain (transentorhinal stages 1 and 2). These stages are thought to be "clinically silent," meaning they are not very noticeable at first. The third and fourth stages are associated with the region of the limbic system (limbic stages 3 and 4) and show incipient Alzheimer's disease development. The fifth and sixth stages are in relation to the neocortical region of the brain (neocortical stages 5 and 6). The disease is deemed fully developed in these two latter stages of the six-stage model of Alzheimer's.

The transentorhinal stages are linked to the entorhinal cortex of the brain. This cortex is located in the anterior (front) part of the hippocampus. A University of Washington website on the neuroanatomy of the human brain shows that the hippocampus, or archicortex, is located in the medial temporal lobe of the brain.[17] Because of its association with the limbic system, the hippocampus plays an important role in the six-stage model of Alzheimer's. The hippocampus is very active while information gets relocated from short-term to long-term memory, and it is also responsible for coordinating the spatial navigation of the Alzheimer's patient. Structurally, the hippocampus is closely associated with the cerebral cortex. Its shape is paired with mirror-image halves in both the right and the left side of the brain.

A report on the diagnosis of dementia suggests that patients going through these stages (transentorhinal 1 and 2) would be far from being clinically diagnosed as suffering from Alzheimer's.[18] However, there is clear evidence of Alzheimer's-related processes in both stages, and thus these phases are diagnostically demonstrative of Alzheimer's disease.

STAGE 1

Braak stage 1 is the stage where tau protein begins to first aggregrate. The process of tau tangles forming is limited to only one particular layer of the entorhinal cortex. This layer is called the prealpha layer. At this stage, the patient fails to display any external symptoms. For that same reason, this stage of Alzheimer's is also referred to as preclinical or clinically silent. Evidence of Alzheimer's-related processes in the shape of tau tangles and neuron decay could be detected only postmortem (after death) in brains examined autoptically (by observation).

A statistical report suggests that Alzheimer patients reach Braak stage 1 somewhere between forty and ninety years of age.[19] The report also states that around 30 percent of fifty-year-old Alzheimer's patients and roughly 50 percent of sixty-two-year-olds who are affected have reached Braak stage 1.

STAGE 2

The same report states that, by Braak stage 2, tau tangles accumulate further and cause some nerve cells to tear apart and die.[20] Mental examination still shows minimal impairment. The report also mentions that brain tangles at this stage are observed in the brains of approximately 60 percent of Alzheimer's patients over the age of sixty-five. The primary location of tau tangles at this stage is found in the cerebral region of the entorhinal cortex. In this region, sensory inputs are filtered before being stored in memory. Neocortical regions are not yet affected by the lethal cell changes, but the initial aggregation of tau proteins and subsequent formation of tangles starts there as well. As mentioned in chapter 2, the cortex region of the brain is responsible for the formation of conscious thought. Notably, Braak stages 1 and 2 relate directly to stages 1 and 2 of the seven-stage model of Alzheimer's to a certain extent, since both models accept the difficulty to diagnose Alzheimer's early on. Both evaluation methods come to the conclusion that a patient in the first stage of Alzheimer's does not present with any cognitive deficits.

STAGE 3

When an Alzheimer's patient reaches the third stage of the six-stage model, tau tangles have initiated the death of neurons in large parts of the brain. Only 10 percent of the patients at that stage will be diagnosed as suffering from dementia. About 45 percent of eight-year-old people in modern society have reached this stage.[21] By the time the third stage is evident, three major regions of the brain are already partly affected. The transentorhinal region is extensively pervaded by tangles of tau protein. The hippocampus is affected, and formation of tangles in that region can be detected. Aggregations of the lethal misformation of protein have even taken over the area of the neocortex. Destruction takes place particularly in layers of the transentorhinal region that are referred to as prealpha, prebeta, and pri-alpha. This process disturbs the forwarding of information to the hippocampus. Looking closely, only the regions designated as CA1 (also known as cornu ammonis or the superior region of the hippocampus) and subiculum (part of the gray structure) are affected by the changes. Light modifications are observed in the limbic regions called nucleus anterior dorsalis thalami (also known as the anterior nucleus of the thalamus), amygdala, nucleus reuniens (thalamus), and nucleus tuberomamillaris (hypothalamus).[22]

For Alzheimer's patients in stage 3 of the Braak model, it can become difficult to classify emotional perception and attribute meaning. Memory stored in the neocortical regions will not be accessed properly, and there can be dysfunctions of the very relevant process of sensually relevant imagery being stored. Access to long-term memory might be impaired, but the effect on the functioning of communication processes in these regions is very small.

LIMBIC SYSTEM'S ROLE

Stages 2 and 3 of the Braak model affect large parts of the limbic system. The term limbic system denotes a composite substructure of forebrain. The term "limbic" comes from the Latin word limbus, for "border" or "edge." The basic functions of the limbic system are (1) to connect other areas of the brain and (2) to provide emotional classification. Most scientists agree in their classification on the limbic regions of the brain being constituted by the following structures:

- Amygdala
- Epithalamus
- Parahippocampal gyrus
- Hypothalamus
- Cingulate gyrus
- Hippocampus
- Septal nuclei
- Anterior nuclear thalamus
- Portions of the basal ganglia[23]

The limbic lobe was first discovered by a French scientist named Paul Broca in 1878 and was originally believed to support a variety of functions including emotion, behavior, long-term memory, and olfaction (sense of smell).[24] The limbic system was originally perceived as the place of emotion and was compared to the neocortex as the supposed home of reasoning and cognition. This segmentation was found invalid and had to be abandoned when damage to the hippocampus, a primary limbic structure, was found to result in severe cognitive and memory impairment. The anatomical changes of both the second and third stages are known to cause behavior that can be clinically recognized as incipient Alzheimer's disease.[25]

STAGE 4

The fourth stage designates a point of development at which an extensive formation of tangles can be observed in the transentorhinal region and in the hippocampus. The isocortical regions start to be affected, marking the beginning of a 100 percent feasible clinical diagnosis of Alzheimer's disease. The hyperphosphorylated tau proteins begin to form ghost tangles, or tangles outside of cells where the host neuron has died. Statistically, 70 percent of patients at this level will be classified as having dementia.[26]

Personality changes will be detected on the emotional level, and attribution and the processing of emotional memory is severely impaired. Evaluation, classification, and storage of new data in the brain structure become difficult for the patient, because the ongoing process of cognition and recognition of existing data that takes place in the hippocampus is severely impaired. Cognition and recognition of contents usually happen to a wide extent based on an ongoing process of comparison with events stored in the long-term memory. Patients encounter major difficulty with attributing any meaning to tasks offered by their social surroundings. It also becomes increasingly difficult to differentiate "familiar" from "unfamiliar." It may be quite normal for them to wrongly attribute importance and significance to information that is actually completely irrelevant to them. Consequently, patients at this stage of the Braak model will behave outside the norms of society. People they interact with may observe strange reactions and behavior. This happens because the process of purpose-oriented attribution of meaning is disturbed. Internal reference is made to memories of the long-term-storage that pertain to the individual biography. Subjectively, patients are unaware of their behavior being strange in front of others because they are really not aware of the way their thoughts and associations are "going down the wrong way."[27] It is quite normal for patients to try to hide the mistakes they perceive as trivial in front of others and to keep acting as if nothing is wrong. As the disease progresses into stage 5 and 6, denying any insufficiencies becomes increasingly difficult, and patients gradually become fully aware of their impairment.

STAGE 5

Superficial and deep layers of the hippocampus are severely affected in this stage. Both the limbic regions as well as the amygdala are completely scattered with the ghost tangles described previously. The hypothalamus and the pars compacta part of the substantia nigra are affected. Around 80 percent of patients with such a high degree of tangles will be diagnosed as suffering from moderate to severe dementia.[28]

Patients suffering from Alzheimer's disease at stage 5 are cognizant of their impairment. All the aforementioned symptoms of dysfunctional communication and inability to attribute impressions become more dominant, gradually resulting in a complete failure to handle even simple everyday routines.

STAGE 6

The primary cortex (motor, visual, and sensory cortex) is affected more in this stage than in the other five. Major parts of the limbic system and the extrapyramidal system, which is primarily in charge of motor functions, are involved. The locus ceruleus is the starting point of the degenerative process. It is important to note that, by the time an Alzheimer's patient reaches the sixth stage, loss of neurons in the locus ceruleus has progressed to between 50 and 70 percent.[29] Patients suffering from Alzheimer's disease at this stage are fully conscious of their impairment. They become unable to find their way within their social environment without the help of others. As destruction of neurons in various parts of the upper brain regions continues, patients gradually become completely unable to take care of themselves. The ability to recognize and perceive is lost to the extent of them having difficulty recognizing even close friends or family members.

NEOCORTEX

The main characteristic of stages 5 and 6 is the complete pervasion of the neoisocortex by tangles. Ghost tangles have taken over the place where neurons used to be. Regions of the brain mentioned in the above stages are now severely contaminated by tangles and include the following:

- Transentorhinal region
- Presubiculum
- Temporal isocortex
- Gyrus dentatus
- Cornu ammonis (Ammon's horn)[30]

RECENT DEVELOPMENT AND OUTLOOK

The Braak stages shed a clear light on the idea that Alzheimer's disease is analogical to an endless river that has its headwater in the very remote regions of young age. For a very long time, the disease was believed to affect only elderly people. Braak's extensive research has revealed though that the illness spreads slowly and systematically, sometimes developing over a period of several decades.[31] The common belief that Alzheimer's comes with old age is a misunderstanding, as the normal process of aging seems to be affecting *all* cells of the human brain. What really makes the weighty difference is that Alzheimer's-related changes in the brain can be detected only in certain cells. While recently conducting research, Braak detected neurofibrillary tangles inside brains of infants and adolescents.[32] In nineteen out of forty-two brains of young people under thirty, he was able to locate early stages of deformed protein structures. After all those years of ongoing research on tauopathies, the place of origin of the malignant changes in Alzheimer's-affected brains seems to be finally identified as the locus ceruleus. Braak refers to this section of the brain as the source and fountain of all Alzheimer's-related changes. The name is derived from the two Latin words *locus* (place or region) and *ceruleus* (blue and sky-like) and was given due to the bluish appearance of the tissue. The locus ceruleus is a tiny section of the brainstem and has to do with physiological responses (the body's reactions) to stress and panic. Braak suspects that nerve cells located in this region send not only ordinary signals to the cerebrum but also error messages of irregularly folded proteins.

MORE ON ALZHEIMER'S AS AN INFECTIOUS PROCESS

In light of the above discoveries, Alzheimer's might well be identified as an infectious process, very much like mad cow disease or bovine spongiform encephalopathy (BSE). One can perceive the illness to be a shadow that gradually spreads out and seizes all of the vital energy from a person and begins to advance in an individual almost entirely on its own. Wherever there is a shadow, there is light, so right at that point the chance for developing a cure seems to be evident.[33] If it were ethically possible to induce early, visible Braak stages of Alzheimer's in humans, it might be possible to stop the persevering process of neuron decay simply by detecting and destroying single neurons contaminated by malfunctioning tau proteins. New therapeutic methods designed to do away with harmful cells would halt the fatal disease at its very origin, thereby nipping it at its bud.

· *10* ·

Seven-Stage Model of Alzheimer's

ALZHEIMER'S DISEASE CLASSIFICATION

As this chapter concludes part IV, it is important to comprehend now the importance of looking at Alzheimer's as a disease that gradually and progressively deteriorates brain function. As such, the classifications that have been developed for categorizing patients take the form of stages, with each stage involving various manifestations that patients exhibit as the problems worsen. The methods of classification (staging systems such as the three-, six-, and seven-stage models) are mainly for determining what kind of care a patient requires and for comparing different patient groups. Classifications can be difficult to us as major prognostic indicators since the rate of deterioration varies greatly from patient to patient.[1] Generally, the younger the person is when Alzheimer's takes hold, the faster the disease will progress. Another factor is usually the presence of a family history of Alzheimer's, in which case, progression is swift, although patients vary immensely in how quickly they deteriorate. When there is a solid family history of Alzheimer's, the rate of progress tends to be much more rapid than if no such history exists.

The seven stages of Alzheimer's disease show the stepwise advancement of the physical and mental symptoms and how it affects the brain as it "travels" through it. As mentioned in chapter 4, a pronounced symptom of Alzheimer's, when in early stages, is memory lapse. It does this by affecting the hippocampus, the structure in which new memories are formed. Over time, memory lapses concerning recent events ensue. The final stages of the seven-stage model are characterized by reduced coordination and balance, and one might even experience difficulty in breathing and have blood pressure complications, functions normally controlled by the cerebellum and the brain stem.[2]

The two most commonly used classifications for Alzheimer's are the three- and seven-stage models. Both classifications overlap in various stages, and some patients do not go through all the stages. Rapid progression of the disease is more often caused by other diseases or other contributing factors. The most obvious difference between the two models is that the three-stage classification has three stages, while the seven-stage classification has seven. This chapter describes each of the following seven stages of Alzheimer's in detail:

- Stage 1: Lacking any major impairment
- Stage 2: Very mild decline
- Stage 3: Mild decline
- Stage 4: Moderate decline
- Stage 5: Moderately severe decline
- Stage 6: Severe decline
- Stage 7: Very severe decline[3]

FROM ROOTS TO STEMS

The seven-phase model of Alzheimer's, also called the Global Deterioration Scale (GDS) or Functional Assessment Staging (FAST) scale, was developed by Barry Reisberg. It was the first model to describe in great detail the crucial symptoms and, in a stepwise fashion, the clinical course of Alzheimer's as it causes damage to the brain. Barry Reisberg is a geriatric psychiatrist, currently a psychiatry professor at the New York University School of Medicine. He also lectures at Canada's McGill University.[4]

Before his residency training, Reisberg studied at Sophia University in Japan and then worked in Nigeria, Turkey, Iran, and India among other countries while enrolled as a medical student in New York.[5] Reisberg has carried out research that has had significant impact in understanding the seven stages of Alzheimer's and their subsequent treatments.[6] In addition, he wrote or cowrote numerous scientific papers in geriatrics, psychopharmacology, and neuroscience, among other related topics. He is also a member of the editorial boards of seven journals specializing in the medical and scientific fields. For his pioneering research work, Reisberg has received many awards and grants from various government, nonprofit, and industrial sources. Key awards include the lifetime achievement award for exceptional research that was presented by the International Conferences on Alzheimer's Disease (ICAD) and by the Alzheimer's Association. The U.S. government has mandated the use of the seven-stage model as a staging tool for Alzheimer's. The system is also utilized widely in some European countries, Canada, and Japan.

STAGE 1: NO COGNITIVE IMPAIRMENT

In the first stage, everything appears to be normal, and there is no notable deterioration in mental, judgment, or reasoning capacity. This can go on for years without being noticed. In this first stage, the person does not experience any memory problems. Even an interview with a qualified medical professional during this stage will not reveal any signs or evidence of dementia.[7]

STAGE 2: VERY MILD COGNITIVE PROBLEMS

At this stage, the Alzheimer's disease affects the part of brain that typically stores memories. The person will experience memory lapse and an inability to think clearly with usual speed and clarity. A person may forget familiar words, places, or the location of normal everyday objects. The patient will shun people and is withdrawn and disinterested. Daily tasks will take longer than normal to accomplish, and handling finances, such as tracking investments and reconciling bank statements, becomes difficult. A medical examination might not detect dementia signs, as even friends, family, or coworkers will be unable to recognize the symptoms and might associate them with the natural process of aging.

STAGE 3: MILD, NOTICEABLE COGNITIVE ISSUES

In the third stage, the symptoms of Alzheimer's will increase quickly, unlike symptoms of aging. The part of the brain that is affected is the temporal lobe, which controls memory and language. The patient may, at this point, start to notice there is something wrong, and people close to him or her might also begin to worry. The patient might even try to conceal the symptoms. At this stage, with a detailed interview, a medical professional might detect the difficulties in concentration or memory. Other symptoms include the following:

- Difficulty remembering names and words, particularly new names, for instance when introduced to someone they've never met.
- Difficulty carrying out routine or normal job assignments. Others start to notice behavioral changes in the patient, especially in social settings.
- Difficulty with writing and general issues of coherence, such as occasionally uttering unusual words.[8]
- Forgetfulness, especially of freshly read material or documents and with losing track of items.
- Deterioration of planning and organizing skills.

At stage 3, most Alzheimer's victims tend to use reminders, calendars, and checklists to make up for their deteriorating symptoms. This stage usually spans two to seven years.[9]

STAGE 4: MODERATE COGNITIVE DISABILITY, EARLY ALZHEIMER'S DISEASE

During this stage, a thorough medical examination is able to detect problems and clearly indicate impairment. Alzheimer's disease at this stage fully affects the frontal lobe, which is associated with short-term memory tasks such as planning and driving. Stage 4 of the seven-stage model of Alzheimer's usually lasts for two years.[10] Symptoms of this stage include the following:

- Inability to remember recent events.
- Deterioration in performing mental tasks, such as counting backward.
- Impaired recollection of personal experiences.
- Difficulties in managing and planning for tasks, such as finances for paying bills and rent.
- Being socially withdrawn or even avoiding mentally challenging situations.

STAGE 5: MODERATELY SEVERE COGNITIVE PROBLEMS, MODERATE ALZHEIMER'S DISEASE

At this stage, the individual requires daily care as there are major gaps in memory function and deterioration in cognitive thinking. The following symptoms occur in stage 5 of the seven-stage model of Alzheimer's:

- Difficulties with—or inability to remember at all—present-day details such as telephone numbers, addresses, date of birth, or the current president, when asked. However, patients might recall an old address, schools attended, or the president twenty years ago.
- Difficulty figuring out which season it is and telling the time of day, the date, the year, or the week.
- Problems performing less complex tasks, including counting backward from forty in intervals of four, or performing mental calculations.
- Need for consistent reminders to change clothes (or they might wear the same wardrobe every day regardless of the climate).

Patients can remember their own names or that of their spouse or children's, but they forget or disregard activities of daily living (ADLs), such as bathing, eating, dressing, toileting, walking, and taking medicine. Simple things can be done in order to help the individual with day-to-day routines. These include the following:

- Providing a safe environment. This can be compared to creating a safe environment for a child. Keeping sharp items such as knives out of reach is very important, and when in use, knives should be handled under supervision.
- Creating a realistic routine. Patients are encouraged to do the same thing every day and at the same time if possible. This will make people with Alzheimer's stay independent for longer.
- Individual chores. Friends and family are encouraged to make patients feel productive by giving them work to do around the house. Chores can consist of dusting, sweeping, and washing. The type of work given should be one that is in a safe environment. Chores such as cutting vegetables and tending to the fireplace should be done under close supervision.
- Physical and mental fitness. For Alzheimer's patients in stage 5 of the seven-stage model, exercises such as jogging and brisk walks will help energize the body. Puzzles and reading will keep them mentally fit.
- Clothing. At the early stages, putting on clothes is not too difficult, but at advanced stages, it might be necessary to get clothes that cannot be easily removed, since in late stages of the seven-stage model, patients tend to undress when it is inappropriate to do so.[11]

STAGE 6: SEVERE COGNITIVE DECLINE, MODERATE TO LATE-STAGE ALZHEIMER'S

The sixth stage is a critical stage, as the individual requires daily care and help with regular activities. There are major gaps in memory function, and cognitive thinking has greatly deteriorated. Some of the manifestations observed in this stage include the following:

- Inability to put on clothes and often requiring help to do this. For example, patients might forget to put on shoes, walking outside in just their socks, or they might have difficulty with buttons and sleeves.
- Urinary issues can be prevented at first by encouraging more visits to the bathroom. Use of bedding and undergarments that are capable of taking in liquids are advised (see chapter 4).

- Problems remembering details such as personal phone numbers, date of birth, address, or the school or college they attended.
- Forgetting names of spouse and children, or often confusing the spouse with the caregiver. Patients might have problems distinguishing faces as well.
- Disruption of normal sleep patterns by sleepwalking, or the inability to fall asleep at night and taking excessive naps during the daytime.
- Inability to respond to simple questions such as: Who is the current president? Patients might recall an old address, school, or a president from twenty years ago.
- Problems with recollecting dates and the current day, time, week, or season.
- Need for constant reminders to change clothes. Patients might wear the same clothes every day regardless of the season.
- Mental changes, such as hallucinations and delusions.
- Compulsive repetitive behavior, such as handwringing.[12] Personality and behavioral changes could be severe and could transform into aggressive, anxious, and even violent actions.[13]
- Wandering (see chapter 11).
- Difficulty speaking and understanding the speech of others.

The Alzheimer's victim forgets or does not pay attention to ADLs such as bathing, eating, dressing, walking, and taking medicine. Simple things can be done in order to help the individual complete simple, everyday routines, such as the following:

- Dressing properly. The patient can make wardrobe mistakes, such as putting on pajamas over daytime clothes or wearing shoes on the wrong feet.
- Regulating the bath water temperature. However, patients can still bathe on their own. As stage 6 progresses, assistance might be needed with bathing, dressing, and general hygiene.
- Helping with toileting (e.g., flushing the toilet, wiping, or disposing of tissue properly).
- Creating a safe environment. This can be compared to creating a safe environment for a child. Knives should be kept out of reach and should be used only in the presence of adequate supervision.
- Creating a daily routine. Patients should try to maintain consistency in their daily routines. This will make a person with Alzheimer's stay as self-sufficient as possible.

- Providing work. People around Alzheimer's victims should help them feel productive by giving them some work to do around the house, such as sweeping, dusting, and washing.
- Helping to stay fit. Exercises such as jogging and speed walking will help energize the body, and mental exercises such as puzzles and reading will keep them mentally fit.
- Dressing. During the early stages of the seven-stage model, putting on clothes is not too difficult, but in the later stages, securely fastened clothing is encouraged, since patients tend to remove their clothing without notice.

STAGE 7: VERY SEVERE COGNITIVE ISSUES, LATE-STAGE ALZHEIMER'S

At this stage, the individual is entirely dependent on a caregiver when it comes to basic daily activities. This is the final stage, when organs begin to shut down. Central nervous system functions are quite deteriorated, and the patient is unable to control most bodily functions and starts experiencing organ failure in some cases. The symptoms manifested in this stage include the following:

- Incoherent speech, although at times, complete words and phrases are spoken. Patients are not able to carry on a normal conversation.
- Frequent incontinence issues. Assistance is needed with toileting and eating.
- Inability to move around without help. The head needs to be supported.
- Impaired swallowing (explained in chapter 17).

During this final stage, patients become incapacitated to the point that they cannot walk without help. They also need support to sit up. They are not able to move their lips to smile, and their head needs to be held up. Patients also are no longer "flexible," meaning movement is impaired as muscles such as those near the elbow slow down. Muscle contractures and joint deformity can occur and hinder the full movement of joints. In this stage, individuals require constant, round-the-clock attention since they are not able to do the majority of essential daily tasks. They have to be assisted with personal hygiene, feeding, and using the bathroom. Patients will also need help sitting up in some instances and will need to be propped up all the time. With sufficient care and life support, patients can live for years in this stage. Pneumonia is the most frequent cause of death of Alzheimer's patients due to breathing problems. Other causes include bedsores, stroke, heart disease, and cancer.[14]

SIGNIFICANCE

The length of detail in the stage-by-stage definitions as well as the symptoms expected in all the seven stages makes this classification system a very accurate guide in identifying and managing Alzheimer's for both medical practitioners and informal caregivers of affected patients. It is a great tool for spouses and close ones of patients since it forecasts what to expect as the disease progresses. A weakness of the seven-stage model is that it is not easy to come up with a universal application for all patients, simply because the symptoms in patients vary widely. As discussed in chapter 3, the disease's progression also varies widely depending on the age and family history of the patient, all of which makes it difficult to devise a standard for all affected individuals. Sometimes, the three- and seven-stage models overlap and are confused. The three-stage model, which uses a time-based approach to classification, is preferred by some since the unique features for each stage are easily distinguishable and therefore make it easy to pinpoint the exact needs of the patient.

V

OTHER MANIFESTATIONS

· 11 ·

Mental Outcomes

$\mathcal{A}$ study from 2001 to 2003 involving fourteen countries showed that mental illness is common and often goes untreated in both developed and underdeveloped countries.[1] Countries that participated in the study were Belgium, China, Columbia, France, Germany, Italy, Japan, Lebanon, Mexico, the Netherlands, Nigeria, Spain, Ukraine, and the United States. The highest rate is found in the United States. These are based on diagnostic surveys in 60,463 homes that showed that mental disorders affect more than 10 percent of people in more than half of the countries that were evaluated.[2]

This study found that mental illnesses are common throughout the globe and that a lot of people do not get treatment while others get treatment they do not need. The prevalence of mental disorders varied widely from country to country. Statistics show that, while 4.3 percent of Shanghai's population has mental illness, it is as high as 26.4 percent in the United States.[3] The findings also showed that serious illnesses were associated with an inability to carry out simple, daily activities. Mental disorders also prove to be disabling on the health and productivity of a country. An article about the global burden of disease shows that mental disorders, including suicidality, rank second in the burden of disease in the United States.[4] Mental disorders have emerged as significant contributors to the burden of disease of elderly patients. However, developing Alzheimer's disease, although common, is not a part of normal aging. Having this illness can be dangerous; people afflicted might need constant supervision to prevent them from inflicting or suffering harm. A larger problem, however, is having Alzheimer's disease and getting diagnosed with another mental disorder as well, creating a much greater disease burden.

DEMENTIA

Dementia is a term used for a set of symptoms of different disorders that affect the brain. People who are affected by it have impairment in their intellectual functioning that interferes with their normal activities and relationships. This disease is diagnosed if two or more of the brain functions are impaired, such as language skills, memory, perception, or cognitive skills (e.g., judgment and reasoning).[5]

The most common cause of dementia is Alzheimer's disease, found in people over sixty-five, and unofficially due to amyloid plaques and neurofibrillary tangles.[6] The brain functions that are involved are memory, language, movement, behavior, judgment, and abstract thinking. Vascular dementia is the second-most common cause of dementia brought about by cerebrovascular problems or strokes. The symptoms of the patient are similar to Alzheimer's disease. However, emotions and personality changes show up late in the disease. (See chapter 4, which discusses dementia in more detail.)

DEPRESSION

Depression has a scientifically proven link to Alzheimer's.[7] This is a mental disorder wherein a person exhibits depressed mood, feelings of guilt, loss of interest in activities, disturbed sleep, disturbed appetite, low energy, and poor concentration for at least two weeks. This can be brought about by stressful events such as death of a loved one, divorce, illness, or loss of a job. It can also be triggered by using certain medications and abuse of illicit drugs or alcohol.[8]

Major Depressive Disorder

Alzheimer's patients can be diagnosed with a major depressive disorder when they experience severe symptoms affecting the ability to sleep, work, study, eat, and enjoy the activities they usually find pleasurable, for a period of two weeks. This can be a disabling disorder that prevents normal functioning. In the United States, severe depression is a major cause of disability.[9] This also holds true for other developed countries. Major depression occurs more frequently in women than in men. Also, more than 50 percent of those who had an episode of depression will continue to have other episodes once or twice a year. This can lead to suicide if left untreated.[10] Research has found a strong link between major depressive disorder and Alzheimer's-related dementia.[11]

Dysthymic Disorder

This is a type of depression where the person experiences depressed mood for most of the time and for at least two years. The symptoms are chronic but are not as severe as in major depression, and the person is able to carry on with daily activities. This disorder gives a person an increased risk of having major depressive disorder and substance-related disorders. Studies have found that dysthymia is associated with probable Alzheimer's disease.[12] Moreover, female Alzheimer's patients are much more likely than their male counterparts to suffer from dysthymic disorder.[13]

Generalized Depression

The Framingham Heart Study investigated late-life depression and dementia for seventeen years.[14] This study had 947 participants and followed their patients from the 1940s. With the average age being seventy-nine, the elderly patients who were enrolled in the study had no signs of dementia, and 125 of the participants were already diagnosed with depression at the beginning of the study. At the end of the study, researchers found that 164 participants had developed dementia, including the 136 participants with a specific diagnosis of Alzheimer's disease. Also, those participants with depression at the beginning had a 70 percent greater risk of developing dementia. Therefore, depression might be a significant risk factor for dementia. According to a follow-up report on this study, it is still unclear whether depression is a risk factor for dementia or if the vulnerability of a person to depression is also what makes the person more susceptible to Alzheimer's disease.[15]

PROBLEMS WITH CONDUCT

Alzheimer's disease has been clinically linked to conduct-related problems during early childhood.[16] Among the many metamorphoses experienced by Alzheimer's patients throughout the progression of their disease include those of changes in behavior and conduct. These changes can be out of character for the patient and alarming to friends and family. Understanding why behavioral changes and problems with conduct can arise will not slow or prevent the progression of Alzheimer's disease, but knowing that such conduct issues might develop helps caregivers prepare themselves and the patients' environments in order to minimize problems and maximize safety. For instance, it is not unusual for even early stage Alzheimer's patients to become less social as they begin to recognize their cognitive deficits. This type of social withdrawal may begin first because of embarrassment as patients forget names of old friends or details pertaining to very recent events. Alzheimer's patients might also become angry and frustrated when they are unable to recall how to perform activities of daily living they know they once performed easily. Anger and frustration, when displayed by an Alzheimer's patient in an unusual manner, are expressions of irregular conduct. Alzheimer's victims' conduct often deteriorates as the disease progresses. In the later stages of the disease, paranoid and hostile behavior may develop as the patients lose more touch with reality.[17]

ANXIETY

Scientific research has confirmed that a correlation between anxiety and Alzheimer's exists.[18] Anxiety is a feeling of worry or apprehensiveness that may be coupled with physical symptoms such as the following:

- Tense muscles
- Numbness
- Headache
- Trembling
- Excessive sweating
- Nausea
- Palpitations
- Diarrhea

Anxiety can be caused by genetics, brain chemistry, or environmental factors. In the context of genetics, it has been suggested by research that family history plays a role in increasing the risk of having an anxiety disorder. Anxiety disorders have been associated with irregular levels of neurotransmitters in the brain, the major organ affected by Alzheimer's disease. These neurotransmitters are essentially chemical messengers that move data from one nerve cell to the next. In the case of environmental factors, trauma and stressful events can bring about anxiety disorders. Examples of stressful events include death of a loved one, abuse, and changing jobs or school. Anxiety also worsens in periods of stress and can be heightened by the use of alcohol, caffeine, and nicotine.[19]

According to a peer-reviewed article, there are about four million people in the United States that suffer from anxiety disorders in a year.[20] These disorders start in childhood or adolescence and are more common in women than men. Anxiety becomes a problem when it gets in the way of performing one's daily activities in the absence of a real threat or when it goes on for a long time after the danger has passed. It can be triggered by stress in one's life, and some people are more vulnerable than others.

Types of Anxiety Disorders

Panic disorder is a type of anxiety disorder wherein the affected person has feelings of terror that occur suddenly and without warning. Another type of anxiety disorder is obsessive-compulsive disorder, or OCD, when the patient is plagued by recurring thoughts or fears that lead him or her to do certain rituals or routines known as compulsions. Posttraumatic stress disorder (PTSD) happens after a traumatic event such as unexpected death of a loved one, sexual or physical assault, or a natural disaster. A person affected by it would have constant, frightening thoughts of the event. In the case of social anxiety disorder or social phobia, there is a feeling of overwhelming worry and self-consciousness about social situations with fear of being judged by others. In specific phobias, there is an extreme fear of an object or situation where the level of fear is usually inappropriate to the situation. Another type is generalized anxiety disorder, which involves having excessive and unrealistic worry even if there is nothing to incite it.[21]

Anxiety and Alzheimer's Disease

Studies show that chronic exposure to extreme anxiety or fear can make a person more susceptible to Alzheimer's disease.[22] A body's reaction to stress has been replicated in mice, where stress led to modified versions of tau proteins known to be the first warning signs of neurofibrillary tangles of Alzheimer's disease.

WANDERING

Unfortunately, wandering in the case of Alzheimer's disease can be so grave that it is sometimes referred to as critical wandering, defined by decreased cognitive ability in an Alzheimer's victim who wanders away from supervised care. According to researchers, wandering is possible when an Alzheimer's disease patient leaves the home or facility unsupervised.[23]

Types of Wandering

Studies on wandering Alzheimer's patients have resulted in numerous new-found theories on the topic. In one study, researchers classified wandering into goal-directed searching, goal-directed industrious, or non-goal-directed behavior.[24] The searching wanderer is when the Alzheimer's patient constantly looks for something or someone that does not exist physically, such as a deceased parent. In the case of the industrious wanderer, the patient has an uncontrollable drive to finish a task or to stay busy with something. The non-goal-directed wanderer walks away aimlessly, following a particular stimulus, but then the patient's attention can be suddenly diverted. Some theories involve using the term "modelers," where the caregivers of their subjects in the study are being actively followed as the caregiver moves about the facility.[25] Other researchers use "critical wanderer" as the term patients who are lost and do not know their specific location.[26]

AGITATION

Agitation can be defined as a state of mind when there is increased tension and episodes of emotional and physical irritability. This can be caused by the following:

- Drugs or alcohol
- Withdrawal
- Depression
- Hyperthyroidism
- Asthma
- Rabies
- Head injury
- Stress
- Sleep deprivation
- Heart attack
- Stroke

More than 50 percent of patients suffering from Alzheimer's disease show agitation.[27] This usually shows up in the middle stages of the disease. Experts have suggested that the best way to manage this problem is through environmental changes rather than medication, which can be the last resort.[28]

REPETITIVE OR SELF-STIMULATORY BEHAVIOR

These behaviors may be exhibited in obvious actions, such as flapping arms or hands, flipping fingers in front of the eyes, making repetitive sounds, jumping up and down, and clenching muscles. Some behaviors may be difficult to detect, such as blinking or eye rolling, hair twisting, or finger tapping. These actions can be performed when people, especially children, feel excited or agitated, but some patients exhibit unusual repetitive behavior at the level that interferes with their ability to perform other activities, common among people diagnosed with autism.[29]

AGGRESSION

Peer-reviewed experiments confirm that mice with Alzheimer's disease have increased levels of aggression.[30] Other research finds that verbal aggression in humans is also associated with Alzheimer's.[31] Aggression or overly aggressive behavior can be caused by substance abuse or any of the following:

- Intoxication
- Personality
- Psychological disorders
- Depression
- Hypoglycemia
- Alzheimer's disease
- Menopause

Aggression may also be confused with other disorders such as epilepsy, multiple drug interaction, attention-deficit/hyperactivity disorder (ADHD), or depressive disorders.[32] Simply put, a patient suffering from Alzheimer's disease may become aggressive.[33] When this happens, it is essential that the caregiver try to understand the cause of the aggression. The aggressive behavior may be in the form of verbal acts such as shouting and name calling or physical acts such as pushing or hitting. The main cause of the behavioral symptoms in this patient is due to the progressive decline of brain cells. Environmental factors can also cause the symptoms or make them worse.

HOARDING

Academic reports suggest a strong connection between hoarding and Alzheimer's, especially when dementia is the primary symptom at hand.[34] Hoarding refers to excessively collecting materials, coupled with the inability to throw them away. This compulsion leads to cramped living conditions wherein homes may be filled to full capacity with only narrow pathways left for walking through stacks of things. Hoarding presents a challenge in the Alzheimer's treatment process since most patients affected do not see it as a problem.[35] Signs and symptoms of people affected by hoarding include the following:

- Transferring things from one pile to another without throwing anything away
- Limited or no interaction with other people
- Difficulty organizing items
- Inability to discard things
- Procrastination
- Feelings of shame or embarrassment when guests arrive
- Keeping stacks of outdated magazines and newspapers
- Acquiring unnecessary items
- Excessive emotional attachment to material objects

The cause of hoarding is unclear, although it is likely that there is a familial tendency wherein genetics and upbringing are important factors.[36]

PARANOIA

Medical studies have proven that Alzheimer's disease patients suffer from paranoia.[37] The primary symptom of paranoia is a permanent delusion that appears gradually. The person afflicted by paranoia has feelings of suspiciousness, irritability, introvertedness, depression, jealousy, and bitterness.

Causes of Paranoia

The exact medical cause of severe paranoia is not known, but there are several diseases that can contribute to it. These include alcoholism, bipolar disorder, dementia, brain tumor, stress, stroke, depression, and drug addiction. If severe paranoia is suspected, patients or their caregivers should consult a doctor as soon as possible. The earlier the treatment is started, the better the outcome.[38]

Symptoms of Paranoia

When Alzheimer's patients suffer from severe paranoia, they can have delusions. Patient might distrust those around them. Patients feel like they are being singled out and might seek evidence to support their delusions. Everyone has some paranoia, but people have severe paranoia, it takes over their everyday life. Severe paranoia can lead to significant anxiety and irrational fear. Paranoia is seen in other medical diseases and psychological disorders. Patients with schizophrenia and multiple sclerosis can show signs of severe paranoia.[39]

Types of Paranoia

The most prevalent kind of paranoia is the persecutory type, sometimes called persecutory delusions or persecutory type of paranoid disorder. In this type of paranoia, the Alzheimer's disease victim believes that everyone around wants to cause harm. Another type is the delusion of grandeur, wherein the person inexplicably believes that he or she is a very important individual. Religious paranoia is when the patient suffers from a delusion that is religious in nature, such as being an exclusive messenger of God sent to "spread the word" to the entire world. Another type is reformatory paranoia, where the Alzheimer's patient believes himself or herself to be a great reformer. Another kind is litigious paranoia, where the patient feels meaningless among others and feels that others are conspiring to commit evil deeds. Hypochondriacal paranoia is the type where the patient thinks he or she is affected by many different diseases at once.[40]

HALLUCINATIONS

Clinical data conclude that Alzheimer's patients suffer from hallucinations, which involve sensing things that are absent from in reality while the person is awake and conscious.[41] These can include a crawling sensation on the skin, hearing nonexistent voices, and seeing lights or objects that are not present. Hallucinations can surface when the Alzheimer's patient uses drugs such as LSD[42] and very potent variations of marijuana, where hallucinations usually involve seeing patterns or halos in the air. Auditory hallucinations, or "hearing things," are common in people with schizophrenia and those taking cocaine, amphetamines, and other stimulants. Some other causes include delirium or dementia, fever in children and the elderly, severe illness, and other psychiatric disorders such as PTSD and psychotic depression.[43]

RESTLESSNESS

Clinical reports note that patients suffering from dementia also suffer from restlessness.[44] To be able to define restlessness, one should know each of the different types. One type of restlessness is an unpleasant state of tremendous arousal, high tension, and irritability. This can occur suddenly or over time and can last for a few minutes, or for weeks or months. Physical agitation, displayed in the form of restlessness, can be increased by pain, stress, and fever. Other types of restlessness include (1) restlessness from excitement, which is really the sensation of amplified anxiety and anticipation; (2) restlessness in the form of alertness, which is a state of watchfulness; and (3) restlessness in the form of restless legs, which is an increased movement of legs during sleep. This is called restless leg syndrome.[45] In summary, restlessness can be caused by factors such as the following:

- Anxiety disorders
- Nervousness
- Hyperactivity
- Sleep problems
- Insomnia
- Attention-deficit disorder
- Medications
- Drug interactions[46]

AUTISM SPECTRUM DISORDERS

Autism spectrum disorders (ASDs) include pervasive developmental disorder—not otherwise specified (PDD–NOS), Asperger's, childhood disintegrative disorder, autistic disorder, and atypical autism. Solid medical research confirms a strong link between autism, which is a very general term that includes ASDs, and Alzheimer's disease later in life.[47] Autism is in fact a form of developmental disability that, upon effect, is evident in the first three years of life. The disorder comes from a neurological disorder affecting the functions of a person's brain that then affects communication skills and social interaction. For those affected by autism, there are problems in nonverbal communication and different ranges of social interaction, such as play or banter.[48] Notably, autism spectrum disorders refer to any developmental disability that is caused by an abnormality in the brain.

Social Skills and ASD

An Alzheimer's patient affected by ASD typically has problems in social and communication skills. This person usually prefers to stick to a set of behaviors and will resist any changes to his or her usual activities. The interaction of a person with ASD is very different from how normal people behave. If the symptoms of someone with ASD are not severe, that person might seem to act socially clumsy, make offensive comments, or fail to get along with everyone else. If the ASD symptoms are more serious, Alzheimer's patients will not be interested in other people at all and will keep to themselves. The usual observation is that the person with ASD makes very little eye contact.

Recognition

With better understanding of the disease and improved health care, there has been an improved ability to detect signs of autism at an early age. More children with autism are taught to look people in the eye, and hopefully, since then, eye contact among people with autism has been improving substantially. A person with ASD might overlook the signal that normal people give to catch someone's attention. In fact, people with ASD might not even know that someone is trying to speak to them. A person with ASD might be interested in talking to a particular person but will not have the same skills as other people to become fully involved in a conversation.

Empathy and ASD

Empathy means understanding and being aware of the feelings of other people. Alzheimer's patients with autism find it hard to understand the feelings of others and have a weaker ability to use instincts to empathize with others. However, if patients are frequently reminded of this problem, they can greatly improve in taking into account other people's feelings. With frequent practice, empathy improves and becomes a natural part of life.

Physical Contact and ASD

Most older people with autism do not want to be cuddled or touched like others do, but many autistic children will hug their mother, father, grandmother, grandfather, brother, or sister without hesitation. The goal for the patient is to anticipate that physical contact is going to happen in life no matter what. In the case of suddenly tickling a normal child's feet, that child will most likely giggle and become happy and excited. However, the reaction will be completely different when tickling the feet of a child with autism, especially if the child does not anticipate that contact.

Speech and ASD

The speech of a person with ASD depends on the severity of the disease. It is possible for them not to speak at all. Some ASD patients will often repeat the words or phrases they hear, a condition known as echolalia.

OUTLOOK

To lower the incidence of mental disorders, the U.S. Department of Health and Human Services has established the National Institute of Mental Health (NIMH). The aim is to reduce the burden of mental illnesses and behavioral disorders within the nation's borders. This is achieved through the support of research on the mind, brain, and behavior. An important goal is to improve the treatment of these kinds of disorders. Through the Division of Services and Intervention Research of the NIMH, they have funded more than one hundred treatment studies in different sites since 2005. The clinical trials that are being conducted are funded by investor-initiated grants, cooperative agreements, and research contracts. It has also been the goal of the World Health Organization's (WHO) Department of Mental Health and Substance Abuse to reduce the burden associated with mental, neurological, and substance abuse disorders. The department has recognized that one of the most effective methods to reduce the burden is prevention. The WHO also published a document on primary prevention of mental, neurological, and psychosocial disorders in 1998.[49]

Diseases Associated with Alzheimer's

$\mathcal{B}$y definition, a disease is any deviation from or interruption of the normal function or structure of any body organ, often characterized by symptoms and signs. The etiology (cause), pathology, and prognosis of a disease may be unknown. As paraphrased from chapter 2, pathology is the study of the cause of a disease, the essential nature of a disease as it causes abnormalities, and the structural and functional changes that result. Diseases such as Alzheimer's can manifest as more than one symptom, and some conditions can be symptoms of other, worse conditions.

General relationships between diseases are common. Oftentimes, simple diseases can lead to other, more threatening conditions if left untreated. Examples include scarlet fever, which could result in heart disease if not treated the right way. Studies have also shown a connection between Alzheimer's disease and other degenerative conditions and metabolic diseases such as diabetes.[1] There are also instances where a particular condition mimics the symptoms of other diseases. Academic research proves that Alzheimer's is associated with thyroid problems.[2] Hyperthyroidism can somewhat mimic the symptoms of Alzheimer's such as memory loss, depression, and irritability. To better diagnose diseases of the endocrine system such as hyperthyroidism, doctors look for other symptoms that are not commonly seen in diseases of other body systems. In the case of hyperthyroidism, symptoms such as constipation, hair loss, and weight gain are common but would not necessarily be present in Alzheimer's disease. Knowing the connections between diseases is very important to accurately give a diagnosis and discover a cure. It could also help in preventing the existing symptoms from worsening and serves as a critical part of early detection. This chapter will take a closer look at other diseases and how they relate to Alzheimer's.

NIEMMAN-PICK DISEASE

Niemman-Pick disease is a group of inherited disorders known as lipid storage diseases that can lead to abnormalities in the brain's white matter, or leukodystrophies. This disease happens when harmful amounts of lipids (fatty substance) accumulate in the spleen, liver, brain, lungs, and bone marrow. This causes the spleen and liver to enlarge progressively. Mental deterioration, anemia, and swollen glands are often observed. Symptoms include difficulty swallowing, slurred speech, enlarged liver or spleen, lack of muscle coordination, memory loss, learning problems, increased sensitivity to touch, and brain degeneration. In some cases, the cornea appears to be clouded, and there is a red halo in the retina. Niemman-Pick disease is often referred to as "childhood Alzheimer's."[3] Symptoms of dementia are common in both of these diseases, and this could lead to misdiagnosis. Niemman-Pick disease, however, commonly occurs in children who have not reached their preteen years.

Niemman-Pick Type A

There are four different variations of Niemman-Pick disease.[4] The most widely known is type A, found commonly in infants. Children diagnosed with this type do not normally reach beyond eighteen months of age. This type is characterized by severe brain damage, an enlarged liver, and yellowing of the skin or jaundiced seizures. Ataxia and eye paralysis are also common. There are currently no universally accepted treatments for Niemman-Pick type A.

Niemman-Pick Type B

The second is type B, which normally occurs in the preteen years. In this type, the brain itself may remain undamaged, but there is significant enlargement of the liver. In some cases, bone marrow transplant has been attempted, as well as gene therapy and enzyme replacement, to cure this type. In both types A and B, there is a significant toxic buildup of a fatty substance in the cell called sphingomyelin. This is due to the insufficient activity of the enzyme referred to as sphingomyelinase.

Niemman-Pick Type C and D

Niemman-Pick type C and D are characterized by the lack of Niemman-Pick type C1 (NPC1) or Niemman-Pick type C2 (NPC2) proteins. These two types can occur at any stages of a person's life. In these two types, the spleen and liver is moderately enlarged, but there is extensive brain damage that causes difficulty in swallowing, an inability to walk and to look up or down, and loss of vision and hearing. Patients who have these types are commonly advised to go on a low-cholesterol diet. Type D often occurs in people with lineage from Nova Scotia and is often referred to as Nova Scotia Niemann-Pick disease.[5]

DOWN SYNDROME

Medical research notes that there are certain factors in Down syndrome that lead to Alzheimer's pathology.[6] Down syndrome is a condition where an extra chromosome causes a delay in a child's development.[7] The extent that Down syndrome affects an individual varies, with some patients requiring extensive medical attention while others live a relatively normal life. The body normally has twenty-three pairs of chromosomes. However, an extra chromosome is present for people with Down syndrome. This causes the physical features and developmental delays that are common in people with Down syndrome. There is no clear reason that Down syndrome occurs, neither is there presently a way to prevent it. Reports show that the risk of giving birth to a child with Down syndrome increases as a woman matures.[8] A woman in her thirties has a one in nine hundred chance, while a forty-year-old woman has a one in one hundred chance of giving birth to a baby with Down syndrome.[9]

There are certain physical attributes common to people with Down syndrome, such as upward-slanting eyes, smaller ears, flat facial profiles, and a protruding tongue. Babies often have low muscle tone, causing them to reach milestones such as sitting, crawling, and walking at a much later time than normal. The baby's growth rate is also slowed. Down syndrome patients often have difficulty swallowing. They also suffer from digestive issues. Although the rate of learning skills may be at a much slower pace, children with Down syndrome do have the ability to learn and can accumulate skills as time progresses. While a large number of people with Down syndrome have no major health problems, others have certain medical conditions that require attention. Statistics show that almost half of babies born with Down syndrome suffer with congenital heart problems.[10] These babies are also more likely to develop pulmonary (lung-related) hypertension, and hearing or visual problems. There is also an increased risk of Alzheimer's disease for people with Down syndrome. This is said to be due to the extra chromosome that people with Down syndrome have. People with Down syndrome age prematurely . They show signs of aging twenty to thirty years ahead of other people. Symptoms of late onset Alzheimer's disease in patients who have Down syndrome appear between the age of forty and fifty, compared to sixty in normal patients.

Studies show that at least 25 percent of Down syndrome patients at the age of thirty-five show signs of Alzheimer's-related dementia.[11] The incidents increase as an individual ages, with the risk of Alzheimer's three to five times higher than normal.

CREUTZFELDT-JAKOB DISEASE

Medical research notes striking similarities between the pathological characteristics of Creutzfeldt-Jakob disease and Alzheimer's.[12] Creutzfeldt-Jakob disease (CJD) is a rare and degenerative disease affecting the brain that can be fatal in some cases. This disease, commonly called "mad cow disease," is really a form of dementia that is not Alzheimer's disease. CJD affects approximately one in a million people each year, with two hundred cases in the United States annually.[13] The most severe symptoms in CJD usually take shape at the age of sixty (much like in Alzheimer's), but patients often die within a year. Early signs of CJD include memory loss, change in behavior, lack of coordination, and visual disturbance. As the condition worsens, mental deterioration occurs, as well as involuntary physical movements. Blindness, weakening of the muscles (especially in the arms and legs), and even a coma can occur.[14]

CJD is a very rare but extremely fatal form of brain damage. Fortunately, CJD is only present in one out of a million people worldwide. It is highly progressive, and patients suffering from this disease have as little as a year to live. CJD starts with memory loss, behavioral and emotional changes, and visual and motor problems. With its advancement, a patient's mental condition rapidly deteriorates, with blindness, weakness, spasms, and maybe even a coma. CJD has three classifications: sporadic CJD, which is the most common type; hereditary CJD, stemming from a family history of this disorder; and acquired CJD, wherein the disease is transmitted through its direct exposure to the brain or nervous system. CJD has long been a rather mysterious disease that can be difficult to identify.

Science has not completely confirmed the full mechanism or isolated a single cause of CJD.[15] The theory is that it comes from an infectious form of prion proteins. Prion proteins are naturally occurring in the body and, for the most part, are harmless. Its infectious form may cause sporadic CJD by changing normal prion proteins. These abnormalities then form clumps that damage neurons and other parts of the brain. In the case of hereditary CJD, genetic mutation causes the infectious prion proteins. Other symptoms of CJD are similar to those exhibited by patients with dementia and other brain disorders, but on a more severe scale and with a faster rate of development.[16]

Types of CJD

There are three major categories of CJD. The first is sporadic CJD. This is the most common type of CJD, accounting for 85 percent of all the cases. In this type, the disease appears even though the patient has no risk factors associated with it. The next one is hereditary or familial CJD. A patient with hereditary CJD has a family history of the disease, and tests have shown that these patients have inherited an associated mutated gene. Approximately 5 to 10 percent of CJD cases are hereditary.[17] The third type is acquired CJD. There is no proof that CJD can be transmitted via physical contact with someone who already suffers from the disease. However, CJD can be due to exposure of the brain or nervous system tissue via certain medical procedures. Since CJD was first exposed in 1920, there have been less than 1 percent of acquired CJD cases.[18] There are several variants of CJD that have been discovered. These variants differ in symptoms and the length of progression of the disease. A variant that is common in Japan, called the panencephalophatic form, has a longer disease course, with its symptoms progressing for several years. Another new CJD variant described in England and France affects younger individuals, often beginning with psychiatric symptoms.[19]

Why It Happens

Patients with CJD will show symptoms similar to those who have other progressive and degenerative neurological disorders such as Alzheimer's disease. Both CJD and Alzheimer's disease are neurological disorders that involve protein misfolding.[20] Proteins have a very specific structure, and misfolding occurs when they fold into a shape outside of the norm. Both CJD and Alzheimer's present with symptoms of dementia. CJD causes unique changes in the brain tissue that can be seen upon autopsy. The disease also causes more rapid deterioration of a person's brain as compared to Alzheimer's. There is currently no known cure for CJD. Current treatments of CJD mainly involve alleviating the effects of the symptoms to make the patient as comfortable as possible.

PICK'S DISEASE

Pick's disease is a rare and irreversible form of dementia. It is similar to Alzheimer's disease, except that it often only affects certain areas of the brain. This is not to be confused with Niemman-Pick disease mentioned above, a disorder that happens when harmful amounts of lipids accumulate in the brain, liver, spleen, and bone marrow. Pick's disease patients have abnormal Pick bodies found embedded in nerve cells in the damaged sections of the brain. An abnormal type of a protein called tau is found in these Pick bodies and Pick cells. This is a normal type of protein found in every cell of the body, but people with Pick's disease have an unusually large amount of tau protein. The exact reason for this abnormality is unknown, but a large number of Pick's disease cases have been found to be hereditary in nature.

Symptoms of Pick's disease can occur in a person as early as twenty years old, but it often begins to manifest between forty and sixty years old with the average age of patients at fifty-four years old.[21] These symptoms include behavioral change, impaired thinking, and speech difficulties that appear slowly but continue to worsen over time. This is due to shrinking tissues on the temporal and frontal lobes of the brain. Other symptoms include movement and coordination difficulty, memory loss, increased muscle tone, urinary incontinence, speech impairment, weakness, and extreme emotional and behavioral changes. The term "frontotemporal dementia" is also used to refer to Pick's disease. It greatly affects cognition, problem solving, analysis, memory, and communication processes. Since the disease is initially caused by damage to the frontal lobe, early symptoms of Pick's disease involve social behavior. Social irregularities include sexually inappropriate conduct such as touching, kissing, or fondling strangers, and regressive behaviors. Frontotemporal dementia is when the frontal lobe, the part of the brain that deals with insight, reasoning, and social comportment, is compromised. As a result, a patient suffering from this kind of dementia goes through personality changes, has hampered social skills, and has little motivation and concentration skills.

HUNTINGTON'S DISEASE

Huntington's disease is similar to Alzheimer's in that they are both degenerative diseases, caused by nerve cells that die and lead to uncontrolled emotional, mental, and physical changes. Huntington's disease primarily affects the basal ganglia. The basal ganglia is composed of a group of nerve cells found at the base of the brain. These nerve cells are connected to the motor cortex, which is the part of the brain responsible for muscle control and motor movements. Because of deteriorating nerve cells, the basal ganglia of a person with Huntington's have smaller structures and form a wider opening. This is why symptoms of patients with Huntington's include jerky movements and uncontrollable muscle spasms.[22]

Huntington's disease is brought about by irregularities in an autosomal gene (not linked to gender), particularly chromosome number 4. A single gene allows for a fifty-fifty chance of acquiring the disease if either parent is a carrier. This means that only one copy of the gene is needed to develop Huntington's disease. This is different from Alzheimer's disease, which can be attributed to two different genes, one being a "risk gene" called APOE-4 (apolipoprotein E4). The second, a "deterministic gene," is rarer than risk genes and are present in only a few hundred families around the world. In addition, symptoms of Huntington's disease will emerge between the age of forty and sixty with an average age of fifty-three. Alzheimer's disease occurs much later in life, although there are early onsets of Alzheimer's disease between the ages of thirty and forty.

Manifestations

Huntington's disease is a hereditary condition that affects certain neurons (nerve cells) in the brain, causing their progressive breakdown. The gene that causes this condition is present since birth, but symptoms often do not manifest until midlife. There are however, cases of juvenile Huntington's disease that occur before the age of twenty.[23] In such cases, the physical manifestations are different and the disease tends to progress more rapidly. Early symptoms of Huntington's disease can include uncontrolled movements, lack of coordination, or balance problems. As the disease progresses, Huntington's disease can affect the person's ability to swallow, speak, and walk. The effects may vary with some patients unable to recognize faces and family members, while others are still aware of their surroundings and can still show emotions and feelings.

Testing

A blood test can confirm the possibility and presence of the gene that causes Huntington's disease. Huntington's disease is often detected via a series of physical, neurological, and psychiatric examinations as well as a review of the patient's family medical history. A doctor might also order brain imaging tests like a magnetic resonance imaging (MRI) and a computed tomography (CT) scan. Images from these tests might show structural changes in a brain that's affected by Huntington's disease. An electroencephalogram (EEG) might also be done in cases where the patients experienced seizures.

Complications

There are certain medical complications associated with Huntington's disease. Once the symptoms of Huntington's disease starts to manifest, a person's functional abilities will continuously but gradually degrade. The progression and duration rate varies, but the time from when the patient first shows signs of the disease to death is normally ten to thirty years. Juvenile Huntington disease, however, can result in death within fifteen years.[24] There is a great risk of suicide among patients of Huntington's disease, due to the depression and psychiatric effects of this condition. Other complications of Huntington's disease include accident-related injuries, pneumonia, and infections and complications resulting from the patient's difficulty in swallowing.[25]

Huntington's disease affects the cognitive, movement, and psychiatric aspects of a person, and these effects vary widely among patients. It is also difficult to tell which symptoms will appear first, and as the diseases progresses, some disorders appear to have a greater impact than others in terms of functional impairment. Movement disorders involve both voluntary and involuntary movements. Patients can suffer from the following:

- Abnormal eye movements
- Involuntary jerking
- Muscle rigidity
- Difficulty swallowing
- Muscle contraction
- Impaired gait, posture, and balance
- Difficulty speaking
- Uncoordinated, slow physical movements

Cognitive symptoms include the following:

- Lack of flexibility
- Difficulty learning
- Difficulty organizing
- Lack of emotional control
- Difficulty focusing on tasks
- Inability to start a conversation
- Slowness in finding words
- Problems with spatial and depth perception
- Emotional outbursts

Psychiatric aspects of Huntingdon's disease include the following:

- Depression
- Lack of interest
- Enthusiasm
- Fatigue
- Insomnia
- Social withdrawal
- Indecisiveness

- Lack of concentration and changes in appetite
- Other psychiatric problems, such as obsessive-compulsive disorders, mania, and bipolar disorder

Treatment

At present, there is no specific treatment protocol that can directly cure Huntington's disease, but certain medications are used to lessen the impact of the symptoms associated with it. This is especially true for those that bring about movement-related and psychiatric disorders such as tetrabenezine, antipsychotic drugs, antidepressants, and mood-stabilizing medications. Psychotherapy, speech therapy, and physical therapy sessions can also be undertaken to lessen the impact of the degenerative symptoms.

PARKINSON'S DISEASE

Parkinson's disease is a progressive disorder targeting the nervous system and affecting movement. It is the second-most common neurodegenerative disease after Alzheimer's.[26] These two diseases are similar in that they are both neurodegenerative diseases.[27] Moreover, studies show that Alzheimer's patients display very similar cortical dysfunctions (problems in the cortex the brain) to that of Parkinson's, which is a gradually developing condition often with barely noticeable symptoms, such as the very subtle trembling of one hand.[28]

Recognition

When seeking information about his or her medical problem, a person with Parkinson's disease should note that doctors refer to it by more than one name. The disease is also known as paralysis agitans. Regardless of the name used by the treating doctor, the resulting degeneration of the central nervous system causes tremors, or involuntary movements in one part of the victim's body. Parkinson's disease symptoms vary from person to person, and early signs can be really subtle and often go unnoticed. Symptoms often begin by affecting just one side of the body and work their way throughout the entire body, with worse effects on the counterside.

Parkinson's Disease and Its Similarities to Alzheimer's

The exact etiology of Parkinson's disease is still unknown, but several factors are attributed to it. One is a specific genetic mutation with both hereditary and environmental factors. Another factor is the exposure to toxins and viruses that might trigger the conditions that will result in the disease. Numerous changes have been found in the brains of both Parkinson's and Alzheimer's patients. These changes are said to cause the escalation of physical symptoms. One of these is the lack of dopamine, which acts as the brain's messenger hormone. This is said to be the likely cause of impaired movements. Another factor is the low norepinephrine level in the nerve endings. This is another brain messenger that regulates the autonomic nervous system (ANS). The ANS controls the body's automatic functions such as blood pressure regulation. The third factor is the presence of unusual protein clumps called Lewy bodies in the brains of those with Parkinson's disease. However, the effects of this are still unknown.

Alzheimer's disease and Parkinson's disease are both degenerative brain diseases. Differences can be found in the causes, symptoms, treatments, and biological and physical manifestations. Alzheimer's disease is really a form of dementia (though the terms cannot be used interchangeably) that is commonly brought about by the lack of acetylcholine, a neurotransmitter in the peripheral and central nervous system. The parts of the brain affected by this are the temporal lobe, parietal lobe, and frontal cortex. In a similar fashion, Parkinson's disease is brought about by the lack of dopamine, a very important neurotransmitter. The disease can be attributed to gender and genetics as most patients afflicted by it are men with a family history of the disease. Multiple concussions and repetitive head injuries are also said to cause Parkinson's disease, especially prior to the patient having dementia pugilistica.[29]

Tremors

This is when the patient's hand begins to shake involuntarily. These tremors are one of the most well-known signs of Parkinson's disease—a sign that can also cause the slowing or freezing of movement.[30] Not every Parkinson's disease patient experiences this, as research has proven that around 30 percent of Parkinson's patients have no tremors.[31] Oftentimes, when the patient's hand is at rest, the thumb and forefinger rub against one another involuntarily. This is known as "pill rolling." Men and women afflicted with tremor symptoms frequently have hands that shake, and as a result, they cannot be counted on for doing simple tasks. The unsteady fingers are unable to even pick up a fork. This inability to complete an expected action results from pathological changes in the brain. Impairment to the nerve cells has destroyed their ability to produce the chemical (hormone) dopamine. That in turn leads to appearance of the back-and-forth motions characterizing the steadily worsening Parkinson's.

Slowed Movement (Bradykinesia)

When a patient suffers from this particular symptom, he or she may find it difficult to make voluntary movements. As the disease progress, the patient finds it more difficult to perform simple tasks. Walking is reduced to slow shuffles, and the feet often "freeze," making it difficult to take the first step. Bradykinesia is a medical condition, and the term is derived from two Greek roots: *bradys* (slow) and *kinesis* (movement), which, when combined, essentially means slow movements. This condition may be a neurological problem or a side effect of medication.[32] Bradykinesia may be caused by basal ganglia diseases, mental disorders, or other illnesses that could have caused inactivity of the muscular system. The beginning stages of bradykinesia include slow movements of the body as well as tremors and rigidity. It normally begins with small muscles, particularly in the fingers, and movement is much slower than the average person. Lack of facial expression is also observed, as well as speech slowness. Although there is treatment for this Parkinson's, there is no cure, and it is not completely diminished by medication.[33]

Rigid Muscles

Muscle rigidity is a very noticeable symptom of Alzheimer's disease.[34] Likewise, Parkinson's disease patients also suffer from muscle rigidity. People with Parkinson's disease would find it difficult to swing their arms when walking. This is due to muscle stiffness that limits the range of movements and causes pain. This makes movement look awkward and affects the patient's balance. Muscle stiffness would also make the affected parts weak and unusable in time. Muscle rigidity is a result of tenseness and stiffness in the body muscles. This negative body effect is felt by those who suffer from both Parkinson's and Alzheimer's disease. Muscle rigidity in Parkinson's is caused by a disorder that is degenerative to the body's central nervous system. Parkinson's results in rigidity of the muscles of the face, and associated symptoms often include a lack of facial muscle control. The patient's face might often feel masklike and stiff. Victims of Parkinson's often experience a lack of blood supply to the brain resulting from contracted, stiff neck muscles that cause the head to pull forward and the jaw lowered.

Impaired Posture and Balance

A person with Parkinson's disease can have a stooping posture and imbalance, although these symptoms usually occur at a later stage of the disease. That is why people with Parkinson's disease require assistance. The patients become prone to potentially fatal accidents. This also limits the patient's ability to perform tasks and rely on themselves. While often encouraged by well-wishing parents, good body posture places the skull's base over the topmost section of the backbone's vertical segments. That in turn decreases the load of the neck muscles but increases the weight loaded onto the cervical and neck bones and muscles. Moreover, good posture puts the foramen magnum directly above the housing for the spine's large bundle of nerves. As neurodegenerative diseases, both Parkinson's and Alzheimer's relate to structural changes in the skull, the spine, and the circulatory system of the brain. Any such change can affect the vertebral arteries that supply the cerebellum. That effect could damage a person's balance and gait. Parkinson's patients often display the effects of such damaging alterations.[35]

Speech Problems

People with Parkinson's disease might have difficulty speaking. They tend to slur or stutter. They also tend to speak rapidly, in a monotone voice or a lot softer than usual. This makes it difficult for patients to convey emotions in their voices. Along with this, patients with Parkinson's disease find it hard to show what they feel with the use of facial expressions. The muscles in the face become difficult to move, resulting in the "masked faces" of Parkinson's.[36]

Dementia

Patients at the later stage of Parkinson's disease suffer from dementia. Their memory and mental clarity suffers similar to those present in Alzheimer's disease. People with Parkinson's disease find it difficult to reason out or to form clear thoughts and put them into statements. It is also strenuous for them to learn things or formulate a plan. These symptoms vary from person to person.[37]

More on Manifestations

Unlike Alzheimer's or Huntington's, Parkinson's does not usually involve the "thinking" parts of the brain. Parkinson's is characterized by uncontrollable tremors and the loss of autonomous movement. What is most affected by this disease is the substantia nigra, the part of the brain that sends signals to the striatum through specialized neurotransmitters called dopamine. This process is responsible for body movements. When Parkinson's infiltrates the brain, the production of dopamine is lessened because of neuron degeneration. This leads to the inability to control movements; difficulty chewing and swallowing; speech and sleep problems; excessive sweating; skin, urinary, and colonic problems; depression; and emotional disturbances. Parkinson's is a progressive disease, developing up to twenty years.[38]

There are many dementia symptoms that can be misconstrued as Alzheimer's. An example is the much-known Parkinson's and, lately, thiamine deficiency. When it comes to Parkinson's disease, the main cause is the sharp reduction of cells that contain dopamine. The reduction mainly occurs in the midsection of the brain, which is also referred to as substantia nigra. No one knows why the cells start to die off in such a peculiar way. As the disease develops, the most commonly noticed symptoms are related to movement and include trembling rigidity, slow responses, and slow movements. There is also a marked difficulty in walking and gait. Therefore, cognitive and behavioral irregularities may arise, with pronounced dementia occurring in those advanced levels of the disorder. Some other symptoms include sensory inefficiencies, lack of sleep, and emotional issues. The diagnoses of the typical cases are normally tied to symptoms, with tests such as clinical neuroimaging used to make a confirmation. Where pathophysiology is concerned, Parkinson's is viewed as a form of synucleinopathy, when an abnormal saturation of alpha-synuclein protein occurs in the human brain and takes the form of the Lewy bodies described in chapter 4.

This is contrary to other similar diseases such as Alzheimer's. In Alzheimer's, the brain ends up building high amounts of tau protein, all in the form of a structure called neurofibrillary tangle. There is a clinical and pathological overlap between the available tauopathies and the synucleinopathies. There is also a high likelihood of coming across irregular neurofibrillary tangles in brains of people affected with Parkinson's disease.[39]

BINSWANGER'S DISEASE

Binswanger's disease is a type of vascular dementia. It is caused by damage to the white matter of the brain, due to the narrowing and thickening of arteries converging on the brain. This happens when cholesterol and other such materials build up on artery and blood vessel walls, creating plaque. When plaque has amply hardened, blood flowing to the brain is blocked, killing brain tissues. Patients with Binswanger's exhibit the following symptoms:

- Short-term memory loss
- Mood swings
- Low attention span

- Inability to make decisions and organize thoughts
- Lack of facial expressions
- Speech and movement difficulties
- Clumsiness
- Changes in personality such as depression and apathy

Compared to Alzheimer's and other such diseases, Binswanger's is a less severe brain disorder. The signs and symptoms, such as forgetfulness, are not as debilitating and are not always present in patients. In some cases, these symptoms just occur as a passing phase.[40]

CEREBRAL AMYLOID ANGIOPATHY

Medical research strongly backs an association between cerebral amyloid angiopathy and Alzheimer's.[41] As explained in chapter 3, amyloidosis can affect various areas of the body, including the brain. If amyloid proteins are deposited largely in the cerebral arteries, it will result in cerebral amyloid angiopathy. It is characterized by seizures, drowsiness, delirium, and dementia. Although cerebral amyloid angiopathy presents with dementia and episodes of confusion, it is largely different from stand-alone Alzheimer's disease. For Alzheimer's disease, a different type of amyloid protein is involved. That protein is called the beta amyloid, which is the fragment and derivative of the amyloid precursor protein (APP). The accumulation of beta amyloid protein results in clumps around the plaques in the brain that will contribute greatly in neural degradation and death. The reason for amyloidosis is really not quite understood. The cause of the deposition of amyloid protein remains unknown. Therefore, there are no exact preventive measures available to avoid its occurrence. Beta amyloid protein deposition into plaques is highly associated with increasing age and the physiological changes of the brain akin to aging.

HYDROCEPHALUS

A clinical report suggests that Alzheimer's patients suffer from a relatively high rate of hydrocephalus.[42] Hydrocephalus is a condition that occurs when excess fluid accumulates in the brain due to a block that prevents proper fluid drainage. The excess fluid causes tissue damage and can compress the area surrounding the brain. If left untreated, hydrocephalus can be fatal. It is often present at birth, although it can also develop later. One out of five hundred children are affected by this condition.[43] Survival depends on how early it was diagnosed and the extent of damage.

Normally, the brain is surrounded by cerebrospinal fluid (CSF) in a certain consistency and pressure. Cerebrospinal fluid flows through the ventricles passing through interconnected channels, and this fluid eventually finds its way into spaces around the brain where it is absorbed into the blood-stream. Keeping a balance in the production and absorption of this fluid is essential. However, hydrocephalus occurs when there is too much production of the fluid or the path where the fluid flows gets blocked or narrows too much.

Normal-Pressure Hydrocephalus

Defective absorption of the fluid by the body causes normal-pressure hydrocephalus (NPH). This is much more common in adults. In this type of hydrocephalus, the excess fluid causes enlargement in the ventricles but does not increase the pressure on the brain. Normal-pressure hydrocephalus can be a result of injury or illness, but most instances have unknown causes. Medical studies prove that surgical shunt implantation can slow NPH advancement for some people, thus allowing for extended quality of life.[44] Normal-pressure hydrocephalus is a rare disorder that is often misdiagnosed as Alzheimer's.[45] Research suggests that, while Alzheimer's is not very treatable, NPH and the dementia it causes, is.[46]

NPH also causes impaired memory and difficulty in muscle coordination due to extra pressure being placed on the brain. The pressure is in the form of fluid that can be caused by any number of reasons, such as head trauma, bleeding, or infections. Unlike the other brain disorders, however, NPH is easier to identify and can be more treatable. Surgery to lessen the extra brain pressure has been successfully conducted on some patients with this condition.[47]

The symptoms of hydrocephalus may vary depending on the age of the patient.[48] In infants, symptoms include an unusually large head (macrocephalus), a bulging soft spot at the top, eyes that are fixed downward, seizures, sleepiness, developmental delays, irritability, and vomiting. In older children and adults, the symptoms include nausea and headache, followed by vomiting, irritability, blurred or double vision, or urinary incontinence. Also common are changes in personality, memory loss, delayed mental development, confusion, and lack of energy. Different combinations of these symptoms can appear, depending on the age group and the cause of the condition. Adults are more prone to normal-pressure hydrocephalus, with incontinence and difficulty in walking. As the condition progresses, the patient develops a type of dementia characterized by slow thinking and difficulty processing information.

Further Complications

Further complications can occur from hydrocephalus. The severity of its effects depends on how soon it is diagnosed. If the condition is at a well-advanced stage upon childbirth, then it may cause severe brain damage and even death. Some cases can be cured, and patients can live a normal life. Diagnoses in babies are done through prenatal and postnatal checkups. For adults and older children, a careful analysis of the patient's medical history is in order, along with a series of physical and neurological examinations that include CT scans and an MRI. Upon diagnosis, a doctor might recommend a shunt placement which is basically an external drainage system to remove the excess fluid. A shunt system might be inserted in a patient for a lifetime, so further surgery is needed to adjust the tubes as the child grows. A surgeon might also perform a ventriculostomy, which is when a hole is made at the bottom of the ventricles to allow the fluid to flow to the base of the brain where it can be absorbed.[49]

Summary

In summary, normal-pressure hydrocephalus in adults has been closely associated with Alzheimer's disease, but the two are in fact very distinct conditions. One similarity between them can be attributed to the occurrence of a certain type of dementia found in both. However, the causes of the two are different. NPH is due to cerebral fluid blockage, causing the ventricles to enlarge, while Alzheimer's disease is induced by the lack of acetylcholine, a neurotransmitter in the peripheral and central nervous system.[50]

HIV AND DEMENTIA

Dementia, typically seen in Alzheimer's patients, also occurs in patients with especially severe cases of HIV infections. Alzheimer's disease patients can test for HIV (see chapter 5), but it is important to know *how* HIV-related dementia manifests in an Alzheimer's and non-Alzheimer's patient. Symptoms can differ individually, but the disorder is collectively known as AIDS dementia complex (ADC). ADC comes from complications of HIV, leading to degenerating functions. This means reasoning and judgment, memory, concentration, and attention are greatly affected. Other symptoms are language and movement difficulties, poor balance and general clumsiness, and altered behavior. As the dementia progresses, other problems such as depression, uncontrollable body functions, vision and sleep disturbances, weakness in the extremities, agitation, hallucinations, and even seizures are manifested. HIV-related dementia is nontreatable but can be controlled with proper medical care and attention.[51]

ANALYSIS

Distinguishing Alzheimer's disease from its related maladies is of utmost importance to ensure the best treatment. While it is only one form of the disorders collectively known as dementia, Alzheimer's disease does account for over 60 percent of dementia diagnoses.[52] Mild cognitive impairment (MCI), Parkinson's disease, frontotemporal dementia, and Huntington's disease are other disorders caused by changes in the brain and should not be confused with Alzheimer's. As evidenced by the above sections, some conditions and diseases closely share symptoms with Alzheimer's. It is very important to see these similarities and relationships in order to come up with a proper diagnosis. This is very important since the specific diagnostic processes for Alzheimer's disease (covered in chapter 5) might be the gold standard for medical procedures and prescriptions essential for treating, if not curing, the disease.

· 13 ·

Pain and Alzheimer's

$\mathscr{P}$ain is closely associated with feelings and sensation. As such, the pain that Alzheimer's patients suffer from is rooted in emotion. In its technical and simplified term, pain is really an unwanted sensory and emotional feeling in response to actual or potential tissue damage.[1] Because of this, pain can either be described as sharp, dull, acute, or chronic. It can be felt in one part of the body, in aggregate parts, or even in the whole of it. While pain is often linked with negativity, one benefit of pain is that it is an "alarm system" for the body. It alerts patients and caregivers about possible problems inside the body. Pain is an indication that something needs to be fixed and requires special attention. For instance, it is painful to touch a body part when it is inflamed or swollen—a signal that a person needs to apply first aid treatment, apply natural remedies, or seek medical advice. Thus, the presence or absence of pain is standard when it comes to uncovering a medical issue such as Alzheimer's disease.

Pain can be described as a fundamental feeling that every Alzheimer's patient obviously tries to avoid. It could be a symptom of physical discomfort or mental distress that he or she experiences. It could also be a sign of inflammation in the body. Physical pain can be identified as the feeling one experiences while burning, stubbing, or getting hurt in any other way. According to reports, pain is both a sensory and emotional experience connected with existing or potential tissue damage.[2] Pain is the warning system of the human body against impending or past injuries or illnesses and can help Alzheimer's victims avoid potentially dangerous or damaging situations, recover from injuries by protecting the damaged parts, and accept treatment for any associated illnesses.

WHY PAIN OCCURS

As all sensations start with the nervous system, pain is born as a sensory nerve response. Specialized nerves called nociceptors activate and pass pain signals to the central nervous system during injuries or potential damage.[3] Based on these signals, the spinal cord initiates bodily reflexes to prevent damage or protect the patient from further harm. The whole process is completed very quickly. After stepping on a sharp object, even if the foot is not critically damaged, one will still pull the leg back from the object before extensive tissue injury takes place.

The study of pain among Alzheimer's patients has been minimal but is gradually gaining ground. The following sections intend to present a deeper understanding of how Alzheimer's patients cope with pain. The sections also summarize the different types of approaches doctors, informal caregivers, and family members can use to manage and improve the comfort levels of the patient.

ROOTS OF PAIN IN ALZHEIMER'S

There are different types of pain from which a patient with Alzheimer's disease can suffer. Physical pain arises from discomfort felt in different parts of the body. Because Alzheimer's is usually common among the elderly population, pain is usually associated with illnesses prevalent in old age, such as arthritis and other painful conditions. When an Alzheimer's patient suffers from unbearable pain, he or she may need assistance while walking, sitting, standing up, and other physical activity. Unfortunately, many of the patients are "glued" to their favorite chair or, even worse, bedridden. In addition to joint pains, the elasticity of the skin among elderly Alzheimer's patients also deteriorates in time. This causes the skin to easily bruise, making it painful for patients to move freely. Particularly in late-stage Alzheimer's, patients can also experience difficulty in swallowing food, making daily eating a challenge for both patients and the caregivers.[4]

PAIN TOLERANCE

Pain among the elderly is often a challenge to diagnose because the patients are unable to communicate pain. For patients with Alzheimer's disease, communication about pain between the doctor and the patient tends to weaken with age. This makes it difficult for elderly Alzheimer's victims to articulate what they are feeling and much more difficult to describe how they feel pain. Another factor that hampers early diagnosis is the Alzheimer's patient's apparent alteration of pain experience and perception when subjected to external stimuli.[5] Peer-reviewed medical studies suggest increased tolerance of Alzheimer's patients to pain.[6] Consequently, patients also have a higher pain threshold. Compared to nondementia patients, pain intensity and effect among Alzheimer's patients are relatively lower and decreased. Because of these factors, pain among Alzheimer's patients is often left untreated and undiagnosed. In addition to guesswork, attentiveness is often needed to determine if a patient is suffering from pain. The caregiver should take note of any sign of discomfort that could be an indication of illness. Examples of these include sores in any part of the body, deteriorating quality of the skin and gums, swelling, or inflammation. All of these need to be relieved at the soonest possible time.

The common assumption has been that Alzheimer's patients do not experience pain or cannot feel pain with the same intensity as do other aging patients. In a study at the University of Melbourne, fourteen patients with Alzheimer's disease and fifteen healthy volunteers (of the same age group) were tested for pain activity in the brain.[7] It was found that pain activity in the brain was just as severe as in patients without the disease. In the case of Alzheimer's patients, pain activity actually lasted for a longer period of time. According to one of the study's lead investigators, patients might even experience increased distress because of their diminished ability to comprehend the unpleasant sensation of pain. Therefore, the physical perception and processing of pain is not reduced in people suffering from Alzheimer's, but the overall tolerance to pain is. As Alzheimer's affects the basal forebrain and the hippocampus areas of the brain that relate to the feelings of pain and memory, patients either forget to feel the pain or simply do not express it. Since verbal cues and expressions are the most widely used methods to recognize and estimate pain, the nature and extent of the pain that Alzheimer's patients suffer from often go undetected.

TYPES OF PAIN EXPERIENCED BY ALZHEIMER'S PATIENTS

Based on various criteria, different categorizations exist for pain. The most common and widely used categorization is that of classifying it into two types, acute pain and chronic pain. Acute pain occurs mostly after a damage or injury to any body part and is usually absent after the injury is healed. It is generally of short duration. Physical expression of chronic pain and its occurrence are much more difficult to comprehend. When the pain persists even after the expected period of healing, it is called chronic pain and is comparatively long term. Pain resulting from a minor burn often disappears within an expected period of time. However, conditions such as rheumatoid arthritis and fibromyalgia lead to chronic pain that lasts for a year or longer.[8]

Other classifications of pain include the nociceptive pain described earlier, which is essentially the pain caused by tissue damage, and neuropathic pain, or pain resulting from nerve damage. One could also experience psychogenic pain, when pain often results from various psychological conditions and factors. Some other types of pain often referred to include the following.[9]

Referred Pain

As the name suggests, this kind of pain is "referred" to another part of the body that is different from the actual source of irritation. When an irritation occurs in an internal organ, the pain is felt in some bodily structure that is distant from the organ. An example is cardiac pain felt in the left arm.

Idiopathic Pain

This is the kind of pain that is felt for no apparent reason. For example, an Alzheimer's patient suffers from back pain, but no actual physical or psychological reasons for the pain exist. The pain is real, however, and often lasts for a long period of time.

Phantom Pain

Originally believed to be just psychological, this type of pain is real and occurs as brain or spinal cord sensations that feel pain coming from outside of the body. This kind of pain is generally felt after an amputation or after removing some other organs. The pain might subside in due time in some patients but might necessitate therapy in others.

Somatic Pain

This is a kind of nociceptive pain. The nerves that detect the pain are situated in skin and deep tissues. When an Alzheimer's patient experiences somatic pain, the pain feels as if the skin is cut or the muscles are stretched too far.

Visceral Pain

Visceral pain is also a nociceptive pain. The nerves that sense this type of pain are situated in internal organs. In other words, this is the kind of pain that results when the internal organs are damaged or hurt. This kind of pain is also known as organ pain.[10]

PAIN MANAGEMENT IN ALZHEIMER'S

Alzheimer's patients are often the elderly who also suffer from other illnesses common in old age. These age-related ailments often get worse as Alzheimer's progresses, adding further pain and suffering throughout the patient's life.[11] These ailments can include the following:

- Vision
- Arthritis
- Heart problems
- Nutritional disorders
- Hypertension
- Hearing problems
- Genitourinary conditions
- COPD (chronic obstructive pulmonary disease)
- Diabetes

The patient's inability to feel, remember, or even express pain often leads to the sad situation of perpetual suffering with no or inadequate treatment. Even when the doctor asks, Alzheimer's patients might not be able to recollect the pain and thus just say they are fine. This is one of the tragic aspects of pain management in Alzheimer's. Caregivers are reliable resources to recognize and assess pain, especially toward the later stages of the disease when patients become increasingly nonverbal. As the sensory-discriminatory method of pain assessment is not possible in Alzheimer's patients, caregivers should opt for the motivational-affective method of assessment. One can suspect the discomfort of pain by observing facial expressions and movements, and general behavior of the patients. The key is to closely watch the facial expressions and movements during painless moments (for example, when the patient sleeps or during his or her waking hours) and then keep these as a baseline to spot any moments of aggression or other expressions of uneasiness. Rapid breathing, frowning, grimacing, bracing the body, moaning, and groaning are some of the vital signals that reveal the patient's suffering. Pain screenings should be done on a daily basis to ensure comfortable living for the patients. Reassessments are required regularly to track and understand any change in the primary disease, which in this case is Alzheimer's.

Another important part of the pain assessment is to keep a history of all the prescription and over-the-counter (OTC) medications the patient has been taking or has taken in the past. Physical examination of the Alzheimer's patient on a regular basis is also necessary; the examination should focus on the usual sites of pain, such as muscles, bones, and the nervous system, and should also take into account the physical functioning of the patient (e.g., the ability to walk about). X-rays and laboratory tests might also be helpful in arriving at a diagnosis and conclusion. When suspecting that an Alzheimer's patient is in pain, caregivers should seek medical intervention. A comforting atmosphere and soothing gestures of touch, massage, fragrance, and music can also alleviate pain in the long run. Effective pain management does have critical significance in improving the quality of life of Alzheimer's patients, especially when in the final stages of the disease. Depending on the nature, underlying causes, or mechanism of pain, as well as the needs of the patient, different methods are used for pain management in Alzheimer's.[12] A combination of two or more of the following approaches is often used in cases of pain today:

- Physical exercises
- Medication management
- Counseling and psychological support
- Diets and other natural methods for pain relief
- Alternative therapies

PRESCRIPTION PAIN DRUGS USED FOR ALZHEIMER'S

Pharmacologic management of pain is a conventional approach where prescription and over-the-counter medications are used for the treatment of physical pain in Alzheimer's patients. The most commonly used pain medication classes are used in the treatment of Alzheimer's pain as well, such as opioids, anesthetics, corticosteroids, nonsteroidal anti-inflammatory drugs (NSAIDs), and muscle relaxants. Detecting and diagnosing pain among the Alzheimer's population remains a challenge. Once pain is detected, it is imperative that the medication or treatment to be given targets the source of pain, or at the very least, lessens the intensity of the pain a patient might be feeling. Since the majority of Alzheimer's patients are elderly, the origin of pain should be investigated thoroughly. Prescription drugs that are normally used to treat and relieve pain among Alzheimer's patients are listed below.

Opioids

One of the oldest drugs in the world, opioids are chemicals that have analgesic (pain-relieving) properties and are commonly included in palliative care for painful and degenerative diseases such as Alzheimer's.[13] Opioids act by binding to opioid receptors in the nervous system and lead to reduction in the perception of pain and greater pain tolerance. In palliative medicine, the field of medicine that deals with life-changing illness, the indication for opioids is moderate or severe pain, regardless of the underlying pathological or physiological mechanism.¹⁴ Both cancer-related and nonmalignant chronic pains are treated using opioids. Some types of pain are considered opioid resistant or opioid insensitive, such as visceral and neuropathic pains. Age is generally not a contraindication for opioid therapy. Commonly found side effects of opioids include the following:

- Gastrointestinal effects such as diarrhea or constipation
- Breathlessness or shortness of breath
- Cough suppression or antitussive effects
- Addiction or opioid dependence

Some other adverse reactions of opioid administration are as follows:

- Confusion
- Dizziness
- Delirium
- Bradycardia (slow heartbeats)
- Skin rashes or urticarial
- Lowering of body temperature
- Muscle rigidity
- Tachycardia (fast heartbeats)
- Urinary retention
- Hallucinations
- Headache
- Flushing

It has also been found that continuous use sometimes compromises the immune system of the patient. Opioids are found in opium, which is a substance from the pod of an opium poppy. These are processed into drugs and are usually prescribed by medical practitioners to manage and relieve pain. The strong pain-relieving properties of opium make it an effective analgesic. In a more basic sense, opioids block the perception of pain. They do this by attaching to opioid receptors in the body, which are specialized proteins found in the brain, spinal cord, and gastrointestinal tract. As with most chemical-based drugs, the use of opioids can have side effects that are harmful to the body or disturbing to the patient. These include drowsiness, nausea, and constipation, and if taken in large dosages, they can depress respiration. Opioids, along with other prescription drugs such as central nervous system (CNS) depressants and stimulants, are said to be one of the commonly abused prescription drugs available today. The addictive quality of opioids increases the risk of overdose among Alzheimer's patients.[15] The usual prescription opioids available in the market include the following:

Alfentanil   This is generally used to manage pain after an operation and to maintain the effect of general anesthesia. It can either be administered as a solution or through injection. The usual impacts of alfentanil on patients include pain relief and sedation. Despite these effects, it also has known side effects. Common side effects observed among patients taking alfentanil include mood swings, dysphoria, euphoria, and drowsiness. It also constricts the pupils, depresses respiratory centers, and improves the cough reflex.[16]

Remifentanil   This is used to relieve pain after an operation and to maintain general and monitored anesthesia for inpatient and outpatient procedures. The drug is administered intravenously in the form of remifentanil hydrochloride. A dosage unsuitable to the patient, given too high or too low, manifests side effects such as short-lived but intense dizziness and intense itching usually felt in the face. If any of these manifestations occur, the patient should seek medical advice from the doctor or other health care professional to adjust the dosage accordingly.

Fentanyl   This is administered intravenously as a painkiller. Fentanyl is also prescribed to improve the effects of local anesthesia during surgical procedures. It is also being marketed as a patch, which gradually releases fentanyl into fats until it is assimilated into the bloodstream, which is more effective compared to other drugs taken orally. Recently, however, fentanyl is being marketed in several forms including lozenges, buccal tablets, inhalers, and nasal sprays. Because it is assimilated directly into the bloodstream, fentanyl provides excellent pain relief. Hence, it is usually given to patients experiencing chronic pain and even in cancer therapy. The common side effect of fentanyl is drowsiness, but skin rash, itching, blister formation, nausea, upset stomach, and difficulties with urinating have been observed among patients taking it.

Meperidine   This opioid is prescribed as a pain reliever to patients experiencing moderate to severe pain. Meperidine relieves the pain quickly; however, patients must be cautious in taking this medication in its tablet and syrup forms. The usual side effects of the drug include drowsiness, dizziness, and lightheadedness. These can also lead to fatal outcomes when used in combination with other drugs. Thus, patients have to inform their medical practitioner if they are taking any other drug alongside meperidine to check its compatibility.

Hydromorphone   This opioid is generally used in the management of chronic pains. Similarly to meperidine, hydromorphone is frequently used to relieve moderate to severe pain usually during and after surgical operations. This is normally used as an alternative medication to morphine for pain relief because of hydromorphone's nonaddictive properties, and thus, the risk of overdose is minimized. Some medical practitioners also prefer prescribing hydromorphone to fentanyl transdermal patches, wherein patients have the possibility to hallucinate. It is oftentimes prescribed as an antitussive for relieving a painful cough. Hydromorphone is a strong analgesic that is administered either intravenously or through an injection. It is also available in other forms, such as tablets, capsules, oral liquids, and suppositories. Drowsiness is a very common side effect.

Corticosteroids

Corticosteroids are chemicals that act similarly to natural steroids made in the human body. These anti-inflammatory drugs are used to control swelling and can also be used to curb certain kinds of pain and increase tissue mobility. Corticosteroids reduce pain in Alzheimer's disease victims by changing the immune response of the body. They can be administered orally, applied locally, or injected into the tissues. Corticosteroids are found to have several side effects that require immediate medical attention, including the following:

- Vision changes or eye pain
- Onset of fresh muscle pain or weakness
- Severe swelling in extremities (hands, feet, and face)
- Rashes that refuse to fade out
- Irregular bowel movements

Other commonly reported side effects, which might not require medical intervention, include the following:

- Dizziness
- Nausea or vomiting
- Sleeplessness
- Headaches
- Change in menstrual cycles
- Skin problems like acnes, redness, or excess hair growth
- Psychological changes such as mood changes, depression, and agitation

Long-term side effects of corticosteroids include the following:

- Cataract or other serious eye damages
- Hyperglycemia (higher levels of glucose in blood)
- Diabetes mellitus
- Insulin resistance
- Osteoporosis (fragile bones due to lack of calcium)
- Anxiety
- Depression

- Hypertension
- Erectile dysfunction
- Hypothyroidism
- Amenorrhea (absence of periods)
- Inflammation of the large intestine and colon

Incidence of peptic ulcer has also been found with long-term use of corticosteroids, especially when administered on a high dose. Corticosteroids can cause some birth defects and should be used in pregnant and lactating women only when absolutely necessary. Corticosteroids are strong anti-inflammatory drugs administered to manage chronic pain and severe swelling of the joints and tendons. These can be administered in the form of injection, pills, or topical (skin) medication. Corticosteroids are usually given to patients who have osteoarthritis, rheumatoid arthritis, synovitis, and tendonitis. Examples available in drugstores include hydrocortisone, prednisone, methylprednisone, and cortisone.

Nonsteroidal Anti-inflammatory Drugs

As one of the most commonly prescribed drugs in the United States, NSAIDs are medications that have fever-reducing (antipyretic) and pain-relieving (analgesic) properties. NSAIDs prevent the cyclooxygenase enzymes, also known as COX enzymes, from working. That in turn slows down the production of hormonelike substances called prostaglandins that cause the feeling of pain. NSAIDs are available as over-the-counter drugs and as prescription medication. The most common indications for NSAIDs are inflammation and pain. NSAIDS are known to relieve pain and reduce fever. When taken in higher doses, its anti-inflammatory actions become more pronounced. NSAIDs are used to manage chronic pain in Alzheimer's patients arising from inflammation. Like corticosteroids, NSAIDs are commonly prescribed to relieve pain arising from osteoarthritis and rheumatoid arthritis. Some also use it to manage migraines and pain after an operation. Examples of such drugs include naproxen and ibuprofen. These are usually purchased over the counter, unless prescribed by a medical practitioner. Most of these drugs are taken by mouth; some can be administered as injections as well. When taking NSAIDs for chronic pain, a short-acting version can be combined with another long-acting drug such as an analgesic or an opioid. Most commonly reported side effects of overusing nonsteroidal anti-inflammatory drugs include renal or kidney problems and gastrointestinal effects such as stomach ulcers. Some contraindications for NSAID administration include allergies to NSAIDs, bleeding abnormalities, impaired renal functions, chickenpox or influenza in children and teenagers, impending surgical or invasive procedures, pregnancy, and lactation.

Below are some of the most widely used prescription NSAIDs in the United States:

- Celecoxib
- Ketoprofen
- Oxaprozin
- Meloxicam
- Piroxicam
- Sulindac
- Etodolac
- Ibuprofen
- Flurbiprofen
- Indomethacin
- Nabumetone
- Naproxen
- Fenoprofen
- Tolmetin

Anesthetics

Anesthetics are drugs that can cause reversible insensibility to pain. These drugs are generally used in surgical procedures and in pain management. While general anesthetics cause loss of sensation to the whole body, local anesthetics create a loss of sensation in only a part of the body while the patient remains conscious. The mechanisms of action (MOA) of general anesthetics are not well understood yet. Local anesthetics act by binding to fast sodium channels from within and blocking sensation in the administered area. Anesthetics are administered through creams and sprays for topical use, as inhalations, and mostly as injections. A combination of these methods could also be used. Anesthesia is usually given to Alzheimer's patients by experienced anesthesiologists or anesthetists before a surgical operation to make them unconscious. While in this state, the intensity of the pain is decreased significantly, thus allowing surgical operations to proceed smoothly. Anesthetics temporarily make the target area numb, making it less possible for patients to feel pain.

There are three different types of anesthesia, depending on the areas targeted for complete or partial loss of sensation: general, regional, and local. General anesthesia affects the whole body. This can be given as a gas, inhaled by patients through a mask, or as an injection. Depending on the dose, this makes the patient completely or partially unconscious throughout the surgery. Regional anesthesia, on the other hand, affects entire regions of the body, such as the lower or upper extremities. Local anesthesia acts on the immediate area of concern to surgery. Much like other medications, anesthetics can have certain adverse side effects on the body. Adverse effects of local anesthesia are known as local anesthetic toxicity, which can affect the whole body (systemic) or only the part where the drug was administered (localized). The adverse effects include cardiac arrhythmia (abnormal rate of heartbeats), which can be resistant to available treatment options and can even lead to loss of functioning and death. When affecting the nervous system, local anesthetic toxicity can trigger agitation, dizziness, confusion, nausea, and vision problems. It can also result in seizures, loss of consciousness, and the collapse of the cardiovascular system. Potential toxicity must be screened before administering local anesthetics. This is especially important for Alzheimer's disease victims who are in later stages of the disease, since they already have problems in other organs such as the brain (see chapter 2).

Examples of commonly used general and local anesthetics in pain management include the following:

- Mepivacaine
- Prilocaine
- Bipivacaine
- Dibucaine
- Procaine
- Chloroprocaine
- Tetracaine
- Proparacaine
- Benzocaine

There are some Alzheimer's patients that exhibit complications from anesthetics. Factors such as age and severe Alzheimer's should be considered before accepting anesthetic drugs. In general, risks to complications from anesthesia are greater for elderly patients and for patients living unhealthy lifestyles that involve drinking too much alcohol, repetitive drug abuse, and excessive smoking.

Muscle Relaxants

Muscles relaxants help treat pain conditions that involve muscle spasms. These drugs affect the central nervous system and result in relaxation of the whole body, concurrently relaxing the tensed muscles to break the muscle-spasm-pain-anxiety cycle.[17] Sedation is a potential side effect, along with vision changes, lightheadedness, dizziness, drowsiness, and dry mouth. Other side effects include the following:

- Hyperkalemia, or exaggerated potassium release from cells
- Bradycardia or very slow heart beat, especially when repeat doses are administered
- Hyperthermia (high body temperature)
- Histamine release

A few prescription muscle relaxants are listed as follows:

- Baclofen
- Benzodiazepines
- Tizanidine
- Methocarbamol
- Orphenadrine citrate
- Cyclobenzaprine
- Diazepam
- Carisoprodol
- Cyclobenzaprine
- Clonidine
- Tizanidine
- Tubocurarine

Muscle relaxants have a sedative effect that relieves pain from muscle spasms and reduces stiffness. However, these drugs target the brain along with the muscles to achieve an overall relaxed body for the Alzheimer's patient.

APPROACHING PAIN NATURALLY

Many believe in using organic and natural remedies in managing pain as these do not cause any serious side effects in the body. This is especially important when dealing with elderly Alzheimer's patients who cannot afford to suffer from any more physical effects and who have difficulty in expressing pain resulting from these side effects. Pain management through medication alone might not be effective in the long run. Also, considering the side effects of medicines, other methods could be employed in the process of pain management along with drug therapy. Dietary changes, food supplements, and even naturally occurring chemicals in the body could prove beneficial in pain management and improving the quality of the patient's life.[18] The following sections list several ways to relieve pain from natural sources found in the diet and within the body, and from alternative methods of treatments such as acupuncture and herbalism.

Diets Known to Relieve Pain

Diets for Alzheimer's patients will be discussed in depth in chapter 16, but there are foods known to relieve some of the pain associated with the disease. Having the right kind of diet is an alternative to chemical-based pain relievers. A well-researched diet will not only ensure a healthy body but also offer a myriad of benefits including pain relief. Studies have now been focusing on certain foods that help manage pain because of its anti-inflammatory properties.[19] These are helpful for elderly patients that suffer from arthritis and other pain disorders emanating from the joints.

Examples of anti-inflammatory foods include cherries and berries that are rich in anthocyanins and resveratrol.[20] The latter molecule is a powerful antioxidant found in naturally produced plants that gets activated when placed in stressful conditions.[21] Antioxidants in the human body function in a similar fashion by protecting body cells from further oxidative damage caused by harmful chemicals and other free radicals that causes stress inside the body. Preventing cellular damage ultimately lowers the risk of developing serious diseases, such as cancer, and slows down the aging process. Similarly, citrus foods such as some fruits, asparagus, and avocados have high antioxidizing properties. Freshly squeezed orange juice is also high in beta-cryptoxanthin, an effective antioxidant that helps repair cells and gets rid of free radicals that would otherwise destroy the cells.

Easily digestible and fresh food items help naturally cleanse, build, and maintain the whole body. Optimal functioning of the body is essential to timely repair any inflammation and damages. It is also believed that certain foods influence pain perception or even mild inflammation. Dietary changes could include avoiding food items that are allergic or unsuitable to the body and its health condition, as well as adding particularly beneficial items to the daily intake. Green veggies, sprouts, and wheat grass are generally found beneficial in reducing certain kinds of pain as the chlorophyll content in them reduces inflammation. In addition, one could also add supplementary chlorophyll sources such as spirulina, chlorella, blue green algae, and dunaliella to the diet plan. Turmeric (a spice grown in South Asia containing curcumin), onions, garlic, flax, yam, ginger, and millet are other food items that could help reduce inflammation and speed the healing of ligaments, tendons, and muscles. Some studies suggest that consuming curcumin could even reduce the risk of Alzheimer's.[22] Fruits with high antioxidant content are really beneficial, and those such as pineapples and cherries can reduce inflammation.

Fats are generally regarded as harmful, but omega-6 fatty acids have been proven to increase inflammation and, hence, increase the risk of painful conditions. However, adding foods rich in omega-3 fatty acids tend to reduce inflammation. Fish oil is a great source of omega-3 fatty acids, as are fish such as mackerel, bluefish, mullet, anchovy, tuna, sturgeon, sardines, salmon, herring, menhaden, and trout. Other food items that contain omega-3 fatty acids include walnuts, almonds, flax seeds, and avocadoes. Omega-3 fatty acids are essential fatty acids that lower the risk of getting heart diseases. Moreover, omega-3 fatty acids are also effective anti-inflammatory agents that relieve pain in Alzheimer's patients who have arthritis, a painful joint disease common among elderly patients. Because the body cannot naturally produce omega-3 fatty acids, the diet should include food sources that are rich in them. Such foods could include fish products such as salmon, halibut, anchovies, pumpkin seeds, walnuts, hazel nuts, and pecans.

Nuts and seeds are another group that can be introduced to the diet of the Alzheimer's patient who is experiencing pain. Peanuts, sesame seeds, sunflower seeds, and hazelnuts are found to be good sources of tryptophan, an essential amino acid component of protein. With strong clinical evidence, tryptophan has been proven to reduce pain in people.[23] Dairy products, soy milk and tofu, whole grains, beans, and lentils are some other good sources of tryptophan. It should always be noted that any supplements or dietary changes should be taken under the supervision of a doctor, to avoid any unwanted complications. This is all the more true in case of Alzheimer's patients, because of the degenerative nature of the symptoms.

Herbs and Natural Supplements

Herbalism, synonymized as an older form of phytotheraphy,[24] is a type of alternative medicine that uses herbs in treating a variety of illnesses. Some herbs are also used in managing pain conditions. Several examples of herbs that provide relief to pain caused by inflammation include white willow bark, capsaicin, boswellia, devil's claw, bromelain, curcumin, and ginger.[25] These herbs are commonly used in treating arthritis, osteoarthritis, and other joint and bone problems typically experienced by the elderly population in different parts of the body. Most Alzheimer's disease victims are elderly, and medical research has suggested a positive link between older patients and bone disease.[26]

In particular, white willow bark is said to be effective in managing pain among patients with gonarthrosis (knee osteoarthritis) and coxarthrosis (hip joint osteoarthritis).[27] Devil's claw relieves pain arising from the back and neck, while bromelain brings comfort to pain arising from musculoskeletal tensions and other inflammation arising from a trauma. Curcumin targets pain related to autoimmune disorders and tendonitis, while capsaicin, a substance found in capsicum plants and hot peppers, alters pain by triggering the release of endorphins that are naturally produced opioids scientifically proven to relieve stress and improve mood in people.[28] Alzheimer's disease patients are no exception to this. Capsaicin is especially useful in relieving pain among patients with arthritis and dyspepsia (indigestion). In general, all these properties make these herbs very good natural analgesics for elderly patients who are at risk for complications resulting from taking synthetic drugs and other chemical-based medications.

Certain minerals and natural herbs or herbal preparations, when taken for a longer period, tend to reduce pain in Alzheimer's patients in different ways. For example, green tea with plenty of antioxidants is found to be quite beneficial to several health conditions and for naturally increasing a person's immunity. Solid medical studies prove that polyphenols in green tea help prevent inflammation and swelling.[29] Minerals such as zinc have anti-inflammatory properties and might be beneficial if administered in recommended dosages. Glucosamine sulfate, magnesium, niacinamide, copper, calcium, and boron are some others that could have beneficial properties in pain management. Valerian root, Jamaica dogwood, wild yam, and black haw are also widely used as muscle relaxants by herbalists. There have not been many studies that could substantially prove the benefits of these supplements or herbs 100 percent, but many of these are used as traditional means to alleviate pain. They can be administered with proper supervision and care.

Vitamins

Vitamins are substances that the body needs in small amounts to achieve balance and maintain functionality. Because the body cannot produce these naturally, vitamins are obtained from diet, sunlight, and synthetic supplements, as well as other sources. Specific illnesses result when the patient is deficient of certain types of vitamins. Examples of these illnesses include scurvy among patients deficient of vitamin C, osteoporosis and rickets from vitamin D deficiency, and night blindness from lack of vitamin A. Besides providing nourishment to the body and ensuring that it remains healthy, there are certain types of vitamins that contribute to pain relief among patients.[30] These include vitamins A, B complex, and D. B complex (B1, B2, B3, B5, B6, and B7) vitamins are water soluble vitamins that can help alleviate chronic back pain. Food sources of B vitamins include meat such as turkey, tuna, liver, and poultry, as well as dairy products, lentils, and green leafy vegetables.

Vitamin C is a powerful antioxidant that protects the body from cellular damage caused by harmful effects of free radicals. It can be found in citrus fruits such as oranges, lemons, and tomatoes, and vegetables such as red and green peppers and broccoli. Vitamin C helps repair broken tissues, facilitates their growth, and promotes healing. As such, vitamin C is given to patients who are recovering from surgery. Scientific research points to the efficacy of vitamin C in relieving pain, especially from bone fractures.[31] This is a significant finding in relation to Alzheimer's because, as noted in chapters 8 and 17, patients are susceptible to falls.

Vitamin D helps maintain healthy bones and thus alleviates chronic pain and fatigue syndromes arising from the musculoskeletal system. Having sufficient amounts of vitamin D in the body can help shield the Alzheimer's patient from painful bone diseases such as osteoporosis, which is prevalent among the elderly, and rickets. It can be obtained from food sources such as dairy products, marine products such as oysters and fish, and especially, egg yolks. Vitamin D is also naturally obtained from exposure to sunlight. Caution must be heeded, though, since too much exposure to the sun can cause skin damage and cancer and quickens the aging process.

Naturally Occurring "Opioids" in the Body

Endorphins are released by the pituitary gland and hypothalamus during intense pain that one might get from strenuous activities, such as long-distance running and bodybuilding. For the elderly Alzheimer's disease population, intense pain can be caused by simple walking exercises when concurrent with joint-related diseases. Endorphins are naturally occurring antidepressants that alleviate the mood and relieves stress. Often referred to as the "happy biochemicals" or "runner's high,"[32] endorphins protect the patient from feeling pain and counteract stress.

Resembling endorphins to an extent, dynorphins are produced by the hypothalamus. They are released in other areas of the body such as the hippocampus (see chapter 2) and the spinal cord. Similar to chemical-based anaesthetics, dynorphins are capable of numbing the body from pain. These substances bring comfort to patients by alleviating mood conditions, and studies show that dynorphins can serve as antidotes to cocaine addiction.[33]

Enkephalins are closely related to endorphins but are produced in the adrenal glands, located near the kidney. Enkephalins have specific points of action that include the brain and the spinal cord. Like endorphins, enkephalins keep patients concentrated and focused on an ongoing activity, ignoring pain signals in the process. Enkaphalins modulate pain arising from the musculoskeletal system, including the joints. Researchers have found that these endogenous opioids are released during strenuous exercises, moments of excitement, and as a response to pain or stress in the system.[34] These function similar to morphine and control pain and relaxation. Further studies in this area might help the medical community to better understand the working of endogenous opioids and how to facilitate their use in better pain management for Alzheimer's.[35]

ALTERNATIVE THERAPIES

The concept of alternative therapies for pain treatment relies on the Eastern philosophies and principles of life, and takes a rather holistic approach to pain relief. Many of these alternative methods or systems have been around for centuries. Such methods include acupuncture, Ayurveda, and Reiki. Differing from the pills, injections, and supplements of the modern dogmas of medicine, these systems offer alternative courses to pain treatment and to life as a whole for the Alzheimer's patient. Accordingly, the mind controls thoughts, actions, and the body itself. Mind, body, and soul should be healthy and fresh for a pain-free life for the Alzheimer's disease victim. It is often advised that alternative therapies should only be used in addition to—but not in place of—modern medicine.

Benefits

The alternative therapies for managing pain in Alzheimer's discussed to this point are safer than taking chemical-based drugs, since the former do not leave behind chemical residues that can have adverse effects on the body, unless the alternative therapies are abused. Vitamins and minerals obtained from healthy food sources bring back the balance in one's nutrition, which helps to increase tolerance for pain. Besides this, they are cost efficient since most of these are naturally produced by the body and are found in many resources such as diet, plants, and sunlight. Chemical-based drugs are often overpriced and cause psychological stress and discomfort to patients who are already experiencing pain. More so, too much dependency on chemical-based pain relievers increases the risk of complications, especially among elderly patients. Alzheimer's patients will therefore benefit substantially from these alternative and natural-based approaches.

Acupuncture

Acupuncture is one of the oldest and traditional practices of treatment from the Chinese system of medicine. This system is very useful in alleviating different kinds of chronic pain. According to the Chinese philosophy behind acupuncture, pain is caused when fluids or vital energy or *qi* (pronounced "chee") are restrained in the body. This restriction could manifest in three different ways, as follows:

- Obstruction or blocked flow of energy—due to swelling, injury, and damage
- Constraint or restrained flow of energy—due to psychic or mental constraints
- Deficiency or weak flow of energy—due to deficiency of qi or blood

Regardless of the cause of pain—obstruction, constraint, or deficiency—acupuncture eases the energy or fluid flow to reduce pain. Specific points of the body are stimulated by way of inserting needles through the skin to regulate the flow of qi. When practicing acupuncture the traditional way, Alzheimer's disease is considered the same as any other kind of dementia-related disease. Alzheimer's symptoms can be treated by acupuncture because of the vitiated mind, disturbed state, and the inability to concentrate associated with dementia. Acupuncture points are selected for the insertion of needles. When done by qualified personnel using sterile needles, acupuncture is generally a safe procedure, but adverse effects might include infection and punctured organs.[36] Though a number of research experiments have been done on the use of acupuncture for treating Alzheimer's, further studies are required to confirm all the benefits.[37]

Ayurveda and Reiki

Massages, as prescribed by the Ayurveda system of medicine, could also alleviate different kinds of pain associated with Alzheimer's. The massage should be administered under the supervision of a qualified Ayurvedic practitioner and certified massagers. In addition to massages, Ayurveda offers oral and topical medications for pain management. Reiki, an ancient system of medicine, manipulates the life energy in the body to heal itself and bring forth favorable feelings of well-being and relaxation. It is used by people across the world to relax muscles, alleviate pain, and induce sleep. Other important methods that could help alleviate physical pain include breathing exercises, meditation, and yoga, when practiced properly with qualified practitioners. It is always important that any alternative approach that an Alzheimer's patient takes is discussed with the consulting doctor and health-care workers well in advance. This helps avoid or mitigate any kind of adverse effects or other issues.

PAIN-REDUCING EXERCISES FOR ALZHEIMER'S PATIENTS

Physical exercise and activity are important in keeping the body healthy and fit across all age groups. In the case of older people, it also helps minimize or retard functional decline seen in Alzheimer's. According to the American Geriatric Society, physical exercises can better the management of pain and increase physical mobility, and should be part of the care program for people with chronic pain.[38] When reading through the following sections on exercise and pain, it is important to keep in mind that chronic pain experienced by Alzheimer's patients can be mental or physical.

Location

Most of the exercises can be done at home or wherever the patient stays most of the time. The simplest of all exercises is walking, which also helps stimulate the patient's brain. In cases of patients with limited mobility, leg lifts and squats could be beneficial. Drawing and folding paper could help keep the hands and fingers mobile. Relaxation exercises such as breathing and shoulder shrugs and muscle- and bone-strengthening exercises such as squatting, heel raises and toe raises, and chair sit-ups can also be performed at home on a regular basis. Exercising at home eliminates the need for travelling to the gym, and thus helps save a considerable amount of time. Flexibility of time and convenience are some other great aspects of exercising at home, in addition to the cost factor. Moreover, one could avoid any embarrassing situations in front of others, especially for people with Alzheimer's or other debilitating ailments. At the same time, lack of company and the absence of an instructor and a structured program might be demotivating and unfortunately lead to quitting. While many simple exercises could be learnt and practiced at home, others such as aerobics need to be done at a training center or gym facility under the supervision of qualified instructors. A gym also provides Alzheimer's patients with an opportunity to go out and be in the company of cohorts. This acts as a great motivating factor for continuing with the program. It also provides one with the benefits of professional and personalized training programs that could be tailored to the particular needs of the patient. It provides continuous monitoring, which might sometimes be scarce at home.

Drawbacks and Benefits

The large barrier to exercising at a gym or similar facility is the cost of membership. Also, gyms do not or cannot always provide Alzheimer's disease victims with the same flexibility as working out at home due to (1) overcrowding, which may be agitating (see chapter 11), or (2) resource crunches. It seems cumbersome to engage elderly patients in exercise programs. Caregivers, therapists, and even family members need to be more patient with patients because exercise has been an effective approach for pain management. Most elderly patients want to rest throughout the day, especially if they are feeling down or any discomfort in the body. While it is true that rest is often an option when feeling pain in the body, it is not adviseable to have prolonged rest because this causes bodily functions to deteriorate. Lack of physical mobility results in stiffness, cardiovascular problems, and gradual deterioration of health. The patient's ability to cope with pain is subsequently decreased. This is where regular execise becomes therepautic among geriatric patients, including victims of Alzheimer's.

Engaging in an exercise regime helps the body naturally release the endorphins mentioned previously, blocking the perception and sensation of pain. Exercise also helps maintain the physical fitness and health of an elderly patient. It improves blood circulation and relaxes the muscles that are subjected to stress. Elderly patients usually feel stiffness in their muscles and joints, which might already be arthritic. Relaxing these areas through the right kind of exercise and physical therapy will help relieve pain.

Diversity

Therapeutic exercise regimes that are widely used in pain management include a range of motion or stretching routines, strengthening programs, cardiovascular aerobic conditioning, specific exercises protocol, and relaxation exercises.[39] These relieve pain by improving blood flow and strengthening and soothing affected muscles and tissues. Exercise helps improve balance in geriatric patients, thereby reducing the probabilties of falling and tripping, both of which are typical causes of broken bones.

ANALYSIS

Pain in Alzheimer's is a phenomenon that includes physical, psychological, spiritual, emotional, and social components. Though undetected or underdiagnosed, pain experienced by Alzheimer's patients is a reality today, accepted and studied by the clinical and research communities around the world. Pain management in Alzheimer's is a developing area of care that needs to take into account all the different aspects of pain. A wide range of skills and approaches are used in the pain management of this disease, starting from conventional medication management to psychological support and counseling activities. Though the foremost goal is to ease the patient's discomfort, it should always be kept in mind that pain treatment should take place under the guidance and supervision of a qualified medical professional. A cautious approach reduces the chances of any kinds of risks, thereby facilitating a better life for those who suffer from pain.

Fragility and Sensitivity

Patients with Alzheimer's disease are fragile in that their body is deteriorating without them being conscious about it. The decrease in pain intensity and the increased tolerance for pain among Alzheimer's patients makes it difficult to immediately identify which part of the body needs attention. This causes delays in diagnosis and hence results in treatments that are administered late. Not treating problems as early as possible aggravates a disease from which the pain arises until it reaches a point that the situation is no longer manageable by simple and nondamaging medications. Caregivers must be extra sensitive and vigilant when dealing with Alzheimer's patients to allow them to easily spot any indication of pain and immediately advise possible approaches for treatment.

Approaches

Pain management proves to be even more difficult because Alzheimer's patients mostly belong to the elderly population. Geriatric (older) patients require more care and attention because of their fragile physical and mental states. For obvious reasons, they are the ones who are usually inflicted with illnesses that are associated with old age, hence planning the right types of treatment for pain relief is very crucial. Family members should also be involved in determining the types of pain relievers that will be given to elderly family members afflicted with Alzheimer's. They know the patient's medical history more than anyone else, especially at a time when the patient has difficulty communicating and articulating what he or she is feeling inside.

In Retrospect

This chapter reviewed the synthetic and natural approaches to relieving pain that might be useful for people who have an elderly family member afflicted with Alzheimer's disease. There are a number of prescription medications given to Alzheimer's patients for pain relief. However effective, these drugs do come with adverse side effects. Because many of the options are addictive, there is danger of these chemical-based drugs getting abused by patients, resulting in drug overdose. As a result, more damage than cure occurs. It should be noted that caregivers must properly consult with doctors and other medical practitioners before administering these kinds of drugs to the patients. The use of alternative medicine has been gaining ground in pain management. These natural-based remedies and strategies are often the better recourse in pain relief, especially among elderly patients. Improving behavioral strategies, such as engaging in an appropriate exercise regime and choosing the right kind of diet, is an effective and promising way of relieving pain, even in the absence of synthetic chemical-based medication that has the tendency to leave harmful chemicals in the body. Engaging in fitness activities naturally produces opioids that provide relief from pain for Alzheimer's disease patients.

VI
MONEY AND RESEARCH

Economic Effects of Alzheimer's

*E*very government has its own budget allocations for the year. Part of this budget includes money for military, education, and social security. Some of the money is allocated to the senior citizens of the country. Alzheimer's is mostly a disease of the elderly, so it is important to first look at the spending for senior citizens.

NATIONAL BUDGETS FOR SENIOR CITIZENS

Based on data gathered on social spending for the elderly by the Organisation of Economic Co-operation and Development (OECD) in 2010, the United States spent 5.3 percent of its gross domestic product (GDP) on public programs for their senior citizens back in 2007.[1]

Many of the benefits that senior citizens receive in America are from social security. According to the Social Security Administration, the U.S. government released more than $659 billion in benefit payments through the Old Age, Survivors, and Disability Insurance program in 2009.[2] Although this includes some disabled workers, survivors, and their families, it is part of the government budget that covers senior citizens through social security funding. In the same year, the government also spent $49 billion through the Supplement Security Income (SSI), which also benefits senior citizens, the blind, and the disabled. In 2010, the funds allocated to Social Security, Medicare, and Medicaid amounted to $701 billion, $446 billion, and $273 billion, respectively.[3] The Social Security Administration estimated that it will be spending over $729 billion through the Old Age, Survivors, and Disability Insurance program, over $52 billion through the SSI, and another $8 million as special benefits for certain World War II veterans in one year alone.[4] These amount to a total of $789 billion, most of which go to senior citizens. Based on President Barack Obama's proposed budget for 2012, the allotted budgets for Social Security, Medicare, and Medicaid are $751 billion, $485 billion, and $269 billion, respectively.[5]

A LOOK AROUND THE WORLD

In Canada, the government spent an average of 3.85 percent of its GDP for their senior citizens from 2000 to 2007.[6] In 2011, it allotted more than $300 million per year for their senior citizens through the Guaranteed Income Supplement (GIS) and more than $10 million through the New Horizons for Seniors Program.[7] The government also anticipates that the enhancement of the GIS will cost around $530 million in the next two years.[8] In Australia, the percentage of the GDP used for programs for the senior citizens was 4.3 percent in 2007.[9] In 2008–2009, the Australian government released $107 million as health assistance to the aged. In the same time frame, they also released over $40 billion as assistance to the aged and almost $7 billion as assistance to veterans and dependents through their Social Security and Welfare program.[10] In 2009–2010, the final budget outcome for senior citizens through the Social Security and Welfare program was over $47 billion. As for France and Japan, their governments spent 11.1 percent and 8.8 percent of their 2007 GDP on senior citizens, while in the UK, the percentage of 2007 GDP used for the same age group was 5.8 percent.[11]

PERSONAL AND GOVERNMENT
COSTS OF ALZHEIMER'S

The costs of caring for Alzheimer's consists of ongoing medical treatment (which includes diagnosis and follow-up visits), prescription drugs, personal care supplies, in-home-care services, adult day center services, and, for some, residential care services such as assisted living and nursing homes. The average total cost of care (from diagnosis to death) for a person with Alzheimer's in the United States is currently around $175,000.[12] The total aggregate cost of health care, long-term care, and hospice for patients with Alzheimer's and other dementia for 2011 was $183 billion, with 70 percent of that being covered by Medicare and Medicaid. The breakdown of this amount is as follows:

- $93 billion from Medicare (51 percent)
- $37 billion from Medicaid (20 percent)

- $31 billion from out-of-pocket payments (17 percent)
- $22 billion from private insurance, health maintenance organizations (HMOs), other managed care organizations, and unpaid care given by family members and friends (12 percent)[13]

For health-care services, the average per-person payments in 2004 from all sources for Medicare beneficiaries aged sixty-five and older with Alzheimer's and other dementia were as follows:

- $9,768 for hospital expenses
- $5,551 for the medical providers (including the physician, other medical providers, laboratory services, and medical equipment and supplies)
- $3,862 for specialized nursing facilities
- $1,601 for home health care
- $3,198 for prescription medications[14]

In 2003, individuals diagnosed with Alzheimer's or other forms of dementia, who were also Medicare beneficiaries aged sixty-five and older, spent an average of $3,455 or 22 percent of their income on health care.[15] For paid care services, there are adult day center services, nursing homes, and assisted-living facilities. The average cost of adult day center services per day was $67 in 2009.[16] In assisted-living facilities, the average cost of basic services in the same year was $3,131 a month or $37,572 a year. Some facilities are able to give specialized Alzheimer's and dementia care that cost an average of $4,556 a month or $54,670 a year.[17] In nursing homes, the average cost of a semiprivate room was $203 a day or $74,239 a year, while a private room was $225 a day or $82,113 annually.[18] If the nursing home had a separate Alzheimer's special care unit, the average cost of a semiprivate room was $214 a day, or $77,998 a year, and for a private room, the average cost was $239 a day, or $87,362 annually.[19] In 2002, individuals diagnosed with Alzheimer's or other dementia, who were also Medicare beneficiaries aged sixty-five and older, had to pay 37 percent of nursing home care costs out of pocket.[20]

The total average annual payment made per Alzheimer's patient with Medicare benefits in 2004 was $42,072, in 2010 dollars.[21] This includes payments from all sources, namely, Medicare, Medicaid, uncompensated (unpaid care given by family members and friends), HMOs, private insurance, other managed care organizations, and out-of-pocket payment. This average annual payment was approximately $3,506 a month and $115 a day. Nowadays, the annual cost of home care for a person with this disease is estimated at $76,000, including medical expenses and indirect costs (i.e., loss of production from unpaid caregivers).[22] That is a total of $6,333 per month and $208 per day. Patients that require an assisted-living facility or a nursing home have to include the annual cost of those as well, which are $37,572 and $79,935, respectively.

Expensive Approaches

As Alzheimer's disease has no cure, there is no realistic end to the pharma-cological and natural treatments given to the patient. The FDA has approved five drug treatments that are given to help manage the behavioral symptoms, improve mental function, and enable some to carry out their daily activities and independent living for as long as possible. The most expensive drug used for treating Alzheimer's today is donepezil, the only approved drug for treat-ing all stages of Alzheimer's, from mild to severe. Prices differ based on the pharmacy selling the drug and the country where it is being sold. Although there are now generic brands of Aricept (donepezil) available, the price of Aricept still remains the same. Some still purchase it because it is the only available drug in their local drugstore.

Another expensive "treatment" for Alzheimer's is proper caregiving.[23] Proper caregiving can be given at home, assisted-living facilities, adult day centers, or nursing homes. Based on a study in 2001, the total annual cost of caregiving for dementia patients in the United States was over $18 billion.[24] Many Alzheimer's patients are cared for by family and friends. Although this is considered unpaid or uncompensated care, it is still considered expensive. In a study in 1999, the national economic value of informal caregiving given by family and friends to ill and disabled adults was $196 billion in 1997.[25] In 2010, unpaid care given to Alzheimer's patients was estimated at $202.6 bil-lion, or 17 billion hours of unpaid care valued at $11.93 per hour.[26]

Caregiving practices impact businesses economically. In 1998, it cost businesses that had employees who were caregivers approximately $25 billion due to missed work, lost productivity, health-care costs, and the cost of re-placing workers who resign to meet the demands of caregiving.[27] In 2002, the cost increased to around $35 billion, and by 2004, it was costing businesses $60 billion a year.[28] The average hourly rate is $21 to care for an Alzheimer's patient at home.[29] For an eight-hour day, that is a cost of $168 a day, $5040 per month, and $61,320 annually. In addition to being expensive, giving care to an Alzheimer's patient is considered custodial care and is not covered by Medicare or most private health insurance plans.[30] There are several factors for the high cost of proper caregiving. Caregiving assists Alzheimer's patients with instrumental and personal activities of daily living.[31] Instrumental ac-tivities include driving the patients around, buying groceries, cooking meals, assisting them with their medications, and following treatment recommen-dations, as well as managing finances and legal affairs. Personal activities include dressing, bathing, toileting, walking, and eating. Aside from the memory loss, Alzheimer's also causes a loss of the ability to understand and communicate, a loss of orientation, and behavioral and personality changes that require more supervision and personal care.[32] All of these create stress on the caregiver and have a negative impact on the caregiver's emotional and physical health. Another factor is the existence of other serious medical conditions in Alzheimer's patients, such as diabetes, coronary heart disease, and congestive heart failure, conditions that the caregiver has to monitor as well.

Direct Governmental Costs for Alzheimer's

Part of the cost for caring and treating Alzheimer's is shouldered by the government. In the United States, around 70 percent of the cost of care for the disease is covered by Medicare and Medicaid.[33] Medicare spent $91 billion on beneficiaries with Alzheimer's and other dementias in 2005.[34] Medicaid, used partially for nursing home care for people with Alzheimer's and other dementia, was estimated at $21 billion in the same year. This program paid for an average of $19,772 per person for Medicare beneficiaries who were diagnosed with Alzheimer's and living in a long-term facility. At the same time, it incurred an average cost of $895 per person for those living in the community.[35] In 2006, the U.S. government spent more than $120 billion to support those struggling with the disease.[36] A report suggests that, by 2025, state and federal funding through Medicaid for nursing home care alone will be almost $38 billion.[37] According to a study done in collaboration with the Alzheimer's Association, total payments coming from Medicare and Medicaid combined for 2011 is estimated at $130 billion.[38] According to the Alzheimer's Disease Research Program, the total national cost of this disease in people over sixty-five years old was $183 billion in 2011 alone. They also estimate that, by 2050, this amount will reach $1.1 trillion.[39] In addition to supporting treatment for Alzheimer's, the U.S. government also spent $600 million for research on the disease.[40]

COST DIFFERENCES IN DEMOGRAPHICS AND STAGES

Cost Differences between Men and Women

While the treatments and care for Alzheimer's patients are the same for men and women, the costs differ. Based on data gathered between 1984 and 1999,[41] a man with Alzheimer's incurred an annual average cost of $9,710. A woman with the same disease, on the other hand, incurred an annual average cost of $16,327. In the UK, costs for women aged sixty-five and over with dementia in 1994 was £5.35 billion while men only incurred £0.95 billion.[42] The reason for this is based on several factors. First, it could be because women spend more time in nursing homes. Based on fifteen years of follow-up, women with Alzheimer's spent around 1.5 years in institutional care, while men spent an average of almost 0.6 years.[43] Gender differences in costs might also be because, when men get the disease, they have family members (women and children) who are able to take care of them at home. When women get the late onset version of Alzheimer's disease, their husbands might no longer be around. Thus, elderly female patients need institutional care. Another factor is that women live longer than men,[44] which means more hours of paid, informal care for women. A harsh reality is that keeping patients alive longer will mean an increase in the severity of the disease, and that in turn leads to increasing expenses.[45]

Cost Differences between Stages of Alzheimer's

Adding to the differences of costs between men and women, the different stages of Alzheimer's also incur different sets of costs. The annual cost of caring for an Alzheimer's patient is $18,408 if he or she has mild symptoms.[46] For someone with moderate symptoms, the annual cost is $30,096, while someone with severe symptoms has a yearly cost of $36,132.[47] Moreover, the costs also change if the patient has other coexisting medical conditions, such as diabetes, congestive heart failure, and coronary heart disease. Based on a research study in 1998, the total annual costs for patients with no coexisting conditions was $19,008.[48] For patients with one or two conditions and those with three or more, the total annual costs were $22,572 and $31,296, respectively.[49]

As mentioned in chapter 8, people who develop Alzheimer's disease and are younger than sixty-five years of age have early onset Alzheimer's. Based on another study in 1998, there were no significant differences in the total cost of illness between patients with early onset dementia and those with late onset dementia.[50] Differences, if any, existed because of the type of service that utilized by the two groups: the younger patients used less of the community resources or services compared to the older patients. The lack of difference in total costs is because the types of care given to people with early onset Alzheimer's did not differ from those received by people with late onset Alzheimer's. Yet, there is a difference when it comes to the out-of-pocket expenditures between younger and older Alzheimer's patients.[51] People younger than sixty-five years of age do not have Medicare. To qualify, a person must be eligible for Social Security Disability Insurance (SSDI) and undergo a two-year waiting period after gaining SSDI.[52] It is also more difficult for people with early onset Alzheimer's to get Medicaid, which helps pay for long-term care. To be eligible for Medicaid, one must meet the low-income and asset requirement, which can be extremely difficult for these people as they have families and spouses who are still able to work and have savings. Another program that helps pay for long-term care is the Administration on Aging (AOA). This covers adult day care, transportation, services to support family caregivers, and meals-on-wheels. This is only for people aged sixty and older, which makes those patients below this age requirement unable to get this benefit as well. Because of such parameters, their out-of-pocket expenditures for health care and long-term care are higher than those for people with late onset Alzheimer's.[53]

According to a very recent report, the out-of-pocket costs for medications for younger patients with Alzheimer's in 2010 were four times higher than those within the same age group who didn't have the disease.[54] Some patients also try to purchase private health insurance, but those who succeed face the additional problem of paying high premiums, deductibles, and copayments. The direct cost of younger people with dementia in the UK was around £132 million a year.[55] For Canadians, the total yearly cost for the same age group was $389.2 million.[56] This may seem small compared to the billions of dollars spent for the total yearly costs of Alzheimer's patients who are sixty-five years old and over. This is because of the small percentage of people who develop early onset Alzheimer's compared to those who develop late onset Alzheimer's.

COSTS OF ALZHEIMER'S BEYOND THE UNITED STATES

Costs also differ between countries. In the UK, it was estimated that the total cost per patient over three months in 1999 was £6,616 for a person with mild Alzheimer's, £10,250 for a person with moderate Alzheimer's, and £13,593 for a person with severe Alzheimer's.[57] More recently, the total annual cost per person with mild Alzheimer's disease living in the community is £16,689, in 2006 prices.[58] Based on the exchange rate of the American dollar to the British pound at that time (£1 = US$1.76),[59] this amounts to $29,372.64. A peer-reviewed article states that, for those with moderate dementia, the cost was £25,877, while for those with severe dementia, the cost was £37,473.[60] The full costs of institutional care, such as hospitals and nursing homes, were estimated at £278.86 a week for mild to moderate illness and £338.38 a week for severe illnesses.[61] Based on extensive research from 2007, the total annual cost of care for people aged sixty-five and higher with dementia in the country was estimated at £17.03 billion, or $29.97 billion in 2006 prices.[62]

In Canada, the estimated cost for a person with dementia sixty-five years old or over was $14,000 a year in 1991. This amounted to a total annual net cost of $3.5 billion. For those who were younger than sixty-five, the total annual net cost was $389.2 million.[63] More recently, the annual cost of taking care of patients with dementia has been estimated to range from $941 per patient with mild disease to $36,794 per patient with severe disease, with an average net cost of about $4 billion.[64]

In Australia, the total financial cost in 2002 for dementia was $6.6 billion, which was over $40,000 per person with dementia each year. In the Asia

Pacific, 78.7 billion was spent on care for dementia patients, which is equal to $32,255 per dementia patient.[65] Comparatively, the costs of caring for Alzheimer's patients in Ireland seem to be lower than those in other countries like the UK and United States. In 1996, the cost of caring for someone with Alzheimer's were between £10,933 and £15,100 per person per year, or £328 million to £453 million in total.[66]

More on Canada and Australia

Compared to America, Canada spent $15 billion in 2008 for the care and treatment of Alzheimer's. They estimate that, by 2018, the total economic burden of the disease will be over $238 billion, and by 2038, it will be over $872 billion, in 2008 dollars.[67] The government of Canada has also contributed $69 million to Alzheimer's research between 2000 and 2005.[68] In Australia, $175 million of federal community services program money was used for people with dementia. Other federal programs in Australia that support Alzheimer's disease patients include the following:

• Dementia Support for Assessment Program ($1.1m)
• National Respite for Carers Program ($87.6m)
• Carer Information and Support Program ($2m)
• National Dementia Behavior Advisory Service ($0.4m)
• Carer Education and Workforce Training Project ($1.1m)
• Dementia Education and Support program ($1.4m budget)
• Psychogeriatric Care Units ($3.5m)
• Early Stage Dementia Support and Respite Project ($1.5m)[69]

More on the UK

In the UK, the total welfare benefits given by the government for the care of dementia patients were around £1 billion in 2005–2006 prices. Aside from welfare benefits, the government also shoulders some of the costs of an Alzheimer's patient through the National Health Service (NHS) and Social Services. For a person with mild dementia living in the community (not in a nursing home), the government covered £7,443 of the £16,689 total annual cost mentioned previously. For a person with moderate dementia living in the community, the amount covered by the government was £8,654 of the £25,877 total annual cost. For a person with severe dementia living in the community, the government covered £10,377 of the £37,473 total annual cost.[70]

SUPPORT FROM NONGOVERNMENTAL ORGANIZATIONS

Support in the United States

As for support from national and international Alzheimer's organizations, the biggest national voluntary health organization committed to supporting Alzheimer's research and giving support to Americans with the disease along with their families and caregivers in the United States is the Alzheimer's Association. In 2010, the organization used the following:

- $28 million for research
- $20 million for public awareness and education
- $5.4 million for chapter services
- $5.3 million for patient and family services
- $4.2 million for advocacy

The total program expenditures that the organization had for the year was $63 million.[71]

Another nonprofit organization dedicated to funding research on Alzheimer's and giving financial help to Alzheimer's patients and their caregivers is the American Health Assistance Foundation. This organization uses 67 percent of its funds for their programs aimed at research, financial assistance, and societal information.[72] In 2009, the organization spent (1) $8 million on research, (2) $3.4 million on financial assistance to patients, families, and caregivers, (3) $3.4 million on educating the public and creating awareness, (4) $1.8 million on helping patients with lifestyle choices, and (5) $616,777 on symptom recognition. Its total program expense for the year was $17.7 million.[73]

Support in Other Countries

The Alzheimer's Society in the UK was able to spend £47.5 million in 2010 for Alzheimer's disease. Out of the £47.5 million, $42 million or almost 90 percent of the expenses were used for the care of patients with dementia and their caregivers, £2.6 million was used for campaigning and raising awareness, and £2 million was used for funding research.[74] In Canada, the Alzheimer's Society was able to release $3 million for their research program and $2 million for public education in 2011.[75] Another organization dedicated to fight Alzheimer's is Alzheimer's Disease International. Based on their financial report in 2010, the organization was able to release $1.2 million for their program services. Their program services include holding conferences, research, member support and development, and providing information.[76] One other organization, Alzheimer's Australia, was able to release $700,000 of their money to fund research in 2010 and promises to release a total of $220 million over the next five years for the same cause. This same organization was able to use $8.5 million and $10 million of their funds for their programs in 2009 and 2010, respectively.[77]

SIGNIFICANCE

Why do people need to know about all the financial impacts of Alzheimer's? In 2005, it was estimated in a report that the worldwide societal costs of dementia was over US$300 billion a year.[78] By 2025, it is estimated that about thirty-four million people in the world will have dementia (of which Alzheimer's is the most prevalent).[79] It has been made clear that this disease places a heavy financial burden on everyone—from the government, to family members, to businesses, and to even the average taxpayer. As the number of people with the disease increases, so do the costs for caring for those who have Alzheimer's. Determining the magnitude of the impact that the disease has on every society will help boost awareness and advocacy.

By informing policymakers of the coming financial burdens that this disease will have, people can make them check the effectiveness and appropriateness of the services given to those with Alzheimer's. It will also stress the importance of creating more health services or programs that will help address the disease better. Informing key decision makers might also result in the production of solutions for the growing problems that result from the prevalence of Alzheimer's in our society, such as losses incurred by businesses. This knowledge will help organizations get more funding for research. Further research into therapies and treatments will allow doctors to get a better idea of how to treat the disease and possibly even cure it. More *specific* research into the health economics of Alzheimer's can lead to promoting a more efficient use of resources in the field of care for Alzheimer's patients. Last, spreading awareness of the economic effects of Alzheimer's will benefit not only those who are associated with the disease but also society as a whole.

Alzheimer's Disease
Research in the United States

STATISTICS AND GOVERNMENT REACTIONS

$\mathcal{A}$side from the attempt to find a cure, one of the most important reasons for Alzheimer's research in the United States is the high number of people with the disease. In the first quarter of 2008, an alarming report stated that 5.2 million Americans were affected by the dreaded Alzheimer's disease, and the numbers continue to grow till today.[1] By way of the report, the Alzheimer's Association projected that at least ten million people of the older population will get Alzheimer's in the succeeding years. Despite technological breakthroughs in treating and preventing Alzheimer's, the report says that one in every American develops the disease every seventy-one seconds. It is also estimated that, after 150 years, the chances of an American getting Alzheimer's will be reduced to every thirty-three seconds. It is predicted that, by the year 2030, a little over seven million Americans will have Alzheimer's and will increase to about nine million more by 2050.[2]

According to the same report, the risk of developing Alzheimer's disease is higher in older women than in men, and one out of six women and one out of ten men develop Alzheimer's somewhere in the ages of fifty-five and above. The report also illustrates the chances of acquiring Alzheimer's disease in the later stages of one's life. More specifically, of the seventy-eight million of the people born between 1946 and 1964 who will be in their midforties to early sixties, approximately 10 to 20 percent of them will develop dementia.

RESEARCH OUTLOOK

Due to the unsettling rise in the number of American citizens affected by Alzheimer's, the U.S. federal government is providing millions of dollars to spend on research for Alzheimer's. A number of experts in the fields of neurology and neuropathology, biochemistry, statistics, and public health are being employed in and out of the country to conduct specialized studies in finding the cure for Alzheimer's or to at least curb the prevalence of the disease. Recent research done by the Alzheimer's Association and the National Institute of Aging (NIA) in 2011 explains the importance of paying close attention to the biomarkers in one's body.[3] The term *biomarkers* is really an abbreviation for "biological markers," which can mean (1) the proteins present in the blood, (2) the pathological status of cerebrospinal fluid (CSF), (3) changes in the genetic information, and (4) irregularities in brain function detected through brain imaging. The research on biological markers as contributors to the development of Alzheimer's disease has still yet to be proven. This involves experimenting with a considerable number of people to finally reach solid ground. At present, there have been no biological markers that would absolutely confirm the future development of this disease in a person within a set time frame, but researchers are continuously carrying out investigations in this regard.

Brain Biomarkers Used in Alzheimer's Research

Researchers focus on detection and prevention of Alzheimer's, which can be accomplished by initial brain imaging. This technique, otherwise referred to as neuroimaging, is the test in which neurologists and neuropathologists check significant changes in brain function through the PET (positron emission tomography) scanning technique explained in chapter 5. By simpler explanations, the brain imaging process is similar to visualizing a written map of the brain. This test is one of the biomarker areas that offer potential in detecting the disease. Brain imaging also involves the use of florbetapir, a radioisotope that binds to the beta amyloids in the brain, and flourodeoxyglycose, a sugar involved in glucose metabolism in the brain. One indicator of nerve cell damage is the depletion of glucose in the brain. Individuals with Alzheimer's have shrunken brains, seen on an MRI (magnetic resonance imaging), and lowered brain glucose levels.

In 2006, the Alzheimer's Association provided approximately two million dollars to the Alzheimer's Disease Neuroimaging Initiative (ADNI).[4] The ADNI is a five-year research project conducted by the National Institute on Aging that laid the standards for procuring and interpreting the images of the brain and its biological parts. Its nationwide goals are as follows: (1) to determine whether the imaging standards accompanied with blood work and psychological tests could identify those individuals who are at a high risk of acquiring Alzheimer's; (2) to encourage early diagnosis; (3) to monitor the progression of the disease; and (4) to keep a close eye on the actions of the experimental drugs that alter the impact of the disease on the individual.

Other Biomarkers Used in the United States

Another commonly used biomarker for Alzheimer's research here in the United States is CSF. This fluid sends nutrients to the whole central and peripheral nervous system. The amount of CSF produced daily in a normal adult is approximately five hundred milliliters,[5] and any noticeable change in the levels of the fluid can indicate a problem. Spinal fluid is strongly associated with the beta-amyloid proteins. Spinal fluid changes can disrupt the level of beta amyloids and, in turn, the proteins release harmful deposits that contribute to the development of Alzheimer's disease. The samples of proteins are carefully studied in different research centers but yield varied results. This problem was solved by having a baseline medical procedure and comparing outcomes in several accredited laboratories. To help with the consistency in studying the proteins, the Alzheimer's Association spearheaded the Alzheimer's Association Quality Control Program for CSF Biomarkers. Through the program (study), experts can compare results with the testing centers in Europe and the United States. In this study, the requirement for individuals wanting to participate is that they have signs of mild, short-term memory loss. One hundred individuals submitted themselves to the study and were closely monitored throughout the course of research.[6]

Other experiments using spinal fluids have been very accurate in determining the presence of beta-amyloid proteins in patients with noticeable loss of memory who then developed Alzheimer's disease.[7] Previously, researchers were only able to accurately diagnose Alzheimer's disease by performing autopsies on deceased patients. Because of this extraordinary discovery of the role of beta-amyloid proteins with regards to the development of Alzheimer's, the experts do not need to wait for years and years before definitive symptoms surface. They now study people at risk for Alzheimer's and get spinal fluid samples from them to test for beta amyloids. After the test, doctors then do the necessary treatments to slow down if not stop Alzheimer's from taking over the brains of the clients. Relying on PET scans, the scientists are able to see visual images of the brain along with the plaques brought about by amyloids. This might well be the accurate way to predict Americans who are candidates for acquiring

Alzheimer's. The latest PET scans are not yet widely distributed throughout the market, but spinal tap tests are available.

With such technological advancements in predicting Alzheimer's in a future patient, scientists are again faced with a major problem on whether to let doctors offer commercial spinal fluid tests, specifically for Alzheimer's, to their patients and whether the latter should consent to it or not. While neurologists *do* take samples of CSF to look for infections, they don't usually take the samples from the brain area while in an outpatient setting. Instead, samples are taken from the back of the patient. Moreover, researchers are considering some safety and competency issues as well as the overall accuracy of test results for the above reasons. Also, the results might vary from laboratory to laboratory. In some cases, memory loss can be attributed to other underlying conditions such as depression and stroke, but not necessarily Alzheimer's.

There is one setback with regard to performing spinal tap tests. The test involves injecting a needle into the epidural space, the fluid-filled space between the bones of the spinal column, and drawing the spinal fluid from there. For obvious reasons, the test can make a patient nervous, and inexperienced doctors can get apprehensive to do perform the test. The procedure is relatively painless for most people, as long as the preoperative preparations are done well. The federal government can help in this process by establishing specialized spinal tap centers that clients can walk into and get tested. A recent experiment involved sampling three hundred clients around the age of seventy, two hundred of whom have memory disorders, with around one hundred of the memory disorders being Alzheimer's.[8] The remaining clients had good memory. The patients were tested for the presence of two specific protein types—beta amyloid and tau. To render unbiased results, the researchers were not informed about who has or does not have the disease. The resulting data showed that almost all of the Alzheimer's patients presented with the typical spinal fluid amyloids, and almost 75 percent of the patients with mild memory defect showed the same patterns. The remaining one-third of clients with normal cognitive function had the proteins as well. The experts made a prediction that these particular people with normal memories will later suffer from the disease. When the scientists reviewed additional data, they discovered that approximately fifty-five of the patients with mild memory loss, whose symptoms worsened as the disease progressed, had the typical protein patterns five years before. The researchers then hypothesized that the presence of the two proteins is a definite determinant of the occurrence of the disease, but they cannot predict exactly when Alzheimer's will come about in a person. The scientists are implying that the proteins serve as a warning sign for Alzheimer's. The presence of the proteins could mean that the person is at risk for Alzheimer's or the condition has already begun and will progress throughout the person's life. Hopefully, (1) once the drugs for treating Alzheimer's show full proof of slowing down or preventing Alzheimer's disease from happening, people will just walk in and have brain scans done as routinely as having X-rays; and (2) experts will not need to do autopsies to detect Alzheimer's disease most accurately.

AMERICAN FACTORS

Genetic Connection

Another potential contributory factor to the disease is heredity. American geneticists and brain scientists are teaming up in order to research the possibility of recognizing inherited Alzheimer's through gene mapping. This procedure involves the collection of anomalous genes with mutations that are seldom present in other genes. With this test, the experts found three abnormal genes and other genes that pose a lowered risk to having Alzheimer's later on in life. Presently, genetic mapping is proving very promising when it comes to discovering defective genes, but eliminating the disease remains undone .

With all the progress that has been going on with the fight against Alzheimer's, researchers go back to the goal of preventing Alzheimer's disease from happening in the first place. The quest for the cure and prevention of Alzheimer's disease goes on and on. The question remains whether Alzheimer's disease can really be prevented. There are surprising breakthroughs in this part but only in the absence of any surefire answers.

Lifestyle Connection

As one can deduce from other chapters, U.S. researchers believe that regular exercise, a balanced diet, and optimum mental health play a vital role in avoiding Alzheimer's. Constant social interaction is another aspect that is essential to mental health. To put it simply, a human being is naturally a social creature and therefore needs to be communicating and engaging in activities with others. Life in the United States is fast paced and can be very stressful. Americans have to be aware of the consequences of leading a stressful life and should balance their careers and their personal lives. Regular exercise is very important to keep the blood and nutrients flowing to the brain and throughout the body.

Research on the Circulatory System

Peer-reviewed reports published in the United States confirm that the circulatory system has a role in Alzheimer's disease since brain performance is largely dependent on healthy blood circulation.[9] The blood is responsible for the distribution of nutrients all throughout the body, especially the brain. If an individual has high blood pressure that eventually results in impaired blood circulation, all vital organs including the brain will get affected. High cholesterol levels cause plaque to form in the blood vessels, thereby obstructing or limiting blood flow to the brain. Decreased blood flow to the brain results in fewer nutrients to its nerve cells. When this happens, some functions of the brain such as memory retention will be cut off or partially impaired. As the human brain ages, there are plaques that form around the areas of the brain. The plaques are not necessarily causing a decrease in memory, but once the brain has vascular disease, the brain will show signs of cognitive impairment.

DRUG TRIALS IN THE UNITED STATES

With regard to finding breakthrough drug therapies to target Alzheimer's disease, scientists have been studying, for a very long time, what makes a healthy brain and what goes wrong in a person afflicted with the Alzheimer's disease. The beta-amyloid protein is a top subject for such research. Experts are digging into the process of how the protein is produced. Because of this, they are now knowledgeable in the process of how beta amyloids are created. They discovered two enzymes that act as catalysts to the production of the protein, namely, beta and gamma secretase. The scientists' goal is to stop the production of beta-amyloid protein that result in the production of plaques in the brain—the typical characteristic of Alzheimer's disease. They are painstakingly examining every step of the beta-amyloid production and are manipulating the protein in order to halt the creation of the plaques even to the point of injecting antibodies to arrest the process. Researchers are also creating experimental drugs that will stop the creation of beta amyloids, but these treatments are currently undergoing clinical tests in the United States.

Clioquinol

An example of the above is the drug named PB-2 (Clioquinol). The pill acts on the beta amyloids in a complex action and prevents it from clumping. In turn, the drug halts the production of plaques. The drug has already completed phase 2 of clinical trials. The results of the trials are positive, and the participants who took the drug showed decreased levels of beta amyloids in the cerebrospinal fluid and received better scores in the cognitive and judgment tests. Research experiments have confirmed the mechanisms behind tau protein and how it affects the toxicity of amyloid-β, which, when coupled with tau, produces symptoms of Alzheimer's disease.[10] This is a significant breakthrough since it has its own implications on how well Alzheimer's disease continues to develop in a patient and how the disease should be treated. As discussed in chapters 3 and 5, the tau protein is the prime component of the twists or tangles that can be features of a defective brain in the disease. Neurologists are searching for methods to control the tau-protein molecules from collapsing or getting tangled.

Methylene Blue

This drug (chemical name methylthioninium chloride, brand name Rember) is another promising substance that is widely used as a dye for staining tissues and to treat malaria. The dye apparently prevents tau proteins from collapsing and entangling, but the total effects are yet to be determined by way of clinical research in the United States.[11]

Varenicline

This is another drug that completed the second phase of research trials and has had favorable cognitive effects on mild to moderate Alzheimer's cases in ages 55 to 65. The drug is normally used for smoking cessation.[12] In one study, researchers used candidates confirmed to have Alzheimer's by the National Institute of Neurological and Communicative Disorders and Stroke and Alzheimer's Disease and Related Disorders Association (NINCDS–ADRDA) and the Diagnostic and Statistical Manual of Mental Disorders (DSM–IV).[13] The experts in that study also chose those patients who scored fourteen to twenty-six in the mini-mental state exam (MMSE).[14] Excluded in the trial were cases of other degenerative disorders of the nervous, circulatory, and respiratory systems. The participants presented with better memory and thought processes than the other control group who were taking a placebo. Trade names for varenicline are Champix and Chantix.

Semagestat

Aside from varenicline, the drug semagestat has undergone extensive research over the years.[15] However, this drug did not become successful because of poor results from different tests. The medicine is supposed to prevent the enzyme mentioned earlier, gamma secretase, from binding to the beta secretase, thereby halting the production of the beta-amyloid proteins in the nervous system. Laboratory tests illustrated the drug's efficacy in lowering the levels of beta amyloids, but the experiments garnered poor results for memory. Instead of cognitive and judgment skills improving, memory loss became more pronounced and the patients became more dependent to care. Some even developed skin cancers. The pharmaceutical company that manufactures the drug had to call off the large-scale research.[16]

It is difficult to know exactly how the drug targets Alzheimer's simply because no one knows the real cause of the disease. Perhaps, the scientists' view of Alzheimer's disease is too focused in just one subject area and there needs to be expanded research on the other factors of the disease's origin. Semagestat had its years of satisfactory and safe results more than ten years ago when it was first given to Alzheimer's patients in the study. The drug showed a significant reduction in amyloid concentrations in the spinal fluid. In 2008, semagestat's manufacturer[17] spearheaded nationwide studies of the drug, and over 2,600 Alzheimer's cases were enrolled.[18] However, the drug suddenly had unfavorable effects on the study participants. This urged the company to stop the research immediately. The participants were then continuously monitored but were not given any more of the drugs. Researchers were convinced of biological activities that they could not define; they are now considering other reasons that might have caused the negative effect of semagestat on the patients.

AN-1792

Swelling in the central nervous system, particularly the brain, is another abnormal characteristic in Alzheimer's disease. It is not yet clear how the brain reacts to and processes inflammation. This is one of the several areas that scientists are currently paying close attention to. An experimental drug called AN-1792, which was supposed to act as a vaccine against Alzheimer's, was discontinued before the investigators even provided conclusive evidence of the drug's effect. The drug contained a type of beta amyloid for the purpose of awakening the body's immune response, but 6 percent of the participants in the research study developed a brain inflammation called aseptic meningoencephalitis, and they were forced to discontinue investigations of the drug.[19]

Insulin

The endocrine system is another system that experts study, specifically insulin resistance.[20] They are getting an outline on how the brain reacts to insulin. The brain must be provided with sugar molecules such as glucose in order to nourish the brain cells, but what happens if the neurons are not getting enough of the energy or rather are consuming too much? This is again connected to the progression of Alzheimer's disease.

STEM CELL RESEARCH IN THE UNITED STATES

Perhaps the most controversial and provocative of all studies is stem cell research. It aims to cure not only terminal ailments such as cancer and diabetes but also Alzheimer's disease, as demonstrated by medical research.[21] Stem cell research involves using stem cells that are still maturing and helping the cells develop into other, differentiated, cells or tissues.[22] In the case of finding a cure for Alzheimer's, stem cells can be cultured into new neurons that bring researchers in the United States a step closer to virtually reversing Alzheimer's and other dreaded illnesses. On the flip side, stem cell research is constantly faced with protests from human rights groups and medical ethics committees, since the process entails using cells of four- or five-day-old embryos or fertilized ovum provided by fertility clinics.

Politics Abound

When cells are extracted from the developing embryo, life is basically taken away. This is the reason for the long-existing legal war on the issue. In 1996, the Dickey-Wicker Amendment bill became law, stopping the U.S. federal government from spending tax money on embryonic stem cell research.[23] The bill confronts the inhumane practice of culturing embryos (growing the cells to multiply and identify their characteristics) and then deliberately killing them in order to get the stem cells needed for the research. The legislation was renewed year after year by the House of Representatives. Not until August 2002 did the then U.S. president determine that tax funds could be used on select stem cell cultures in the United States, provided the samples were extracted from embryos already preserved.[24]

The battle did not stop there. Congress was overwhelmed with political rivals and the unwavering cries of people suffering from illnesses for whom stem cells might be the only possible escape from their diseases. By 2007, the predominantly Republican Congress passed on similar bills, but not enough to exceed the then president's veto.[25] When President Barack Obama came to office, he overturned the veto when he signed an executive decree to fully support stem cell research. Currently, the heated debate on stem cell research funding remains on the hot seat.

Adult stem cells, which can be differentiated into a number of varieties of tissue-specific cells, are still the main focus of many recent studies on neurological issues such as Alzheimer's disease. In 2008, research showed that neural stem cells are available in parts of an adult patient's brain.[26] The same research revealed that adult stem cells actually help *prevent* multiplication since there are chemical signals from astrocytes that bar them from doing so. Using the brain's own ability to regenerate its own cells helps this version of treatment to gain credibility since it is a more natural strategy to cure brain disorders or the effects of severe brain injuries. It works the same way for Alzheimer's disease. Studies show that scientists can utilize neuronal stem cells that exist in adult animal brains to improve brain disorders.[27] This helps develop more advanced nerve cells if intranasal methods are used to deliver the nerve growth factors. Medical research has also proven that it is possible to use adult neural stem cells to uncover better ways of administering treatment to people suffering from blood diseases.[28] Many other diseases such as Alzheimer's may follow suit in the United States.[29]

RESEARCH BREAKTHROUGHS

It is still unclear why patients known to have Down syndrome or trisomy 21 continue to have a higher likelihood of getting Alzheimer's disease upon entering late adulthood. Women with Down syndrome will always have a greater risk of suffering from Alzheimer's compared to their similar-aged male counterparts who are forty to sixty-five. In broader terms, research on Alzheimer's disease, learning disabilities, and stunted growth has received less attention from policy-making organizations on how care providers should conduct their business. In part, there have been continued trends of reduced life expectancy since the risk of dementia will continue to revolve around people of a certain age group. This is gradually ending as survival into more advanced age or old age is becoming more common for most people who have Down syndrome. Mild forms of dementia remain a common problem.

Research Breakthroughs and Diagnosis

It is important for patients and caregivers to understand that diagnosing Alzheimer's disease based on techniques discovered via research in the United States will often be inclined to change. Experts can report changes that they witness in someone's ability to continue doing certain crucial body tasks. There will often be changes in language flow and day-to-day behavior, and crucial life skills will continue to slowly decline. The internal processes of Alzheimer's will take years longer to diagnose in a precise fashion, so research on the disease is very likely to improve the lives of many. Diagnosis of people with signs of Down syndrome or many other forms of mental disability will frequently involve one or more practitioners who work side by side with service providers due to the nature of care that the mentally disabled are supposed to receive.[30]

Research Breakthroughs and Treatment

Caregivers do not directly address the main neurodegenerative processes in the brain. It would be sufficient to have a natural medication (described in chapter 7) that would completely protect the brain cells from loss, while concurrently causing the brain to continue producing the crucial brain messenger chemical called acetylcholine. On a more positive note, there is already a natural medication that works in this manner. This medication is referred to as nerve growth factor. The idea behind improving the prognosis of Alzheimer' disease cases lies heavily on the fact that nerve growth factors are proteins naturally produced by the human brain. Research companies in the United States are beginning to unearth tricks to isolate all the human genes that cause nerve growth factor and then use this same gene to come up with large amounts of the potentially remedial protein to treat people with Alzheimer's disease. The problem occurs when the nerve growth factor is too large, such that crossing from the blood circulation into the brain is a problem. Medical researchers are therefore on their toes trying to find a means of correcting that "transportation" problem. A major research center in Minnesota suggests that certain therapeutic proteins can be administered through the nose (as nose drops) and can make the way into the brain directly instead of having to be ingested through the blood.[31] This is made possible since there is a direct link existing between one's brain and nose, via olfactory nerves. The nerves are capable of sensing certain distinct odors.

The U.S. Department of Commerce has given the Minnesota research facility a patent for a new drug and is treating it as a new method of delivering drugs into the body. This has roused a lot of excitement since researchers believe that, if there is a decreasing level of nerve growth factor in aging rodents, the animals can end up developing symptoms similar to Alzheimer's and bear the pathology similar to that of humans. The use of intranasal nerve growth factor reverses brain degeneration in mice. Thus, even with Alzheimer's pathology, loss of memory can be partially recovered.[32]

Extensive research has also showed that different types of nerve growth factors, such as the insulin-like growth factor-1 (IGF), are able travel to the brain using the same intranasal means of ingestion.[33] This administration through the nose shows that growth factor has unmatched potential as a practical treatment for head injury and mental disorder patients, not only Alzheimer's disease victims. The growth factor works well in reducing brain damage and also helps improve neurological functions of the brain. Progress has been made in the area of intranasal delivery, but there is still much room for improvement. Much can still be done to improve intranasal delivery of nerve growth factors as this method is now accepted as being able to effectively protect brain cells from damage.

PARTICIPATING IN ALZHEIMER'S
RESEARCH IN THE UNITED STATES

For obvious reasons, patients and caregivers hope that one day a curative drug will be discovered and that such a medication will make a difference. Before that happens, drug companies should at least try to develop and safely test run a number of prototypes on humans who have volunteered for trials—these volunteers being patients of Alzheimer's disease. Volunteers make a generous contribution to research knowledge, but it is crucial that they and their families understand the related dangers. They have to know the requirements of the study and what it entails, right up to what results and improvements are expected but not guaranteed.[34]

The Right Candidate

From a logical standpoint, anyone suffering severe impairments would not be the right candidate for Alzheimer's research here in the United States since there is very little chance of recovery. Also, people who are in the early stages of the disease might see little or no improvement, or at times might see remarkable and substantial development. Either way, they should know that the drugs might cause deterioration. Commonly, people who take part in research and testing are not told if the desired medication being taken is just a placebo or if it is indeed a drug being given to counteract the actions of Alzheimer's disease in the body. Placebos are inactive substances that can sometimes fool the person in believing that he or she is taking real medications. Placebos are used so that there will be a clear demarcation between the people genuinely going through change and others who are not taking the actual drug.[35]

Information and Preparation

It is important for Alzheimer's disease patients in the United States to find out, prior to volunteering, the main purpose and rationale behind which the study is being conducted. It is all about awareness. Therefore, there needs to be an indication of the potential side effects. People need to know what expenses will be incurred so they are well aware of the requirements of taking the study. They need to be informed about who is paying for any expenses involved. It is always good to check the researchers and their credentials to make sure the study is not being done by unqualified individuals. Researchers should always give a basic description of how the study is to be carried out. Thus, informed consent from the patients will be certain, and it is only then that the safety and dosage that has been chosen will be mentioned and the administration can begin. The researcher normally has a distinctive approach, which the people taking part in the study should be keen to review.[36]

An Alzheimer's patient looking to participate in a research study in the United States should know everything about the safety procedures aimed to protect the participant. A recent research on a likely Alzheimer's vaccine released by major pharmaceutical corporations is proving to be a good example of tests being carried out in good practice. Studies point out that, even though there have been benefits to people who have volunteered for the clinical trials, such trials have also caused notable brain swelling among participants.[37] When this problem was noted, the study was discontinued so that lives were not risked. However, the surveys and experiments themselves were kept since the findings could end up benefiting someone else's research in the future. The practice of volunteering for research here in the United States contributes in one way or another to the existing body of knowledge. It also ensures effective treatments are developed later down the road.[38]

ANALYSIS

Americans belonging to the geriatric age group are faced with the dilemma of possibly getting Alzheimer's, but it is a relief to know researchers here have made tangible progress in accurately diagnosing the disease. The road to encountering an exact cure in the United States by way of research is rocky and full of obstacles, and while the upcoming part VII is titled "The Personal Quest," patients should nevertheless understand that they are not alone in the struggle to eradicate the disease.

VII

THE PERSONAL QUEST

· _16_ ·

Diet and Alzheimer's

$\mathcal{A}$n introduction to Alzheimer's disease for patients and caregivers would be incomplete without the inclusion of brain-strengthening diets. Diet is generally defined as the food and drink that a person consumes on a regular basis, and more specifically as the kind and amount of food and drink that is prescribed to a person for a special reason. Diet is also defined as a regimen of eating and drinking sparingly in order to reduce one's weight.[1] Therefore, diet might refer to the inclusion as well as the exclusion of certain foods and drinks in an Alzheimer's disease patient's daily consumption, with a need for moderation in the quantities consumed. Eating properly requires the right balancing of both the contents of each meal and the intake of food throughout the day.[2] Diet is important for Alzheimer's patients because it helps to maintain their fitness and health. Proper diets assist in maintaining normal bodily functions, while poor diets have been linked to certain diseases. For instance, diets containing plenty of vitamins have been associated with a healthy brain, while diets that are high in cholesterol increase the risk of stroke and brain damage.[3] To increase its effectiveness, a healthy diet needs to be combined with regular physical exercise.[4]

BEST DIET FOR A HEALTHY BRAIN

Since the brain is the major organ affected by Alzheimer's disease, it is important to consider the best meals for proper brain health. The best diets for a healthy brain are those that contain omega-3 fatty acids, fruits, vegetables, and whole grains. The following is a look at foods in these categories.

Omega-3 Fatty Acids

Omega-3 fatty acids are polyunsaturated fatty acids, considered "good" fat, and provide several health benefits including the building of brain cell membranes as well as helping to control blood clotting. Omega-3 fatty acids are classified into two major types: (1) docosahexaenoic acid (DHA), which is found in oily fish such as salmon, tuna, trout, swordfish, sardines, and mackerel, and (2) alpha-linolenic acid (ALA), found in vegetable oils, which include canola oil, walnuts, flaxseeds, and soybeans. ALA can also be found in some vegetables, including spinach, kale, salad greens, and Brussels sprouts. While it has not yet been established whether DHA and ALA are equally valuable, an Alzheimer's disease patient should include at least one source of omega-3 fatty acids in his or her daily diet. For instance, one might have a serving of oily fish, add a handful of walnuts to the morning cereal, or use a tablespoon of canola oil in cooking. Although it is more beneficial to get omega-3 fatty acids directly from food, omega-3 supplements may be taken by people who do not eat foods that have omega-3. Both DHA and ALA omega-3 supplements are available.[5]

Fruits and Vegetables

Research has shown that the vitamins E and C found in fruits and vegetables contain antioxidants that help to protect the brain.[6] Antioxidants assist in preventing or lessening the oxidative damage caused by the byproducts produced when oxygen is depleted in the body.[7] Oxidative damage may lead to diminished brain function and has been linked to several diseases such as Alzheimer's, diabetes, and cancer. Dark vegetables and dark-skinned fruits have the highest levels of antioxidants.[8] In addition to the vegetables mentioned in the omega-3 fatty acids category, other vegetables rich in antioxidants include broccoli, alfalfa sprouts, red bell peppers, eggplant, corn, onions, and beets.[9]

Whole Grains

Whole grain foods have minerals such as vitamin B1 (thiamine) that help to increase blood flow to the brain, leading to better brain function. Unlike processed foods and sugary foods that are digested quickly once consumed, causing blood sugar levels to spike, whole grain foods are digested slowly, which helps keep the body's blood sugar levels stable, keeping the patient energized for longer periods of time. Foods in this category include the following:

- Whole wheat
- Bran
- Brown rice

- Oatmeal
- Whole grain breads
- Barley[10]

WORST DIET FOR A HEALTHY BRAIN

The worst diets for the brain are those that contain trans fats and refined sugars. The following is a look at the foods in these categories.

Trans Fats

Trans fats are considered the worst kind of fat for the brain, and they should be consumed in limited quantities. Trans fats are detrimental to one's health because they reduce the level of good cholesterol. In addition, they increase bad cholesterol levels in the body, leading to a buildup of fat in arteries. This restricts the proper circulation of blood, including that within the brain, and can lead to brain damage.[11] Trans fats are found in several foods, including processed snacks such as chips and fried food, baked foods such as cakes and cookies, and hydrogenated vegetable oils such as stick margarine. Also, many restaurants prepare their food using trans fats. It is therefore wise to avoid any fried foods on the menu, including French fries, fried onion rings, chicken-fried steaks, and fried fish. It should be noted that even foods that have "zero trans" indicated on them are allowed to contain up to 0.5 grams of trans fats per serving.[12]

Refined Sugar

Refined sugar has all of its fiber, minerals, protein, fats, and enzymes depleted, leaving only empty calories. As a result, the body needs to take away nutrients such as calcium, sodium, potassium, and magnesium from its healthy cells to be able to metabolize the sugar. If the body lacks the nutrients it needs to metabolize sugar, the waste produced builds up in the brain and nervous system, causing damage. When sugar is consumed regularly, it causes the body to have too much acid. In an attempt to restore the acid-alkaline ratio, the body uses up its stores of vitamins and minerals, depriving the brain and other structures of these minerals.[13]

Sugar affects the processing of other compounds in the body. For instance, when sugar is consumed, it kills some good bacteria found in the intestines that are responsible for manufacturing vitamin B compounds that help in the processing of glutamic acid, a compound found in vegetables. If glutamic acid is not processed due to the level of vitamin B compounds declining, a decrease in brain function and sleepiness occurs.[14]

Several foods and drinks contain refined sugars, including the following:

- Soda
- Energy drinks
- Fruit juice mixes
- Candy
- Sweetened cereal
- Jams
- Jellies
- Baked goods
- Frozen pizza
- Spaghetti sauce
- Canned fruits
- Canned vegetables[15]

BEST DIET FOR IMPROVING AND MAINTAINING SPECIFIC BRAIN FUNCTIONS

The brain is responsible for coordinating vision, hearing, and speech. As substantiated by medical research, all three qualities are impaired in Alzheimer's disease. The following sections review the best diets for these brain functions.[16]

Best Diet for Vision

A diet containing vitamins A, C, and E; the B vitamins; the minerals zinc, selenium, chromium, magnesium, taurine, lutein, and zeaxanthin; and omega-3 fatty acids contributes to overall healthy vision.[17] The following are foods that contribute to healthy eyes. Yellow and orange vegetables contain vitamin A, sometimes referred to as beta carotene. Beta carotene helps to protect the eyes from sun damage and is also good for the eye's retina. The retina is the lining located in the inner eye surface and is sensitive to light. Foods in this category include carrots, pumpkins, squash, and sweet potatoes.[18] Eggs supply a lot of nutrients, including vitamin A, the B vitamins, and zinc. Eggs help to raise the blood levels of lutein and zexanthin, two nutrients that help to prevent eye damage and cataracts. The yolks of the eggs contain the most nutrients, and the darker the yolk, the more nutritious the egg. Eggs that are produced by pasture-raised chickens are the best because these chickens consume a nutrient-rich diet.[19] Garlic and onions maintain a healthy blood circulation in the body, which helps to protect the eyes. The two are also rich in sulfur, a compound that the body needs to produce glutathione, which is an antioxidant beneficial to the lens of the eye.[20]

Best Diet for Hearing

A diet rich in vitamin D and manganese helps to maintain good hearing. Vitamin D is important because it enables the absorption of calcium by the body, which is vital for building bones. A lack of vitamin D can lead to a condition known as osteopenia, which causes the bones of the ears to harden and become porous. Some of the foods that contain vitamin D include fish oil, cod liver oil, egg yolk, and liver.[21]

Manganese is necessary for normal brain and nerve function. A deficiency in manganese has been associated with hearing loss and tinnitus (ringing ears). Foods that contain manganese include pineapples, apples, apricots, beans, raisins, celery, and legumes.[22]

Best Diet for Speech

To maintain healthy speech, one should consume a diet that contains fruits, vegetables, and whole grains. These foods contain vitamins A, E, and C, which help prevent slurred speech and loss of speech. In addition, these foods help to keep the mucus membranes that line the throat in a very healthy state.[23]

FOODS TO AVOID WHEN IMPROVING AND MAINTAINING PROPER BRAIN FUNCTION

The worst diets for brain function are those that contain trans fats, excessive sugar, excessive salt, and monosodium glutamate (MSG). Foods in these categories include the following:

- Fast foods
- Processed foods
- Prepackaged foods
- White bread
- Potatoes
- Pasta
- Syrup
- Sugar

The next sections look at the effects of these foods on brain function.

Sugar Substitutes

Since the brain requires glucose as the main source of energy,[24] proper sugar balance is important for Alzheimer's patients. Sugary foods are considered high glycemic index foods. The glycemic index measures how much certain foods raise blood sugar levels. Clinical research notes that foods that rank high in the glycemic index are digested quickly and result in blood sugar levels spiking rapidly.[25] This causes problems with brain function such as making the eyes susceptible to age-related macular degeneration (AMD), which affects the retina of the eye and is the top cause of vision loss in the United States.[26]

Sugar substitutes might not be any better than refined sugar after all. Aspartame, a low calorie sweetener, is used in several diet sodas and other diet foods. Aspartame leads to damage to the nervous system because, when it is digested, it releases a compound that excites brain neurons, causing them to fire repeatedly until they eventually die. This interferes with normal brain function. It is also possible that, when aspartame is digested, it releases methanol in the small intestines. Methanol causes visual problems by interrupting the retina and optic nerve transmissions. While formal studies have not been done on the effect of aspartame on vision, there have been thousands of reports of visual problems from people who drink too many drinks containing aspartame.[27]

Monosodium Glutamate

MSG is a salt that is used as a preservative and a flavor enhancer in food. It is found in processed and prepackaged foods such as processed meats and canned foods. When MSG is consumed, it breaks down into glutamate in the body. Glutamate has the same effect as Aspartame, as it is an excitatory neurotransmitter that triggers the firing of neurons, causing damage to the nervous system and interfering with normal brain function.[28]

Excess Salt

Salt is an important component of daily diet as it helps in maintaining proper water levels within body cells. However, when salt is consumed excessively, it restricts the blood vessels and interferes with the proper flow of blood in the brain, ears, and eyes. Most processed and prepackaged foods contain high levels of salt. For instance, a can of prepackaged soup has more sodium than the recommended daily amount for an adult.[29]

BEST DIET FOR PEOPLE WHO ARE AGING RAPIDLY

When Alzheimer's patients age rapidly, there is a decrease in the body's metabolic rate and an increase in the risk of contracting diseases such as cancer, heart disease, and diabetes. As a result, a change in diet may be required.[30]

Mediterranean Diet

The traditional diet of people who live in some Mediterranean regions such as Greece, Spain, and Italy has been linked to lower rates of disease and longer life for the elderly. The Mediterranean diet is rich in fresh vegetables, fruits, cheese, yogurt, garlic, onions, protein such as fish, and legumes such as beans, peas, and lentils. This diet also consists of whole grain foods and healthy mono-unsaturated fats including those from olive oil and fish. Foods in the Mediterranean diet are consumed mostly in their natural state. Red wine, consumed in moderation, may also be included in the Mediterranean diet. Red wine contains components such as polyphenolic compounds and resveratrol, which have been found to significantly reduce the risk of strokes and heart diseases.[31] According to a 2005 study, older people who followed the Mediterranean diet increased their lifespan by between 8 and 14 percent.[32] Medical research proves that resveratrol reduces plaques seen in Alzheimer's disease.[33]

Micronutrients

Vitamins B12 and D are important for older Alzheimer's patients. Vitamin B12 helps to keep the nerves and blood healthy and is found in foods such as trout, grain breakfast cereal, and trout. Vitamin D can be obtained from sunlight and foods such as milk and eggs. When a person such as an Alzheimer's disease victim gets older, the need for vitamins B12 and D increases as these vitamins are not absorbed efficiently by the body. Older people might also need to take supplements for these vitamins. Calcium is an important nutrient for the aging as it helps to keep the bones strong, while vitamins A, C, and E are good sources of antioxidants and help to protect older patients from diseases such as cancer and heart disease.[34]

Fluids

As the Alzheimer's patient ages, the mechanism that signals thirst declines and can result in older patients going for longer periods of time without drinking fluids.[35] It is important for older people to keep themselves hydrated in order to decrease the stress on the kidneys and to ease constipation, which are common problems for the elderly. Water, green and white teas containing flavonoids, and foods such as soups and fruits with high fluid content should be included in the diet.[36]

Herbs and Spices

Herbs and spices are used as food flavor enhancers and have medicinal properties as well. Herbs usually come from plants' leaves, while spices come from the seeds of plants, such as cumin; the plant's buds, such as cloves; the roots, such as ginger; the berries, such as peppercorn; or the bark, such as cinnamon. Herbs and spices are a good source of antioxidants and provide minerals such as sodium, calcium, potassium, iron, magnesium, and vitamins A, B, E, C, thiamin, riboflavin, and folic acid. Herbs and spices can be used for natural remedies. For instance, ginger and turmeric have anti-inflammatory properties, which might help to reduce the risk of Alzheimer's disease and provide relief for other age-related problems, such as knee pain from arthritis.[37]

WORST DIET FOR PEOPLE WHO ARE AGING

The worst diets for the aging are those that contain nitrates, frozen meals, saturated and hydrogenated fats, excessive sugar, high fat, high sodium snacks, and soda pop. The following is a look at some of these food categories.

Nitrates

High levels of nitrates are found in cured meats such as hot dogs. Nitrates are used to preserve color and to prevent bacteria from forming in these cured meats. Nitrates are harmful because they can convert to nitrite in the body, which leads to the formation of nitrosamines, chemicals that can cause cancer. Alzheimer's disease victims are no exceptions to this effect. Cured meats should be replaced with nitrate-free organic meats, and if foods containing nitrates must be taken, then extra vitamin C should be consumed since it prevents the conversion of nitrates to nitrosamines in the stomach.[38]

Soda

Soda contains sugar or artificial sweeteners, and may contain caffeine, artificial flavors, and colors. Soda is a poor source of fluids and can lead to diseases.[39] Having an occasional soda may not be harmful to one's health, but regular consumption will produce negative effects. One can of soda contains approximately eight teaspoons of sugar, while the amount of sugar that is recommended daily is approximately six teaspoons for women and nine teaspoons for men.[40] Research experiments suggest that the phosphoric acid contained in soda can take away calcium from the bones, leaving aging people at the risk of developing osteoporosis, a condition that makes bones fragile and leads to otherwise avoidable fractures.[41]

Frozen Foods

The hurried and busy lives of many people encourage methods of getting a meal ready quickly. Any frozen foods that can be heated in a microwave oven help to satisfy that need. However, the men and women who consume such items could develop an unhealthy brain. Freezing traps glucosides (a type of glycoside) and galactosides in vegetables. When a plant-based food becomes exposed to microwaves, those stored sugars undergo a marked alteration of their own makeup. That, in turn, reduces the vegetable's nutritional characteristics that would otherwise be reserved for the patient's brain. It increases the level at which important substances break down. By the same token, microwave ovens interfere with the brain's electrical impulses. They disrupt the junction potential of the cerebrum, and the altered mind fails to function as well as it should. While frozen foods may not be bad for the body if they have the right ingredients, they prevent a person from eating natural and fresh foods, which contain more nutrients and fiber.[42]

Sugar

The effects of sugary foods become more detrimental as people age. As people grow older, there is a loss of bone density, a reduction in body mass, and a body fat increase around the heart and other organs. With all these changes, sugar can be damaging since it targets the liver, heart, and pancreas. While it is not harmful to have an occasional sugary snack, consuming meals high in sugar on a regular basis can cause problems such as obesity. Being overweight as an elderly person places strain on the muscle and bones.[43]

BEST DIET FOR MEMORY

The best diet for memory is one that contains the B vitamins and vitamins A, E, and C. The following is a breakdown of the nutrients and foods in these categories.

Vitamin A (Beta Carotene)

Beta carotene is described above as a nutrient that helps vision. It is a yellowish compound found in yellow, green, or orange vegetables. Beta carotene is converted to vitamin A in the liver and in the small intestines but helps to prevent memory loss. A twenty-two-year clinical study demonstrates that this beta carotene helps people to retain the ability to think, reason, and remember.[44]

Alzheimer's patients are no exception to this. Beta carotene can be found in foods such as cantaloupe, carrots, turnips, sweet potatoes, and spinach.[45]

B Vitamins

The B vitamins, particularly B6 and B12, are important to maintain proper memory function. These vitamins help to lower levels of homocysteine, an amino acid that has been linked to impaired memory and reasoning.[46]

Foods rich in vitamin B6 include the following: (1) fruits and vegetables such as spinach and bananas; (2) meats such as chicken and trout; and (3) nuts and cereals such as walnuts and wheat bran. Folic acid can be found in (1) vegetables such as lettuce and spinach; (2) fruits such as grapefruit, oranges, bananas, papaya, and cantaloupe; and (3) in other foods such as beans, asparagus, avocado, and broccoli. In 1996, the Food and Drug Administration (FDA) suggested that folic acid be added to certain food products to help reduce birth defects that occur due to a deficiency in folic acid. These foods include breads, pastas, cereals, orange juice, and cornmeal. Vitamin B12 is found only in food derived from animals, including lean meat, eggs, skinless poultry, and low-fat versions of dairy products such as yogurt and milk. Also, some breakfast cereals are fortified with vitamin B12.[47]

A diet rich in vitamin B12 significantly reduces the onset of Alzheimer's. Research done in Scandinavia, where experts analyzed blood specimens of around 270 people aged sixty-five to late seventies who consumed a diet of fish and enriched cereals, presented no evidence of memory impairment.[48] The scientists tested the blood for existence of vitamin B12 and for homocysteine, a kind of amino acid that is closely connected to an increased incidence of Alzheimer's and even cardiac circulatory diseases. Vitamin B12 and its derivatives, when present in large amounts in the blood, showed decreased levels of homocysteine. After seven years had passed, the seventeen research participants got diagnosed with Alzheimer's disease. There were also the people with high homocysteine blood levels. The occurrence of the disease was reduced to 2 percent in the individuals who had plenty of the vitamin B12 in their blood. Eating foods with plenty of B vitamins such as leafy green vegetables, fish, and fish oils make a difference.

The ties between the vitamin B12 levels, homocysteine, and Alzheimer's disease are complicated and are more noticeable in elderly people. At the moment, the role of vitamin B12 in stopping Alzheimer's disease from occurring is still yet to be fully understood in the absence of further investigation. The mechanism of vitamin B12 for lowering the homocysteine levels in the blood is really an important milestone for a healthy cardiovascular system. While the efficiency of adding folate to food is still vague, it is still preferable for people at risk for Alzheimer's disease to get blood work done regularly to check the levels of their folate and vitamin B12.

Vitamin E

Scientific studies have shown that vitamin E (tocopherol) is an antioxidant that reduces memory loss.[49] Vitamin E can be found in (1) green vegetables such as spinach and broccoli; (2) polyunsaturated fats, which are found in liquid vegetable oils including sunflower, canola, and olive oil; (3) seeds such as sunflower seeds; and (4) nuts such as almonds, peanuts, and hazelnuts.[50]

Salad dressings that are oil based are rich in vitamin E. Vitamin E is one of the potent antioxidants that fight free radicals in the body and help maintain overall health. Vitamin E is a component of nerve cells, and in the case of Alzheimer's disease, there is in parts of the brain randomized neural death that leads to a chain of cognitive problems. Also rich in vitamin E are foods based on nuts such as peanut butter and others that fall into the whole grain categories. It is important to note that a number of beneficial results stem from eating a proper diet and not necessarily from taking supplements.

Vitamin C

In addition to strengthening the immune system of the Alzheimer's patient, vitamin C keeps blood vessels strong. This helps to keep proper blood circulation, ensuring that the brain receives adequate nourishment that results in improved memory. Vitamin C can be found in foods such as oranges, red pepper, strawberries, tomatoes, green leafy vegetables, and kiwi fruit.[51]

WORST DIET FOR MEMORY

Excessive Alcohol

Excessive consumption of alcohol, particularly binge drinking, is harmful to memory function, causing memory loss and confusion. Research suggests that drinking alcohol excessively increases the risk of memory loss.[52] However, mild drinking improves blood flow in the brain, boosting memory.[53]

Alcohol has a sedative effect because it acts as a depressant to one's central nervous system. Alcohol can affect a person's memory, even if the person has consumed only a few drinks. People might have blackout episodes in which they forget what happened when they were intoxicated. The memory loss associated with severe alcoholism happens because alcohol inhibits the breakdown of vitamin B1 (thiamine), even though a person might be consuming an adequate amount of this vitamin. Also, excessive alcohol consumption can cause damage to the hippocampus, an internal brain structure that is involved in converting short-term memories to long term.[54]

Excessive Saturated Fats

Saturated fat intake should not constitute more than 7 percent of an Alzheimer's victim's calorie intake. Of a woman's daily intake of 1,500 calories, saturated fats should not exceed 17 grams.[55]

Recent research has found that excessive saturated fats result in the inflammation of the brain and cognitive impairment.[56] Saturated fats increase the level of harmful cholesterol in the blood. Cholesterol is a waxy, fatlike substance needed for building body cells and for metabolizing fats and vitamin D. The body naturally produces the cholesterol it needs, but it also absorbs it from dietary sources. There are two types of cholesterol: high-density lipoprotein (HDL), considered good cholesterol, and low-density lipoprotein (LPL), considered bad cholesterol. High cholesterol levels are harmful for the Alzheimer's patient's brain and have been linked to memory loss as the arteries become blocked, restricting normal blood flow to the brain and other organs. Saturated fats can be found in animal products such as red meat, poultry, and full dairy products, and in oils such as palm oil and coconut oil. Red meat is especially high in saturated fats and can be replaced with fish, lean poultry, or vegetarian sources of protein such as nuts and beans, as well as reduced-fat dairy products. As one can see, the worst diets for memory are those that contain excessive alcohol and excessive saturated fats.[57]

BEST DIET FOR IMPROVING AND
MAINTAINING PROPER COGNITIVE ABILITIES

As mentioned throughout this writing, cognitive decline is one of the major symptoms of an Alzheimer's patient. Neurons, which are the nervous system's specialized cells, are responsible for cognitive functioning in the brain. Neurons form networks that connect cells, enabling these cells to generate thoughts and emotions, as well as to perform problem-solving exercises.[58]

The best diets for maintaining such proper cognitive abilities and neuronal health include vitamins, foods that have a low glycemic index, omega-3 fatty acids, and proteins. The following is a look at food items that fall into such categories.

Vitamins

Vitamins B12, D, and E help to maintain proper cognitive abilities. Vitamin B12 helps to keep myelin, a nerve coating that enables proper neuron communication in the brain, healthy. Myelin is vital for cognitive functions, and a deficiency in vitamin B12 has been shown to cause defects in myelin, causing neurological symptoms that impair cognitive functioning. Vitamin B12 can be obtained from eggs, milk products, and poultry. Vitamin E acts as an antioxidant in the brain, helping to protect the neurons against oxidative damage that is linked to a decline in cognitive functioning. Cooking with oils such as olive and corn oils increases the amount of vitamin E in one's diet. Vitamin D regulates calcium levels in the body. Calcium is important for cognitive functioning as it helps nerve cells to transmit electrical impulses. Vitamin D can be obtained through exposure to the sun and from consuming foods such as salmon and mackerel.[59]

Low Glycemic Index Foods

The glycemic index assesses the amount of blood sugar raised by consuming food. Low glycemic index foods help to provide the brain with a steady supply of energy, maximizing cognitive function and preventing the harmful rapid spiking and dropping of blood sugar levels. Fruits, vegetables, legumes, and grains are considered low glycemic foods. Some examples of food items in these categories include cherries, oatmeal, chick peas, and soybeans. The consumption of low glycemic index foods throughout the day ensures that the brain receives a steady supply of energy in addition to maintaining steady blood sugar levels.[60]

Protein

Amino acids—the "building blocks" of protein—are necessary to develop neurotransmitters in the brain that help to maintain mental alertness and cognitive function. Foods that are rich in protein include seafood, eggs, and meats. Wild fish and game meat provide higher-quality protein than farmed fish and domestic meat, respectively. Plant sources of protein include nuts, seeds, and grains.[61]

WORST DIET FOR COGNITIVE ABILITIES

The worst diet for maintaining proper cognitive function includes high glycemic index foods and hydrogenated fats. Foods in these categories cause blockage in the circulatory system, which reduces blood flow in the brain, depriving the brain cells of oxygen and important nutrients necessary for maintaining proper cognitive abilities.[62]

High Glycemic Index Foods

Foods that rank high in the glycemic index include highly processed simple carbohydrates found in the following:

- White flour
- Foods made from refined flour, such as white bread, donuts, and cakes

- Starchy foods such as white rice
- Sugary snacks such as frosting and candy
- Sugar- and syrup-sweetened drinks such as cola and juices[63]

Hydrogenated Fats

Hydrogenation adds hydrogen bonds to fats, which makes fat more solid at room temperature. As a result, hydrogenated fats contain tightly packed molecules that restrict blood supply to the brain, and therefore affect proper cognition. When fats are fully hydrogenated, they are referred to as saturated fat, and when they are partially hydrogenated, they are referred to as trans fat. Frozen packaged foods such as pizza and pot pie; snacks such as chips, dips, and crackers; and fats such as cake frosting, shortening, and stick margarine all contain partially hydrogenated oils.[64]

SUMMARY OF BENEFITS AND IMPORTANCE OF DIET

Fish, including salmon and tuna, have naturally occurring omega-3 fatty acids and DHA or docosahexaenoic acids. These elements present in the fish are essential in maintaining the perfect condition of the nerve cells in the nervous system. If one goes on a seafood-exclusive diet, the lack of red meat consumed will mean a lesser risk of getting the arteries clogged. While the vitamin B12 in red meat has its benefits, it is found elsewhere as well.[65] Red meat has proteins in it that pose a threat to normal blood circulation.[66] Green leafy vegetables, guacamole, sunflower seeds, and berries are all rich in vitamin E and folic acid that helps to maintain a healthy nervous system. Clinical studies have revealed that moderate intake of red wine lowers the risk of getting afflicted with Alzheimer's disease.[67] Red wine is also rich in resveritrol, a compound present in grapes that facilitates weight loss and normalizes the blood circulation. Scientific experiments have proven the positive effects of resveratrol in Alzheimer's patients.[68]

Diet plays a critical role in an Alzheimer's patient's overall health, including maintaining the proper functioning of the brain. As deliberated in this chapter, certain items have been linked to memory loss and the interference of other brain functions, while others have been found to enhance brain development and prevent or reduce the risk of cognitive impairment. Moreover, maintaining a diet that is healthy for the brain and combining it with physical and mental activity will help to protect brain cells and slow down the progression of Alzheimer's disease.

· 17 ·

Alzheimer's and Exercise

$\mathscr{T}$he word "exercise" is derived from Latin roots, meaning "to keep" and "to ward off." In reality, exercise is any form of physical activity that is practiced repetitively in order to improve and maintain both the health and fitness of one's body. Exercise is also a very important tool in the physical rehabilitation of an Alzheimer's patient and has the added benefit of enhancing mental and emotional well-being.[1]

Many different forms of exercise exist, ranging from activities that increase muscle strength, to others designed to keep joints mobile and pain free or increase overall fitness and cardiac health. Some exercises are vigorous and require a substantial amount of energy, while other forms of recommended activity are designed to gently stretch and tone the various muscle groups in the body. Exercise is beneficial for everyone, no matter the age or health of the individual, provided the right form of physical activity for the person's age, health, and general physical state is adhered to. The human body is a marvelous and intricately designed piece of "engineering" that needs to be given both time and attention to function at an optimum level. Neglect or abuse from an Alzheimer's patient on his or her body results in impaired function, physical discomfort, and reduced mobility. It is therefore sensible to take part in the right form of exercise on a regular basis in order to maintain health and well-being, and to slow down the effects of the disease.

As deducible in chapter 2, the brain is the command headquarters of the body and requires an appreciable amount of blood circulation in order to function properly. Any moderate aerobic activity that increases heart rate and the flow of blood to the brain of the Alzheimer's patient is beneficial, an example being walking into an outdoor environment. Shallow breathing results in reduced oxygen in the blood and therefore deprives the brain of vitally important fuel needed for it to run smoothly.[2] Science has demonstrated that a body that is inert or goes without physical activity for long periods of time will have less production and transmission of vital neurotransmitters in the brain than a body that exercises regularly.[3] Since neurotransmitters are responsible for communication between the brain and the body, it is easy to comprehend that continual inactivity has a detrimental effect on an Alzheimer's patient's brain. Practicing correct posture and deep breathing daily, thus utilizing one's full lung capacity every day, is helpful to the brain. Research has shown that aerobic exercise also stimulates the growth of new brain cells and improves one's ability to learn and to remember.[4] Scientists are not sure exactly why aerobic exercise has this effect on the brain, but it is thought that the increased blood flow and a rise in certain hormone levels may contribute to this positive result.[5]

Although stretching and toning is beneficial in maintaining the flexibility of muscles and joints, it does not increase pulse rate significantly and therefore is not the best exercise to partake in if one is focusing specifically on brain health. Still, stretching is an important part of a balanced exercise routine to keep the body supple and agile.[6] A well-rounded exercise program will result in all-around health and fitness for both the body and the brain, no matter the age of the Alzheimer's patient.

IMPROVING AND MAINTAINING
PROPER BRAIN FUNCTION

As previously stated, exercise is extremely important for proper brain function. In the 1960s, the then U.S. president-elect determined that fitness should be a priority for every American,[7] but today's sedentary lifestyle is precipitating an ever-increasing health crisis. The culture of computer and video games and watching endless hours of television produces sluggish blood flow in the body and to the brain and therefore inefficient functioning in every part of the delicate communication system between brain and body.

A patient's brain can only function efficiently when it receives adequate oxygen and glucose, and the less sedentary one's lifestyle, the better it is for his or her brain.[8] Inadequate exercise habits developed in youth are usually carried into adulthood and old age, unless a person becomes aware of the exponential negative effects of such a lifestyle and makes the necessary changes. Beginning a healthy exercise routine produces numerous benefits, both physically and mentally, including the avoidance of the onset of any form of senile dementia and, more particularly, Alzheimer's. When one gets older, activities such as watching educational programs, reading, and doing crossword puzzles all assist in maintaining cognitive ability to a certain extent. A brisk walk in the fresh air has an equally, if not more powerful, positive effect on overall brain function.[9] Studies have shown that aerobic exercise has a markedly beneficial effect on the prefrontal and frontal areas of the brain that are involved in cognitive function.[10]

A lack of regular physical exercise is a known contributing factor in the onset of all forms of dementia including Alzheimer's, so it is imperative to develop a habit of daily moderate aerobic exercise to both delay the onset and reduce the severity of cognitive impairment and memory loss in later years. Water aerobics and dancing are both forms of exercise that require concentration, coordination, and the learning of different movements, all of which contribute to the maintenance of brain function. These disciplines are favorable both in warding off the onset and slowing down the progression of cognitive dysfunction experienced in Alzheimer's disease.[11]

It is important however, to avoid excessive and aggressive exercise as this can cause injury in older people who have not performed any exercise for a long time. Peer-reviewed research maintains that too much physical exercise leads to irregular shaping of the muscles.[12] The best approach is to start gradually and then increase the exercise time and difficulty as the patient becomes accustomed to it. The muscles also get stronger and more toned as the heart responds to the slowly increasing intensity of aerobic exercises. The idea is to improve the fitness and flexibility of the body without causing undue strain on joint and muscles. If dancing is the exercise of choice, learning new dance moves is an excellent way of stimulating the brain to produce new memory pathways as well as using muscles in a different way and improving balance.

Under no circumstances should an Alzheimer's patient be left to exercise unsupervised, since poor form, balance, or technique can often lead to injury. Alzheimer's patients also tend to forget what it is they are doing and wander off. A supervisor or caregiver must accompany the patient at all times when seeking to improve fitness and establish a regular exercise routine. Supervision is also vital to ensure patients conduct the movements properly in order to avoid hurting themselves. Sometimes, patients suffer from other health problems beside Alzheimer's. It is important for a health care professional to assess the patient and recommend an exercise regime suited to the individual's needs.

EXERCISE AND AGING

As one gets older, there is a tendency to become less physically active, and those who have not developed a regular exercise routine experience faster aging and a loss of mobility and agility as the years go by.[13] The saying "If you don't use it, you lose it" becomes all too relevant during the senior years, but it is never too late to begin an exercise routine. Physical exercise has been shown to protect the brain and a wide range of mental processes. Those who are inactive are twice as likely to develop Alzheimer's compared to people who participate in exercise three or more times a week.[14] Even patients who simply do light exercises, such as a slowly walking around the block, reduce the probability of mental decline.

There is a difference in the benefits of aerobic versus nonaerobic exercise in the elderly. Participation in gentle toning and stretching classes helps with flexibility, but studies have shown little improvement in brain and cognitive function as a result. However, regular brisk walking, an exercise that speeds up the heart rate and blood flow, results in a significant improvement in the results of mental tests. Other medical studies have found that even when a person is elderly, regular cardiovascular activity has a positive effect on the brain based on past experiences.[15] This would also apply to older Alzheimer's patients. It is important to vary one's exercise type and to learn new exercises as this promotes better prefrontal cortex function. Since water aerobics consist of a variety of different exercises, the brain is stimulated in the process of attaining and remembering the various movements performed. Research proves that bicycling is also an acceptable form of aerobic exercise that also benefits the patient emotionally as he or she rides through the neighborhood and views different landscapes.[16] Bicycling also improves muscles strength and balance and is therefore recommended as long as it is supervised and takes place during the early phases of Alzheimer's. Once the disease has advanced, disorientation makes bicycling difficult, and falls can result in injury and even cause accidents with vehicles or other cyclists.

EXERCISE AND ITS RELATION TO COGNITIVE IMPROVEMENT

The ability to think logically, respond during conversation, and absorb new information are all critical in functioning socially and maintaining independence as one gets older. Regular aerobic exercise plays a large part in helping the brain to keep functioning efficiently in the areas that control and maintain cognitive ability. When discussing aerobic exercise, Alzheimer's patients must keep in mind that this involves continuous and repeated rhythmic use of the large muscles of the body for at least fifteen minutes, preferably three or more times a week. This must also produce an increase in resting heart rate to approximately 60 percent of the maximum.[17]

Activities such as walking, swimming, or riding a bicycle all help build endurance and improve the health of the circulatory system, the carrier of the absolutely essential oxygen to the brain cells. By way of research, nonaerobic exercises such as resistance training have also shown cognitive benefits when practiced alone.[18] However, this produces greater effects when combined with aerobic exercise. It has also been found that music-based aerobic exercise produces significant improvements in cognition in patients who suffer from Alzheimer's and other forms of dementia.[19] Studies show that ambient music has a strong but temporary calming effect on Alzheimer's disease patients.[20]

Although the loss of memory is the most common early symptom of Alzheimer's, deterioration in other cognitive functions also signals the onset of the disease. Cognitive function is extremely important in maintaining basic daily activities such as housekeeping, shopping, meal preparation, and money management. Healthy visuospatial functioning helps with accurate face recognition.[21] Navigating one's environment and visuomotor skills control movements such as correct toilet procedure, making a phone call, and dressing oneself.

Neurogenesis, the Creation of New Brain Cells

Scientific experiments suggest that neurogenesis is associated with improved cognition.[22] The brain is capable of producing new brain cells that are used to maintain already existing connection pathways necessary for long-term memory and allowing the acquisition of new memories. Physical exercise is an important role player in stimulating and protecting the brain, but mental exercise also plays a helpful role. Those who keep their brains active by playing cards, reading, and completing crossword puzzles are 50 percent less likely to develop Alzheimer's disease.[23] Even during the early stages of the disease, such activities play an important role in slowing the progression of Alzheimer's and increasing cognitive ability.

Mental Stimulation

Clinical studies prove that the game of bingo provides mental stimulation.[24] Bingo also very therapeutic for patients with Alzheimer's disease. Those working with the patients as part of the study noticed they were more alert and aware for hours after playing. There are also computerized training modules that are useful for improving cognitive abilities in healthy adults.[25] Even when diseased, the brain has the ability to form new neurological connections. Because a computer game has different stages of difficulty, it can be adjusted to function at the level of the patient who is playing, and it is this precise thing that makes it useful in treating and delaying the progress of Alzheimer's. When it is used in conjunction with psychomotor stimulation, the benefits extend for weeks after its use. The term "psychomotor" refers to when mental activity initiates movement. Researchers also point out that older people who engage in little social activity have an increased risk of contracting Alzheimer's disease.[26] Mixing socially and visiting with friends, partaking in activities at clubs, and doing hobbies together with others all help to reduce the risk of cognitive decline. Some older people even learn a new language as a challenge that helps grey matter function.

EXERCISES FOR THE PHYSICAL
SYMPTOMS OF ALZHEIMER'S

Those suffering from Alzheimer's disease experience many different physical symptoms as well as mental deterioration. Various exercises can relieve these symptoms.

Exercises for Incontinence

One of these distressing symptoms associated with Alzheimer's is urinary incontinence.[27] There are exercises to train and strengthen the muscles that control urine output. These are called Kegel exercises. Designed for both men and women, these movements involve the contraction of pelvic floor muscles, which support the urethra, bladder, uterus, and rectum. To locate these muscles, one can try to stop the flow of urine during urination while keeping other muscle groups relaxed. Preferably, this is done in a seated position. Once the muscle group has been isolated, the exercise consists of sitting or lying with knees together, tightening the muscles, holding for a count of four, and then relaxing for a count of four seconds. This should be carried out twice a day for five minutes at a time.

Kegel exercises are used to treat stress incontinence and urge incontinence, the latter being the need to urinate that is so strong one cannot reach the bathroom in time.[28] The muscles to be exercised are called the pubococcygeus muscles. It is easy to compensate for weak muscles by using the abdominals, buttocks, and thighs. These muscle groups must be kept relaxed as the exercise is performed. An Alzheimer's patient can practice these very beneficial exercises on the couch in front of the TV, when stuck at a traffic light, or even lying in bed. If Kegel exercises are practiced regularly, the person can ward off any urinary incontinence, thus retaining dignity and independence for much longer in old age. Older people who learn to do the Kegel exercises can override the signals from the brain telling them they need to use the bathroom. The muscles, the brain, and the exercise all work together to prevent incontinence.

Exercises for Difficulty Swallowing

A loss of brain cells can also interfere with swallowing mechanisms in patients going through the later stages of Alzheimer's, as substantiated by medical research.[29] Difficulty swallowing in this instance is called dysphagia,[30] which makes taking medication hard and absorbing sufficient nutrition to keep healthy a challenge. In order to prevent choking in the later stages of Alzheimer's, it may become necessary to instruct the patient when to chew and when to swallow. Keeping the person upright for half an hour after eating helps to prevent choking. Eventually, food in liquid form has to be given to the patient as their swallowing ability becomes limited to liquids. Choking and swallowing problems can lead to pneumonia because the person inhales liquid or pieces of food into the lungs.

Exercises for Breathing Difficulties

According to a peer-reviewed scientific report, pneumonia is a frequent cause of death in Alzheimer's patients.[31] Elderly people with pneumonia might not display fever or complain of pain and might have little coughing. In general, they seem weak and confused due to insufficient oxygen reaching the brain. Of course, with Alzheimer's patients, they are often unable to communicate discomfort effectively; so it is up to the caregiver to notice the increased disorientation and weakness. Treatment for pneumonia always involves a hospital stay and antibiotics. In some cases, liquid nourishment intravenously helps to prevent further weight loss.

Options to avoid pneumonia, besides vaccines, include deep breathing and coughing exercises.[32] A forced cough followed by holding the breath for three to six seconds and simple exercise, such as a walk around one's room, can be enough to stop pneumonia from setting in. Normal, healthy people take approximately four deep sighs every hour. This ensures that the parts of the lungs not normally used in breathing get exercised. A slow, deep breath through the nose, followed by holding one's breath for five seconds and slowly exhaling, exercises the lungs and gets secretions moving. If this is done ten times, followed by forced coughing, it greatly reduces the risk of contracting pneumonia. Depending on symptomatic status, Alzheimer's patients can manage to do these simple exercises.

Exercises for Improving Balance

When brain cells degenerate, the body's ability to identify where one's limbs are in space is affected. Thus, Alzheimer's patients get disoriented[33] and lose their balance and fall,[34] resulting in broken limbs and even head injuries. Changes in the brain, slower reaction time, and difficulty gauging the height of steps are all things that precipitate falls. An Alzheimer's patient may not remember that there is a step in front of the door and, therefore, trip over it. Help with this problem can be as simple as providing a walker or a cane, but an Alzheimer's patient must be reminded to use the device. The loss of cogni-

The loss of cognitive functioning and the feeling of being disorientated are very unnerving for the patient, and so care must be taken to avoid falls as much as possible since it adds the fear of repeating the fall to their list of many preexisting struggles. Balance training repairs the connections in the nerves associated with balance and muscle control. This type of training also helps to develop fine motor control in arms and legs. Exercises can be done to improve balance in the comfort of one's home. A simple exercise consists of standing next to a countertop and lightly touching it with one's hand, then lifting one foot off the floor and maintaining balance for a count of ten seconds. This whole process is repeated with the other leg. To progress further once this is easily achieved, one does the exercise without holding onto the counter. The most advanced form of this exercise consists of performing the movements with both eyes shut. Using an exercise ball under guided instruction is also an excellent way of improving balance. It is very important that an Alzheimer's patient does not attempt to exercise on the ball when alone, as severe injuries can result. An organized exercise class with a trained professional is the best way to approach ball exercises. It is beneficial to take a break from the exercise ball to do other minor workouts such as a walk in the garden or around the block, with a helping hand at the patient's elbow to provide support and balance.

Alzheimer's and Gait

Gait disturbance is prevalent in those suffering from Alzheimer's disease.[35] Patients who suffer from gait problems move slowly, experience muscle rigidity, and shuffle when they walk. A stooped posture is also typical of Alzheimer's patients. Lack of balance and muscle strength contributes to frequent falling. As previously stated, low-impact aerobic exercise, perhaps at first in the safe environment of a treadmill indoors where one can hold on to a handle in the beginning stages, develops strength and balance. When deemed safe, simply sitting and standing unaided develops the said abilities and helps the brain to function properly. Strengthening one's back and core muscles via exercise can improve posture. Deep, even breathing during exercise ensures adequate oxygen to the parts of the brain being used at the time. Standing on one foot while holding onto a counter and extending the other leg in small movements up and down exercises the muscles normally employed in balance and gait. In essence, there are numerous exercises that can be performed to improve the typical gait of those with Alzheimer's, and the added advantage of these activities is that the cognitive and motor areas of the brain are stimulated, thereby retarding the degenerative process.

Exercises to Strengthen Bones

Medical research has found that Alzheimer's patients have weakened bones.[36] Weight-bearing exercise is any form of activity where one's bones are supporting body weight. It does not have to be a high-impact exercise such as jogging, which is of course dangerous for Alzheimer's patients as fast motion, coordination, and balance are difficult to attain. Weight-bearing aerobic exercise such as walking, dancing, stair climbing, gardening, or even exercising in water all help to strengthen the muscles and bones in the spine and body. The stronger a muscle, the greater force it exerts on the bone it is attached to. It follows that, when patients strengthen their muscles, they are also strengthening their bones. Strength training on land also helps to reduce mineral loss in bone, especially in postmenopausal women. Since more women succumb to Alzheimer's disease than do men,[37] it is especially important that older women have regular, varied exercise routines. Exercises that are beneficial for bones include the following:

- Water aerobics
- Step aerobics
- Walking
- Dancing
- Hiking
- Swimming
- Low-impact martial arts

Exercises to avoid include running, basketball, tennis, and weightlifting.

Exercises for Improving Vision

Poor eyesight is clearly one of the symptoms of Alzheimer's disease.[38] This is often due to deterioration not so much in the eye itself but in the brain connections that control cognitive function and recognition. Medical research has also shown that people who stay moderately active and participate in exercise regularly as they age tend to suffer less from age-related macular degeneration of the eyes.[39] Being able to see properly is a requirement for most activities that are known to lower the risk of suffering from Alzheimer's. Reading, interacting socially, and all physical activities require adequate vision. According to a study from the University of Michigan Health Department, elderly patients with untreated vision problems are significantly more likely to suffer from Alzheimer's.[40] It is therefore important for elderly people with poor eyesight to visit ophthalmologists and to have their vision problem diagnosed and treated, to avoid dementia. Treatment could include surgery to remove cataracts and treatment for glaucoma.

Exercises to Improve Hearing

There is a connection between hearing loss and the onset of Alzheimer's. Research done at the University of Washington found a very strong correlation between the extent of hearing loss and the degree of cognitive deterioration.[41] Hearing loss contributes to social isolation, which in turn produces depression. Depression is known to be a significant risk factor in developing senile dementia. If hearing loss is corrected, social interaction can resume and mental health improves.[42] Quite a large portion of the brain is used in processing information received from the inner ear. Input from a person's ears allows the brain to comprehend surroundings. Hearing loss often goes unnoticed since other Alzheimer's symptoms already exist and therefore produce a masking effect. Once a hearing aid is fitted, communication becomes easier and patients are often more cooperative and aware of what is going on around them. Even if a patient already has Alzheimer's disease, correcting hearing loss decreases memory loss.[43]

SUMMARY

This chapter explained the benefits and drawbacks of exercise for an Alzheimer's disease patient. Research has thoroughly proved that exercise plays a vitally important role in prohibiting or delaying brain deterioration observed in Alzheimer's.[44] Those who have regular exercise routines that include various types of aerobic and nonaerobic exercises have a significantly smaller chance of developing any form of senile dementia. As the human brain directs and controls all bodily function and movement, including thought processes, it is imperative that both men and women begin exercising early in life and continue the habit, adjusting the type of exercise to suit age and fitness level right into old age. Exercise plays a vitally important role in preventing and treating neurological disorders such as Alzheimer's because it increases oxygen and glucose delivery to the brain. This helps the brain to develop both new brain cells and new connection pathways, slowing the process of brain deterioration. Old age then becomes a period of one's life to look forward to rather than to dread.

· 18 ·

Finding Motivation to Cope with Alzheimer's

$\mathcal{A}$lzheimer's disease is a progressive, degenerative, and irreversible neurological disorder that not only inflicts physical suffering but also saps the patient's willpower and motivation. The disease is characterized by gradual changes that get worse as time passes. Upon hearing the diagnosis of Alzheimer's disease, heavy emotions and concerns can follow, putting an enormous burden on the patient and his or her family. As covered in preceding chapters, feelings of shock, denial, depression, anxiety, and all other emotions akin to loneliness and despair is expected to occur. In fact, studies show that apathy in Alzheimer's disease is associated with decreased blood flow to the brain, an organ with a very critical and obvious role in finding motivation.[1]

Knowing that Alzheimer's is associated with incurable memory loss, disorientation, and decreased cognitive and motor function may make the patient want to give up easily and end his or her life rather than endure the pain and hardships.[2] If the patient stays hopeless in the absence of any motivation and is unwilling to cooperate, then the medical management originally aimed to delay Alzheimer's disease progression and prolong the life of the patient will be of no use. In the treatment process, the patient, family, caregivers, and physicians must work together and help each other for it to be effective. Alzheimer's patients need to cooperate and find motivation because they are the ones who play the largest role in fighting their own symptoms.

DIFFICULTY FINDING MOTIVATION

Old Age

The chance of getting Alzheimer's disease increases with age and mostly affects the elderly. As of 2010, 35.6 million people worldwide have suffered from the disease.[3] In the United States alone, around 4.5 million people are diagnosed each year,[4] putting the disease in the top 10 of all mortality-causing diseases in the country.[5] The demographic relationship of old age to the causes for lack of motivation among patients is highly significant. After all, the relationship exists due to the feelings and concerns found among the elderly. Unfortunately, patients might go to extremes and prefer to give up completely, considering that they have already come of old age. Believing they are too old and weak enough to help themselves during the course of the disease is a major hindrance in gaining cooperation once Alzheimer's disease treatment begins. Patients might consider suicide acceptable since they have already lived long, fruitful years. Feelings of contentment and satisfaction with the number of years that they have lived give them a reason to stop fighting and admit defeat. The normal degenerative changes that occur with aging make the patients lose confidence and motivation even more. Loss of the desire to move forward will contribute to hopelessness and an inability to surpass the effects of the disease. These feelings are too strong for the patients to overcome, leading to negativity and frustration. If these feelings are not changed, motivational strategies can be ineffective.

Unruly Personal and Family Relationships

Facing Alzheimer's disease means to turn to a new page in one's life and a new beginning where the greatest challenge is yet to unfold. While clinical evidence suggests that Alzheimer's disease places a significant amount of stress on the family, the patient is not alone on the journey since the motivational process involves the family members and loved ones as well.[6] Knowing that a family member is diagnosed with Alzheimer's requires a great deal of responsibility in understanding and providing emotional support to the patient. Family members who bestow emotional support can boost the patient's self-esteem.[7] This gets the patient motivated and encourages him or her to strive hard to fight the disease. If surrounded with negativity and conflicts, the patient's situation can worsen and the patient can get more depressed and less motivated.

Certain changes and conflicts that disrupt family relationships will occur as soon as a family member has been clinically diagnosed with the disease.[8] Every member of the family has varying suggestions and solutions on how to appropriately deal with the distressing situation. Also, they cope differently due to feelings of grief and loss over the patient: Some might be avoidant or go into denial.[9] Some might seek out counseling and gather more information pertaining to the disease. The diverse emotions and opinions between relatives will consequently lead to conflicts, confusions, and disharmony. Family relationships will be in turmoil and inflict additional burdens that break the patient down even more. If the Alzheimer patient's family goes through a conflict, it is recommended that everything get resolved quickly for the benefit of the patient. Instead of prolonging disagreements, the family should band together and be closer to the patient than ever. This will yield a strong family bond and provide motivation for the patient battling Alzheimer's disease.

Low Physical Activity and Lack of Motivation

Physical activity normally declines with age, but for those who never exercised much, this decline leaves them with little or no exercise at all when older. Studies have revealed that performing exercise regularly, which often requires motivation,[10] will greatly improve strength, flexibility, endurance, and cardiovascular fitness, which reduces the risk of acquiring diseases and disabilities that develop as people grow older.[11] Physical activity also enhances musculoskeletal strength, which helps to avoid falls, fractures, and difficulty with walking and climbing that is common among the elderly. Loss of function and mobility associated with aging is largely due to physical inactivity. Lack of physical activity is also a precursor for major health problems such as diabetes, heart attack, hypertension, stroke, and many others. In summary, the importance of the motivation needed for physical activity cannot be ignored and must be continued as Alzheimer's disease victims age.[12]

Older patients deemed physically inactive prior to diagnosis need not worry since it is never too late to achieve the motivation necessary to perform exercises. Those who are physically active will prevent numerous health problems and yield significant effects. Patients must remember that performing exercises and engaging in sports can still be done by older patients provided that they do it the right way. According to the World Health Organization, moderate physical activity should be performed for 150 minutes throughout the week.[13] To attain this, it is best to allot thirty minutes of moderate activity such as walking, gardening, dancing, or any preferable activity for five days. It is also essential to perform activities of moderate intensity since exercising too vigorously will lead to certain health problems. Older Alzheimer's disease victims can only perform activities moderately due to normal physiological effects of aging. However, the normal physical and mental degradation of the body that occurs with aging should not keep an older Alzheimer's patient from performing exercises and participating in sports.

Physical activity can yield significant improvements in older people suffering from chronic diseases. This also holds true for Alzheimer's disease patients. Patients need to be physically active and perform exercises that they can do to improve their motivation and delay the progression of the disease. Physical activity can improve one's self-confidence, thereby reducing anxiety and depression among patients. Knowing they can still be physically active despite the disease will boost patients' motivation even further.[14] It also delays the progression of the disease by preventing more complications associated with sedentary lifestyle. For patients who are physically inactive and prefer to remain sedentary, the effects will be the exact opposite compared to those who are still active.

Negative Environments

The environment in which Alzheimer's patients live reflects their lifestyle.[15] The environment influences personality, culture, beliefs, and quality of life, including the person's health condition. It impacts the health and emotional well-being of an Alzheimer's disease victim. The environment has to have the following attributes to bring motivation to the patient:

- Enlightening
- Nurturing
- Inspirational
- Comfortable
- Satisfactory

If the environment is not ideal for the patient, the patient is likely to suffer. Today, high living cost is coupled with technologies unfamiliar to older people. Family ties are much different than in the past since there is a lot more focus on work. This essentially leaves older Alzheimer's patients behind. These factors are not considered part of the Alzheimer's patient's comfort zone and will therefore disrupt his or her environment and create a sense of loneliness and depression.[16]

Negative, uncomfortable, and unsatisfying environments that the patients live with will make them lose the motivation and personal drive necessary to face the disease properly. To correct this problem, patients with Alzheimer's disease must have an environment according to their preferences. It should allow them to move, participate, control, and maintain their level of functioning for as long as possible. The environment must also be simple, comfortable, organized, neat, and most importantly, safe. The families and loved ones of patients with Alzheimer's disease must show their support, love, and compassion, and be as close as possible to each other. Environments can pose influence over the lives of patients with Alzheimer's disease. Implying negativity will make the problem worse, but providing an environment that is inspiring will benefit the patient.[17]

Mistreatment and Abuse of the Elderly

There is an overwhelming amount of scientific evidence that elderly people are mistreated by society.[18] As senior citizens strive to be healthy and live longer, cases of abuse and neglect have been increasing substantially. According to statistics, about two million older people suffer from all forms of abuse and neglect in the United States.[19] The exact number for those who suffer from abuse and neglect could not be identified due to the fact that most cases remain hidden and unreported to authorities. This means that approximately two million people have lived to the end of their lives suffering from elder abuse and neglect. Most cases remain unreported due to fear of the abusers and hopelessness, making the patient suffer until death.[20]

Medical research has found that Alzheimer's disease victims face abuse.[21] Patients diagnosed with Alzheimer's disease who also put up with abuse or neglect from their families and caregivers go through a lot of problems when it comes to treatment protocols. Reports suggest that Alzheimer's caregivers go through much stress and fatigue, and this does not ease the process of finding motivation from the patient's standpoint.[22] Alzheimer's patients have endured the emotional burden introduced by their situation, so abuse or neglect will make them feel even more frustrated and worthless. The resultant anguish will cause a drop in motivation, making patients withdraw from treatments and give up. Rather than abusing and neglecting the patient, caregivers must treat Alzheimer's patients with respect and let them live the remaining days of their lives happily and peacefully.

CAREGIVING

Personal Caregivers

In the early stages of Alzheimer's disease, families might choose to care for their loved ones with the disease at home. The personal caregiver is normally a member of the family or a close companion. Sometimes however, patients will hire a professional caregiver to live with them. Before making a decision to be a personal caregiver, one must understand what the job entails since being one requires an enormous amount of patience, compassion, and hard work. A caregiver can be rewarding and beneficial to the patient in all aspects. They (1) provide physical assistance in all day-to-day necessities; (2) initiate activities that add to the patient's productivity; (3) administer prescribed medications; and (4) render continuous social and emotional support. The caregiver's role is critical in helping prevent complications and to delay the progression of the disease. Caregivers are responsible for the patient's physical, emotional, and social well-being. The holistic care that they provide, when done correctly, can help the patient find motivation.

Having a personal caregiver tend to the needs of the patient can also create potential problems that will hinder the overall progress and disrupt motivational tactics. The demanding and overwhelming tasks that a caregiver carries out twenty-four hours a day creates an unbearable amount of stress. Some caregivers will lose patience and understanding for every dramatic change that every patient undergoes. The caregivers may give up and stop caring for the patient, and as a result, mistreatment occurs. Intense emotional feelings such as anger, guilt, grief, and depression related to caregiving are felt at any point of the disease process, and soon, problems may arise. Caregivers face a lot of struggles alone in giving holistic care to Alzheimer's disease patients, making the role extremely difficult. Family members and loved ones should provide continuous support and encouragement to the main caregiver to prevent the several drawbacks of caregiving. They should assist and help with the many tasks that need to be done to help the Alzheimer's disease patient get motivated. This eases the heavy physical and emotional burden felt by the caregiver. Allow the caregiver to have some rest, and let him or her engage in caregiver trainings and support groups so that there will be a better understanding of the disease and proper interventions will be known and applied to the patient. If these steps are done the right way, effective caregiving will be implemented on the patient and motivation will be there.

The Role of Nursing Homes in Finding Motivation

As discussed in part IV, the physical and mental capacity of the Alzheimer's patient will deteriorate over time. This makes the management of caregivers insufficient when it comes to matching the needs of the patient. If and when this occurs, the patients are usually transferred to nursing homes. These patients need careful evaluation, assessment, and monitoring and require the help of health care professionals to look after them twenty-four hours a day.

Transferring patients to nursing homes provides several advantages in addition to finding motivation. First, some nursing homes have licensed physicians with expertise in Alzheimer's disease to continually supervise the medical management of the patients, although a research report suggests that this can be quite a challenge.[23] These doctors are responsible for continually assessing, monitoring, and evaluating the patient twenty-four hours a day. Any problems that may come about must be attended to immediately.

Professional nurses, caregivers, occupational and respiratory therapists, and social workers are always on the premises to take care of the patients. These people are specially trained to care and manage Alzheimer's disease patients. Knowing this will make loved ones feel secure as they transfer the patient to the nursing home, which will provide the motivation needed to withstand the symptoms. Second, nursing homes are uniquely structured and designed to promote safety and provide a healthy environment for the patients. Adequate lighting, specialized rooms, recreational areas, and places for the patient to safely go about should be made available. Third, recreational activities such as exercising, singing, dancing, and drawing are usually conducted for the patients to actively participate and enjoy. These are specifically formulated programs that are suitable and appropriate for the patients. This way, patients will not feel bored and worthless as they get to do activities that they enjoy. Fourth, nursing homes uniquely provide the highest level of appropriate medical services to the patient. Patients living in nursing homes will find motivation and inspiration because they feel that they have gone through the right treatments.

Despite all the benefits, transferring an Alzheimer's patient to a specialized nursing home creates an emotional transition between the patient and his or her loved ones. Patients and their families will once more endure the hardships of separation, acceptance, and adjustment as a new phase of life takes shape. Heavier burden is placed on the patient since living in a new environment without the family is extremely difficult. Some patients might not understand the why they are being transferred and feel anger and worthlessness. These feelings make the patient once again lose his or her motivation and hope. It is recommended that physicians, nurses, and caregivers at the nursing home make patients feel at ease and help them adjust and adapt to their new surroundings.

Rehab Facilities

Rehabilitation facilities offer the same services as that of nursing homes. Alzheimer's disease is a chronic, degenerating disease that requires long-term therapy, part of which may take place in rehab centers. It is up to the family to decide where to best transfer the patient for effective long-term care. The benefits and drawbacks to placing patients in nursing homes are quite the same for those placed in unique rehabilitation facilities.[24]

Moreover, Alzheimer's is a terrible disease that is currently affecting millions of people around the world. Fortunately, there are many rehabilitation centers in existence dedicated to helping people cope with this serious mental condition. Families will not have any difficulty in finding a center within or close to their area.

Motivation through rehabilitation centers is one of the keys to help-ing Alzheimer's patients. Medical research shows that motivation provided through rehab facilities can improve the memory impairments associated with the disease.[25] Rehabilitation of Alzheimer's is a very serious issue that each staff member of the institution is not supposed to take lightly. The staff at memory clinics and Alzheimer's disease rehabilitation centers is trained to motivate patients to complete their everyday tasks on their own. This measure is taken in order to move patients to a point where they can have normalcy in their life.

THE ROLE OF FAMILY MEMBERS

Family members provide an integral part in building a patient's confidence and motivation to fight Alzheimer's. There should be a tremendous amount of support, compassion, love, and strength offered by the family throughout the course of the disease. Upon hearing the final diagnosis, the patient will be in extreme denial and sadness. It is crucial for the family to counsel and provide guidance to the patient right away to prevent further psychological distress. As discussed previously, the environment can be a major influence in building either positive or negative emotions about oneself . Therefore, one must try to alleviate the anxiety and despair of most patients by creating a calm and peaceful environment first. This can be accomplished by getting rid of noises, bright and glaring lights, and other disturbances typically found inside the home. The people around the patient should also try to remain calm to avoid instilling unnecessary fear and misery in the patient.[26]

The patient should be encouraged to express feelings. After the patient has calmed down, the caregiver can ensure that the patient is ready to talk about his or her feelings. Once the patient is ready, the caregiver should allow the former to vent and discuss any suppressed feelings that may be brewing inside. As a member of the family, it is advised to listen carefully as the patient talks about his or her emotions. Attention and interest should be shown to let the patient ex-press openly. A tap on the shoulder, a hug, or a kiss afterward may be necessary to boost the patient's mood. The caregiver should remind the patient that the latter is still the same person and is not crazy as noticeable mental and behavioral changes will occur only in the early stages of the disease. At this time, it is best to constantly remind the patient that nothing has changed and he or she is still the same person. This will put things in ideal perspective.[27]

Family members should help patients fight off their symptoms and get motivation while the patients battle against the disease. All family members should give their support, strength, and positive vibes to encourage the patient into feeling the same way. The patient needs motivation to be an active par-ticipant in fighting and striving hard to win the battle, and family members ought to initiate measures to let the patient remain optimistic. This is especially important during the difficult times of the disease. Doing so will make the disease more manageable. Planning ahead will often lead to a greater chance of the patient getting directly involved in his or her improvement. It is recommended to include patients while still possible, with regard to treatment and other plans concerning the disease. One should also involve the patient in his or her daily activities. Restricting them from doing activities that they can still perform will lessen their confidence and make them feel worthless.

Let the Games Begin

Daily activities such as eating, bathing, dressing, walking, playing sports, and doing household chores with the family should not be kept from the patient entirely but should be encouraged instead. It is important to allow Alzheimer's patients to continue doing what they enjoy, while they still can. These activities will help maintain their motor and cognitive skills and promote independence as long as possible. If the patients continue to carry out the different activities, it will remove their depression, increase their motivation, and give them a sense of accomplishment as they complete every activity. The activities are healthy ego boosters and will enable patients to enjoy any motivational techniques.

Activities to be performed by the patient require careful planning and assessment. Games designed for the patient should match mental and physical capacities and be simple yet enjoyable. Patients should incorporate activities such as household chores, gardening, sorting, reading, writing, painting, dancing, singing, and many others that utilize old hobbies and abilities. They should also invest in games that match their interests. Certain games are designed specifically for Alzheimer's disease. These games are made to stimulate certain areas of the patient's brain and improve memory and rational thinking capabilities. Studies have revealed that exercising the brains of Alzheimer's disease patients by playing mind-boosting games can slow down the progression of the disease.[28] Not only will these games be fun and enjoyable, it will be healthy as well. Suitable games include the following:

- Crossword puzzles
- Word find
- Scrabble
- Trivia games
- Checkers
- Chess
- Puzzles
- Dominos
- Card games

Games can be improvised and personalized, as long as brain stimulation remains the primary objective.

Visitations

Patients greatly looking forward to having visitors during the day. It helps them interact with the loved ones they miss the most and gives them a sense of fulfillment by letting them know they have not been abandoned by their families. Visitation also provides motivation to the patient since he or she knows they will still get the support and strength to carry on with the next phase of the disease. Family members and friends have the right to visit the patient every day as long as it does not force the patient to do something against the patient's consent. Initially, family members and friends who plan to visit the patient must first make an appointment with hospital staff members, informing them of their intention to visit on a specific date. In exchange, the hospital will let the patient know and ask for the patient's approval. If the patient is no longer capable of making decisions, staff members are responsible for fixing the time and date for personal visits in accordance with the rules and regulations of the institution. The visitors will then be briefed about the "dos and don'ts" of visiting, such as placing an excessive amount of stress on the individual. The visitors are reminded about the proper approach, and communication techniques are occasionally taught prior to the visit. Visitors can bring photos, memorabilia, and old possessions that are particularly helpful in stimulating memory. They are provided with quality time with the patient to allow for bonding and socializing. Most importantly, families and loved should always keep their appointments; failure to stay on schedule may upset the patient.

FROM PATIENT TO PATIENT

Since Alzheimer's disease victims' perspectives on their own medical status have largely been ignored throughout the years,[29] it is important for a patient to discuss his or her problems with others who are going through the same experiences. Sharing experiences, ideas, and coping mechanisms with other patients suffering from Alzheimer's disease provides an exchange of additional emotional support that is useful in boosting motivation. Other Alzheimer's patients have a better understanding of the current situation compared to loved ones, and they can truly relate to the needs and adjustments in connection to Alzheimer's. The development of coping strategies is met once successful interactions among copatients occur. Patients who cope very well with the disease and are happy can enable others in the same boat to maintain a positive outlook. Getting to talk with other Alzheimer's patients also provides a sense of relief, knowing they are not alone in battling the disease. Therefore, caregivers should encourage them to open up and talk with their peers so they can be fully motivated in fighting Alzheimer's disease.

STRENGTH IN NUMBERS

Motivation through Focus Groups

Clinical experimentation has demonstrated how symptoms improve through support groups.[30] These groups are normally comprised of members who share the same pathology as those around them. Patients get together from time to time and discuss their tough situations, feelings, and ideas without the concern of getting judged by anyone. Participating actively in support groups will help an Alzheimer's patient deal with disease-related problems effectively. The primary purpose of support groups is to let everyone know that that the patient is not alone. There are a variety of support groups of specific conditions and experiences, such as groups for cancer patients, rape victims, and many others. Alzheimer's disease also involves different support groups that aim to provide benefits for all members. Letting a patient join support groups that are specifically designed for Alzheimer's disease will result in numerous benefits,[31] many of which are listed below.

- Support groups allow every patient to vent all their feelings, struggles, and challenges among other Alzheimer's disease victims trying to find motivation. This scenario is not typically found among family members and friends.
- Support groups provide a deeper and a thorough understanding of Alzheimer's disease and its emotional burden, thus motivating the patient even further.
- Sharing coping strategies and solutions to handle the disease effectively will help patients adapt. Seeing patients who are managing Alzheimer's well will inspire the others and eventually convince them to try different techniques.
- Each patient receives sincere emotional support from all the members, and this makes the patients feel motivated to reject the symptoms associated with the disease. It enhances their motivation to strive hard in facing the disease.
- Support groups give everyone a chance to be an advocate and a counselor, to help each and every patient out of his or her misery. It brings on a sense of camaraderie and fun throughout an Alzheimer patient's path to finding motivation.

For patients with Alzheimer's disease, it is extremely important to continuously provide positive emotional reinforcement, and letting them join support groups is a great way for this to happen.[32]

More on Friends and Family

Friends and family constitute approximately 75 percent of all the care given to Alzheimer's disease victims.[33] Through familial motivation, Alzheimer's disease patients can let go of their feelings of hopelessness that disallow them to get them anywhere when it comes to the prolongation their lives. Feelings of isolation and solitude in facing the disease must be stopped through the help of their respective families, friends, and support groups. Severe Alzheimer's disease patients may not be ready to face all their symptoms on their own. It is simply too much for one person to handle. Therefore, family members should shower the patients with utmost support, compassion, guidance, and love as these will enable the patient to move ahead and gain motivation. Family members should contact all of the patient's friends and colleagues to give their support and care through letters, e-mails, gifts, and visitations. They should initiate supportive measures periodically to constantly remind the patient that he or she is not alone. The more people who stand behind the patient to offer their support and love, the more motivation the patient will have throughout the course of the disease.

· *19* ·

Alzheimer's at Home

$\mathcal{T}$he statement "There is no place like home" can apply when trying to figure out the right approach to any degenerative disease. People with medical conditions such as Alzheimer's tend to feel isolated and insecure at home. The home has always been a venue that provides a sense of security and belonging. Therefore, approaching the treatment of diseases in general at home is an excellent option to consider. Neurological conditions are the result of physical or chemical impairments in the brain and nervous system. The nature of neurological diseases such as Alzheimer's causes the sufferers to lose the ability to perform daily tasks and live comfortably. This will mean that they are much more prone to feeling isolated and insecure. Alzheimer's patients will also require more understanding and care compared to patients of other diseases, making the disease an ideal one to be treated at home.

Proper care of the Alzheimer's disease patient is really not a simple matter, though. The progression of the disease and the various factors involved in the care amidst the variety of symptoms expressed by Alzheimer's disease requires professional supervision. It is important to consult a psychologist or an equivalently licensed medical professional for a list of things to be observed in the Alzheimer's patient. The list may include the various therapies and medications that are available for the patient at home, tips on how to conduct them, and discussions about regularly scheduled checkups.

TAKING CARE OF CHILDREN AT HOME

Parenting is a very important role that an Alzheimer's disease victim might decide to undertake at some point in his or her life. Its importance lies in the proper shaping and upbringing of another human being, and such an important role comes hand in hand with occasionally tedious responsibilities. Being an Alzheimer's disease sufferer and a parent adds a whole new dimension to life while raising kids, which involves catering to needs that change over time as the child grows. At the same time, Alzheimer's disease, being a progressively degenerative problem, will incite varying levels of disability over time as the disease progresses. The stages of a child's growth consist of *infant, toddler, school-age children,* and *adolescent.* Each stage of growth allows for a new set of needs of the child and of responsibilities to be undertaken by the parent suffering from Alzheimer's.

Newborns and Infants

When in the first month of life, an infant is considered a newborn. The parent's responsibilities really begin at this stage. The parent will have to provide food, comfort, sleep, and hygiene—all of which are basic needs of an infant. For obvious reasons, the infant is fully dependent on the parent. This will put the Alzheimer's disease patient under a lot of stress while concurrently placing the infant at possible risk for neglect. The infant will require feeding almost every two to three hours, causing a disruption to the sleep cycle of the parent who has Alzheimer's. The patient may suffer confusion, restlessness, and memory loss, so it would be beneficial if they had sufficient and proper sleep cycles. Infants normally develop an attachment to their parents around six months and respond to caressing and cuddling. Alzheimer's disease patients might display some levels of emotional apathy and thus fail to bond with the child sufficiently.[1] Attachments formed early in life influence the quality of the relationships that an infant will create later. Infants will learn to walk at approximately one year of age; afterward, they will be considered toddlers. During this time, they are fully dependent on their parents for mobilization. Toddlers are carried in the arms of a guardian or transported in carriages and strollers. It is a concern that an Alzheimer's victim may forget about the infant during trips outside the home, or even misplace and forget the location of the child.

Toddlers

Toddlers are normally capable of walking. They begin to explore their surroundings by themselves and they are much more active than they were when they were infants. This new level of activity will require the parent to always keep the child in check. These newly instated "demands" may overwhelm an Alzheimer's disease patient whose issues might have progressed into much more frequent memory loss. Toddlers further develop their emotions at this stage. They will also further develop their communication skills and widen the scope of their vocabulary. Toddlers begin to understand social order and proper etiquette. This massive repertoire of skills is acquired by mimicking adults, specifically parents. This is a predicament for Alzheimer's patients as some of the symptoms presented by their disease present inappropriate behavior or present an inefficient level of verbal communication for the toddler to replicate.[2] These symptoms can include the following:

- Impaired communication
- Poor judgment
- Problems with language
- Restlessness
- Loss of initiative
- Social withdrawal
- Changes in personality and behavior
- Inability to follow directions
- Emotional apathy

Toddlers are very curious about their surroundings and are enthusiastic about learning about the world around them. Toddlers try to accomplish new activities and challenges in a bid to establish a sense of independence. In the course of their endeavors, toddlers are likely to encounter setbacks and are prone to be frustrated by them. Faced with frustration, the toddler is likely to burst out in an episode of tantrums. This period of frequent episodes of tantrums is known to many as the "Terrible Twos,"[3] the age at which the tantrums begin. The tantrum can be caused by various minor setbacks, some of them as simple as the child not being able communicate properly. This period in the child's growth can be stressful and demanding for an Alzheimer's disease patient already prone to confusion and restlessness. Parents take the role of guide and teacher during the toddler years. They are expected to establish basic routines (e.g., washing hands before meals or saying "thank you" or "sorry"), thereby slightly increasing the child's responsibility. Alzheimer's disease sufferers may be frustrated during this stage when they themselves are already forgetting basic routines that they are supposed to relay to their children.

School-Age Children

School-age children are more independent than when they were toddlers. Having established a little more independence and confidence from exploring the world and facing new challenges and experiences, the school-age child will now have grown to make decisions on what to do when certain situations arise. These situations involve searching for a playmate or playing all alone when experiencing boredom. Toddlers will also be able to create their own simple, personal opinions, so an Alzheimer's patient must try to avoid the symptoms of irritability and aggravation discussed in chapter 4. By this point in time, the child will also be old enough to enroll in an educational institution. This new phase in life, wherein the child is expected to enter school, will bring new responsibilities to the parents in overseeing, preparing, and disciplining the child for an academic environment. The child will soon start forming friendships. These friendships and the child's ability to create his or her own opinion may lead to stigma (for the Alzheimer's disease), in both child and parent.

Alzheimer's patients at this stage of a child's growth are expected to encourage their child to interact with others and display appropriate social behaviors. This can pose a problem, since Alzheimer's disease patients are sometimes withdrawn from society, either because they are unable to conduct proper social behaviors or because they are afraid to expose their situation to the public. This would mean that Alzheimer's disease patients are unable to facilitate and encourage their children's social interactions. A large portion of the child's learning at this stage of growth is taken from participating and assisting in activities inside (household chores) and outside (outdoor games) of the home. Children enjoy being helpful and able. The child of an Alzheimer's disease patient may have decreased opportunities to learn from such activities as the patient is unable to participate in indoor or outdoor activities. Additionally, the Alzheimer's disease patient will have decreased opportunities to communicate and to offer guidance to the child.

Parents are expected to make responsible decisions about the future education of their child. When it comes to education, parents differ in their levels of involvement, with some parents becoming heavily involved in coordinating activities and early learning programs. Other parents choose to let the child grow with very few organized activities. Children normally begin to learn responsibility and consequences of their actions with the help of their parents. Parents also teach their children about hygiene, overall health, and eating habits through instruction and example. Parents who establish a good relationship and means of communication with their child at this stage in their child's life are usually able to maintain an excellent relationship with their children as they mature. The Alzheimer's disease patient will be unable to fully guide, or set an example for, their children due to the neurological symptoms displayed by the condition. The quality of their relationship with their children might be of poor quality.

Adolescence

Aspirations, identities, beliefs and values, career goals, and sexual orientations are shaped during the adolescent stage of growth. As such, adolescence is correctly labeled as the identity vs. role confusion stage or the fifth stage of Erik Erikson's Stages of Psychosocial Development.[4] Adolescents are heavily influenced by friends and adults outside of the family as guides and examples for their own behavior. Parents have to screen and look into the influences and activities coming into their child's life and often feel isolated and alone when parenting adolescents,[5] more so for an Alzheimer's patient who is already less involved with the development of his or her child. Patient might be unable to properly guide their children at a point in life that could drastically change the children's futures.

Simply put, the adolescent stage for offspring of the Alzheimer's disease patient is a high risk and volatile stage because children have a new level of freedom for themselves upon becoming a teen, and these decisions can drastically change their future for the better or worse. Children with lack of freedom in the previous stages of growth might become rebellious teenagers, making them difficult to deal with at this stage. Adolescents who are still trying to establish their own identity might not want to identify themselves with a parent who is an Alzheimer's disease sufferer, because teens might feel the parent's condition define their own futures. Regardless of the child's stage of development, whether an infant, toddler, school-age child, or an adolescent maturing into adulthood, it is always accompanied by a certain degree of difficulty for both parent and child, but it is always good to be optimistic and patient. It is important to keep in mind that the disease really affects both the parent and the child. The children will always be greatly concerned with the parent's condition and may also fear that they will develop the disease themselves. It is important for the parents to openly discuss their Alzheimer's-related symptoms and the future with the child, so they understanding each other and stay on common ground. Decisions regarding the disease that will affect the whole family need to be explained to the child if and when appropriate. Alzheimer's patients can join support groups and encourage their children to participate as well. For younger children, it may be a good idea to record thoughts, feelings, memories, and lessons that Alzheimer's disease patients want to pass on to their offspring. Patience and understanding is needed from both parent and child to develop and maintain a healthy parent-child relationship.

THINGS ONE CAN DO AT HOME TO TREAT ALZHEIMER'S

There are two modes of care for treating Alzheimer's disease patients; namely, pharmaceutical assistance and psychosocial intervention. This applies to all dementias including, but not limited to, Alzheimer's.[6] Pharmaceutical assistance and psychosocial intervention at home work in tandem. The medications have an increased excitatory effect on neurons, allowing continued function and delayed cognitive decline. Psychosocial interventions, on the other hand, provide adequate mental activity for the patient. Provision of adequate mental activity suitable for Alzheimer's disease patients is important as some tasks only serve to frustrate the sufferer.

Psychosocial Interventions

These interventions should be implemented in a day-to-day schedule, and home care should seriously be considered, with the guidance of a psychologist or an equivalent licensed medical professional. Psychosocial interventions can further be subdivided into behavioral, emotional, and cognitive interventions, and stimulation therapy. There are certain advantages in taking care of an Alzheimer's disease patient at home. Behavioral interventions involve close observation of the patient's behavior. An accurate account of the patient's behavior can be established in the home where the caregivers do not have to focus on a whole population of other patients that need to be observed. Emotional interventions involve invoked feelings of familiarity and security, usually through a conversation. These interventions also involve care at home, which greatly fosters these feelings. Cognitive interventions involve submitting the patient to simple puzzles and thinking exercises. This type of intervention requires minimal supervision, making it easy to practice at home. Stimulation therapy involves simple repetitive activities for recreational purposes and physical exercises. They are easily conducted at home or within the community. Various therapeutic activities can be done daily at home and in the community with relative ease, and some are usually implemented without realizing they are beneficial activities. However, there are day-to-day activities that are counterproductive for the Alzheimer's disease patient. Some beneficial and counterproductive activities will be discussed below.

Swimming

Recreational activities such as listening to music, arts and crafts, playing with pets, and various other activities and exercises are stimulatory activities beneficial for the patient. Recreational activities that have a repetitive and rhythmic nature induce a soothing feeling among Alzheimer's disease sufferers. They also establish variation in the Alzheimer's disease patient's routine, which is the central purpose of these therapies.[7] Swimming is an excellent form of exercise for an Alzheimer's disease patient among many other exercise options.

According to a factsheet, exercise metabolizes the adrenaline acquired from stress.[8] Exercise signals the brain to produce endorphins, which promotes a positive mood. That in turn increases energy levels, produces a healthy appetite, and promotes better sleep. Swimming provides a full body workout. The rhythmic nature of swimming and the sound and sensation of gliding through the cool water gives a calm and soothing feeling. This calm and soothing sensation is helpful in improving an Alzheimer's disease patient's mood. It can be an equally beneficial form of stress relief and physical exercise for anyone who accompanies the patient throughout the exercise. It is necessary for a significant other or guardian to accompany the patient in swimming and other physical exercises used in the patient's therapy as the patient's level of mental decline may lead to self-injury if left without guidance. Swimming is a valuable and very enjoyable activity for many Alzheimer's patients.

Reading

Reading is a daily activity that is taken for granted very easily. In fact, reading is an effective and versatile tool in therapy, especially for Alzheimer's disease patients. Reading sessions can be scheduled during the time of day when the patient seems regularly moody, as a calming and distracting activity; this makes it an option for behavioral therapy. Reading books can be a calming activity for a patient. When reading a favorite book from the past (or being read to by a close relative or friend), reading can provide feelings of security and familiarity as a form of emotional therapy. Also, depending on the level of reading and comprehension that the patient is still capable of and the type of book being read, reading offers varying levels of critical thinking and stimulation, making it a plausible cognitive intervention and venue for stimulation therapy. Alzheimer's disease patients in the early stages of the disease may still be capable of relating to books for their age group, but Alzheimer's disease sufferers in the later stages may only be able to comprehend books at the level of a child in second grade, and reading these books can be frustrating for some patients. Certain books that cater to Alzheimer's disease are written at a level that would make them appropriate for schoolchildren, yet the content and story line is suitable for elderly readers.

According to a landmark study, higher levels of literacy in the elderly made them less likely to develop Alzheimer's.[9] Reading books at home renders a more active brain.[10] The selected participants of this study possessed diaries detailing their personal histories, which were later evaluated. Those whose diaries contained higher idea density and grammatical skill had decreased chances of developing Alzheimer's. Maintaining heightened levels of literacy as people age can curb cognitive decline related to Alzheimer's and, as such, can be helpful in its treatment. Reading maintains literacy and is therefore useful in treating Alzheimer's. It should be noted that literacy is better achieved by reading early in life, making it a potent preventative measure against Alzheimer's later in life.

Too Much TV at Home

A study investigating the recreational habits of various elderly people at different points in their life has shed light on a relationship between watching television for extended hours and an increased likelihood of developing Alzheimer's.[11] Watching television is said to be a mind-numbing activity where the viewer is rendered into a semiconscious state, but it is not watching TV itself that increases the likelihood of developing Alzheimer's. Watching television serves as a distraction from much more productive physical or mental activities. Both physical and mental activities keep various parts of the brain active, and a decrease in such activities hinders the brain from developing further to prevent or delay the onset of Alzheimer's. Alzheimer's is not primarily caused by watching television. Instead, Alzheimer's is partially attributed to an inactive physical (or mental) lifestyle.

As an Alzheimer's disease patient, it is advisable to limit the hours of watching television.[12] Patients should watch programs that have short bursts of action or humor to induce a reaction, instead of shows with deep plots that can keep an Alzheimer's disease patient in a static state of mind. The patient should also be accompanied when watching television. Some Alzheimer's disease patients cannot discern what they see on television from reality, therefore it is best if they have adequate guidance.[13]

HOW TO DEAL WITH
ALZHEIMER'S-RELATED STRESS AT HOME

Stress is the human body's natural reaction to change. It is an important part of the adaptation process that the human body will have to go through to adjust to the changes and adversities it faces.[14] Stress can also be destructive if the body fails to adapt to the stress and adversities it is presented with. The same definition and effects of stress are applicable to the human body, as well as groups and units of human society such as family. Stress can trigger a myriad of emotions including fear, depression, confusion, and anger. It is therefore important that stress is addressed before it becomes a destructive factor. Stress relief can generally be attained in two ways: first, by finding a recreational activity to distract from the stressful issue at hand, and second, by tackling the issue causing stress through action or discussion. A blend of both is ideal to deal with stress; together, these methods help the patient adapt, which is a positive way to deal with stress.[15]

Inside the Minds of Family Members

The symptoms of the disease place the patient's family in a state of mind similar to a long goodbye. In lieu of an absolute cure, home-care options provide comfort and maintain functions the Alzheimer's patient might still be able to keep. As such, the family will have to provide years of care, and along the way as the patient displays another level of degeneration, it brings more stress and grieving. The patient will, one by one, forget (1) the names of those who are important parts of their own life, (2) why the people were important in the first place, and (3) the nature of the relationship the patient and significant others used to have. The Alzheimer's disease sufferer may not even want to see a doctor, be assisted, or be taken care of by relatives.

Alzheimer's disease can create major stresses in the family.[16] A person could even be famous, but that person's own parent who is an Alzheimer's disease sufferer would not take notice of their famous child when the latter enters a room. Family members would seem like complete strangers and would need to introduce themselves as a son, daughter, or significant other. The family members might want to talk to the Alzheimer's disease sufferer and discuss their day, but they find that the patient does not understand and that they can only give their love, care, and support instead. The family members can only accept the Alzheimer's victim for what they are. It is important to address conflicts in the family together to be able to concentrate on much more important issues regarding the care of the family member suffering from Alzheimer's.[17]

Conflicts at Home

Conflicts tend to be rampant as family members try to deal with various situations, whether in or out of the context of Alzheimer's disease. To reduce these conflicts, it is best to address the issues together with the patient. In a bid to minimize these conflicts, the following tips in dealing with family conflicts are advised.[18]

Responsibility   Each family member has his or her own life to live, but they all share the same burden and responsibility in caring for a family member with Alzheimer's.[19] It is important then to consider each family member's preferences, resources, and abilities.[20] Some family members may be able to be much more involved in the Alzheimer's disease patient's care, while others may be only available for emergent tasks such as household chores or errands, and some may only be able to handle financial responsibilities. It is important to keep in mind that each family member does want to help in the care within the limits of their daily schedules. It is important to organize and assign each one's capabilities to maximize resources for the benefit of the family member affected by Alzheimer's.

Meetings at Home   Alzheimer's is a progressively degenerative disease, and as the disease progresses, the treatment and care of the patient will undergo many changes and will need to be fine-tuned to proceed smoothly. The burden of caregiving can lead to misunderstandings within the family. It is then advisable to schedule regular face-to-face meetings of the family members, especially those who are part of the caregiving team and are directly responsible for the family member with Alzheimer's. Each person's caregiving responsibilities should be defined or redefined if needed. Each one should be able to voice any challenges or difficulties experienced in the caregiving process. If family meetings tend to turn into arguments, a counselor, social worker, or other professional can be asked to moderate. It is important to keep in mind that all this is done for the family member affected by the disease. This means the regular meetings are not a venue for bickering, imposition, or a show of superiority and inferiority. The goal of these meetings is to achieve a consensus that will be equally comfortable for all involved.

Zarit Burden Interview   The Zarit burden interview,[21] also called the Zarit burden inventory,[22] is a self-reporting questionnaire designed for caregivers of the elderly, which can include home-based caregivers helping out the Alzheimer's disease population. The questionnaire originally had twenty-nine questions and was later scaled down to twenty-two items. Each question requires a caregiver to respond to a series of statements with different levels of agreement. The options for responses range from "nearly always" to "never." This particular interview questionnaire reportedly has a somewhat unclear factor structure, and many researchers cite a particular two-factor model as the most accurate. These two addressed factors are designated the *role strain* and the *personal strain*.

The model of the Zarit burden inventory was endorsed by Réjean Hérbert, Gina Bravo, and Michel Préville in 2000. These researchers have so far provided information that is cited frequently as the most reliable existing data for the validity of this questionnaire. Their comprehensive study of 312 caregivers shows that the set of questions is reliable according to established statistical measurements.[23] The study examined common factors in scores based on criteria that are unrelated to employment or marital status, age, locale, language, or living situation. Ending statistical results showed a positive correlation between elderly adult patient behavior problems and adult caregiver rates of persistent depression. Criteria for measuring depression rates were taken from the Center for Epidemiological Studies Depression Scale.[24]

Questions from the Zarit burden survey are intended to measure caregivers' perceptions of the elderly patients in their care. Caregivers are asked if they regularly feel they are required to help more than necessary. They are also asked about the demands that their tasks place on their time, their daily stress levels, and any existing feelings of anger or embarrassment toward their charges. These attitudes have particular significance when the caregiver and patient are relatives.

Many respondents to this questionnaire reveal uncertainty about their relative's futures and feelings of resentment over lost privacy or strained relationships with other family members. Increased senses of dependency and mental stress are often key contributing factors to a heightened likelihood of depression. Topics covered in the survey include the following:

- Lack of control over life due to the relative's condition
- Wish to hand over the care of the relative to someone else
- A frequent sense of uncertainty about what to do with the relative from one day to the next
- Doing a poor job of taking care of the relative
- Life becoming unmanageable or even uncontrollable since taking care of the relative
- The need to be doing more for the relative
- A frequent sense of being burdened with the responsibility for the relative
- Feeling that the care of the relative has become a financial strain on available resources
- Feeling one's social life has declined since caring for the patient
- Feeling unspoken tension around the relative
- Feeling the relative is more dependent on one than before
- Feeling the relative would not accept help from anyone else besides oneself, the designated caregiver

The overall purpose of the Zarit burden interview is to gauge when a situation is becoming negative for both a caregiver and the elderly relative who is no longer able to function fully independently due to an ailment such as Alzheimer's disease. Caring for a relative can have unintended effects on the mental health of the caregiver in many cases, leading to increased chances of further problems for both.

SUMMARY

The treatment of Alzheimer's at home is a viable option to consider when taking into account the sense of isolation some patients have. Home-based approaches apply sensible and involved managements to treat the disease. However, home care should not be confused as an independent mode of treatment. Home care for an Alzheimer's disease patient is done in conjunction with the advice and prescriptions of an appropriate licensed medical professional so the symptoms can be dealt with safely and appropriately within the home. Alzheimer's disease has a variety of symptoms, levels of degeneration, and speeds at which the disease progresses. This means that the modes and options for management or treatment will also need to be varied. The descriptions, treatment guides, and options described in this chapter are offered as a general discussion of Alzheimer's and may not necessarily reflect the current status of every Alzheimer's disease sufferer.

· *20* ·

Conclusion

$\mathcal{A}$s the end of this comprehensive journey to uncover Alzheimer's disease nears, the reader should now understand that this disease is a problem in the brain wherein the memory of a person decreases gradually until he or she is unable to properly reason, communicate, and learn. The disease also prevents them from properly completing daily tasks. People who have Alzheimer's suffer from hallucinations, abnormal patterns in behavior, and anxiety. Patients also have difficulty performing basic tasks and could even cause danger and harm to themselves.[1] Furthermore, there is no drug that can cure Alzheimer's. All the above factors comprise the reason that (1) hope, (2) patience, and (3) confidence are needed when dealing with Alzheimer's disease.

IN LIGHT OF HOPE

Getting diagnosed does not mean the end of the world. Even after the disease has been identified in a person, "life goes on." Patients and caregivers are still breathing, and the life that they still have should never be wasted. They still have the chance to be with their loved ones and to enjoy life. Alzheimer's disease is degenerative and irreversible, but that is not valid reason to surrender to it. Patients must have faith in delaying the progression of the diseases in order to continue carrying the beacon of hope.

In the end, however, the patient cannot deal with the disease alone.[2] Alzheimer's disease victims need their families, loved ones, friends, and other significant people to be with them, especially when times are difficult. Relatives of people suffering from Alzheimer's must not forget to show their care and support. A simple hug or a tap on the shoulder works wonders when it comes to providing hope.

IMPORTANCE OF PATIENCE

Sincere appreciation of what an Alzheimer's patient is able to do successfully should be present throughout the course of treatment. It is usual for patients to feel despair, isolation, and frustration, so it is critical they receive constant appreciation and care from family members and loved ones. However, verbal dishonesty needs to be avoided, since offering sufferers unrealistic hopes and burdening them with falsehood will not help their problems and will only hinder their abilities to build patience.[3] In the end, Alzheimer's disease victims could inadvertently feel they are a burden and cause deterioration to their own physical health. Patience is important for tending to the physical needs of elderly patients since these patients are very much dependent and vulnerable.[4]

All in all, patience is needed because there are times when patients will do irritating things they themselves might not be aware of.[5] The caregiver should remain calm and try to keep the patient's environment quiet and away from loud noises. It is easy to feel tired, frustrated, or angry for both patient and family.[6]

Alzheimer's disease is a devastating disorder, robbing the patient of memory and the ability to communicate and understand. For people who take care of patients with Alzheimer's, it can often be very difficult to let that person know that the best is wanted for them. Sometimes, even the best caregivers will feel frustrated that their efforts do not always seem to have the right results. Patients also need to be assisted when they go to the bathroom and when they are eating and drinking. When a patient is wandering, it is a sign that he or she needs something. Involving the patient in some form of physical activity helps.[7] Patients can play board games or go out for a light walk. These activities help keep their mind off distress. As a result, they feel the relaxation needed to develop the patience to address their problems.

An end-stage Alzheimer's disease patient would have lost control over many elements in life. Alzheimer's disease affects the cognitive powers of an individual. As such, he or she may lose the ability to remember objects, people, and events. The patient may also forget the right words needed to communicate properly. In spite of all this, developing patience is not impossible. The key to remember when helping a person with Alzheimer's disease to develop patience is that the sufferer is not at fault. Try as they might, patients may not have the ability to say, think, or do whatever it is they want to do. Their medical status is not the result of stubbornness or the refusal to communicate—it is just that the patients have simply lost the ability to act and do as they once did.

The caregiver should remember what the patient means to him or her at all times. The person suffering from Alzheimer's may be a family member, a friend, a colleague, or simply a stranger who has become a patient. Regardless, it would help if the caregiver remembers the relationship with that person and how he or she feels about the patient. If it is the mother, for example, the caregiver should keep in mind how much they love her and care about her well-being. Since the caregiver wants only the best for her, it is the gift of patience that she will need most.

Caregivers should remember the professional background of the person. Alzheimer's disease can strike anyone—a housewife, a teacher, an athlete, and even a scientist. The disease changes the way the person behaves, and such a change can be difficult to accept for people providing care. When developing the patience needed to approach Alzheimer's, one must keep in mind that the person who now sits in the corner not remembering much is still a person, albeit a different one in the context of mental capabilities. An Alzheimer's disease victim is still someone's child, brother, sister, father, mother, or friend who needs everyone's understanding.

CONFIDENCE

Caregivers who are in charge of a patient with Alzheimer's disease need to have confidence in order to develop and follow a regular, everyday routine. Such routines need not be set in stone. Activities can be flexible according to the patient's condition. Consistency is important, and familiarity and structure are equally critical. The time a patient wakes up, bathes, eats, dresses, sleeps, and receives visitors must be consistent each day as these help patients remain oriented. The caregiver should also allow the patient to know what he or she is to expect. For instance, an open curtain in the morning means that the day is about to begin. In the evening, putting on quiet music could be used as a reminder that it is time to sleep. Caregivers could help patients tie their shoes or place their clothes into a hamper.

Body Language and Communication

Research suggests that body language is very important when addressing Alzheimer's disease.[8] Incidentally, understanding people's body language helps to build confidence in both patients and caregivers of virtually any illness.[9]

Eye contact should be practiced as much as possible. The caregiver should try to relax by taking deep breaths if he or she feels tense, irritated, or anxious. Unnecessary tension could make the patient feel more flustered. Taking deep breaths can help make everyone feel at ease. If the caregiver feels relaxed, it is highly likely that the patient will feel more confident. As Alzheimer's develops, physicians and other caregivers might notice a change in the way a patient communicates.[10] Patients might have difficulty finding words and be confused easily. When this happens, the caregiver should call the patient by his or her name and ask only a single question at a time while giving the patient enough time to respond. Questions should be repeated gently. Paying attention to the patient's body language is important. As the disease progresses and patients cannot remember the name of an object, the caregiver should encourage the patient to gesture or point to the object instead.[11]

All in all, it is important for caregivers and family members to have confidence when they feel overwhelmed by any difficult behaviors a patient is prone to expressing. Caregivers should feel free to ask for support and help from medical teams or to reach out to fellow caregivers for support.

How to Develop Confidence

Alzheimer's disease can be a difficult disease to deal with. It is truly challenging, not only for the person experiencing it but also for the caregivers. Some patients with Alzheimer's live in a home where they can receive professional, specialized care, while others still manage at home with their family and friends helping to look after them. Regardless, both patient and caregiver need to understand how to appropriately live when there is a disease this challenging involved. The two essential steps in gaining confidence are (1) learning how to develop and maintain self-control and (2) learning to avoid getting stressed out and overwhelmed by the situation. As patients deal with Alzheimer's, the disease progresses and they begin to feel more symptoms directly associated with the disease. Life becomes more difficult, and the patients can feel sad, lonely, depressed, confused, and even helpless. They may also feel so troubled and emotional because there are things going on with their bodies they are generally unable to control. In order to start building confidence and to keep confidence levels high, Alzheimer's disease victims first need to research the disease. The more patients read and find out information on the disease, the more in control they will feel. Patients start to understand the different symptoms and why they are experiencing them, which in turn helps them to (1) develop confidence and (2) come to terms with what they are feeling and dealing with at such a point in life.[12]

Field studies conclude that community awareness and knowledge about Alzheimer's in the general population are not too great.[13] When it comes to building confidence, it is important that caregivers have a firm grasp on the disease and try their best to understand what the patient is feeling. Patients do not necessarily need caregivers to exhibit pity or sadness toward them, but rather, Alzheimer's disease sufferers need caregivers to be there to support, help, and let them know they are not alone. Whether a person is a family member or a professional caregiver hired to take care of the patient, there must be kindness, caring, and understanding. Together with confidence and control, someone suffering from Alzheimer's can live the happiest, healthiest life possible.

THE FAREWELL

In the final analysis, it is important that patients consult with the appropriate, licensed medical practitioner for specific details on a course of treatment appropriate for each individual patient. This avoids any misunderstandings and complications. As an additional reminder, Alzheimer's disease sufferers and caregivers should get second opinions before accepting any management or any variations thereof in a set treatment course. Doing so along with motivation, patience, and confidence will allow patients and caregivers to understand fully the nature of Alzheimer's disease.

Appendix A:
Alzheimer's Disease-Related Links

www.ahaf.org/alzheimers/about
www.ahaf.org/alzheimers/resources/memorygames.html
www.alz.org/alzheimers_disease_what_is_alzheimers.asp
www.alzfdn.org/
www.alzheimerbc.org/
www.alzheimers.org.au/understanding-dementia/alzheimers-disease.aspx
www.alzheimers.org.uk/site/scripts/documents.php?categoryID=200120
www.alzheimersdisease.com/
www.alzheimers-disease.net/
www.alzresearch.org/tensigns.cfm
www.bupa.co.uk/individuals/health-information/directory/a/alzheimers-disease
www.cdc.gov/features/Alzheimers/index.html
www.chestandards.org/diseases/alzheimer-disease-information.html
www.diet-and-health.net/diseases/alzheimerdiseaseinformation.html
www.emedicinehealth.com/alzheimer_disease/article_em.htm
www.mayoclinic.com/health/alzheimers-disease/DS00161
www.medicinenet.com/alzheimers/focus.htm
www.medicinenet.com/alzheimers_disease_causes_stages_and_symptoms/
    page4.htm#risk
www.medterms.com/script/main/art.asp?articlekey=2940
www.nia.nih.gov/Alzheimers
www.ncbi.nlm.nih.gov/pubmedhealth/PMH0001767
www.ninds.nih.gov/disorders/alzheimersdisease/alzheimersdisease.html
www.northernstar.com.au/story/2011/08/18/laugh-off-your-alzheimers
www.psychcentral.com/lib/2006/areas-of-research-into-alzheimers-disease
www.utsouthwestern.edu/utsw/cda/dept23589/files/46161.html

Appendix B:
Research and Training

Aging and Alzheimer's Disease Center
Oregon Health and Science University
3181 SW Sam Jackson Park Rd.
Portland, OR 97239
(503) 494-6695
www.ohsu.edu/research/alzheimers

Alzheimer's Disease Center
Bolton University
VA Boston Healthcare System
Neurology Service (127)
150 South Huntington Ave.
Boston, MA 02130
(888) 458-2823
www.bu.edu/alzresearch

Alzheimer's Disease Center
Emory University
Wesley Woods Health Center, 3rd Floor
1841 Clifton Rd.
Atlanta, GA 30329
(404) 728-6950
www.med.emory.edu/ADC

Alzheimer's Disease Center
Ralston House
3615 Chestnut Street
Philadelphia, PA 19104
(215) 662-7810
jason.karlawish@uphs.upenn.edu
www.uphs.upenn.edu/ADC

Alzheimer's Disease Center
Rush University Medical Center
Armour Academic Center
600 South Paulina St. Suite 1028
Chicago, IL 60612
(312) 942-3333
www.rush.edu/radc

Alzheimer's Disease Center
University of California, Davis Medical Center
4860 Y St. Suite 3700
Sacramento, CA 95817
(916) 734-5496
Fax: (916) 703-5290
www.alzheimer.ucdavis.edu

Alzheimer's Disease Cooperative Study (ADCS)
University of California, San Diego
9500 Gilman Dr.
La Jolla, CA 92093
(858) 622-5880
brainlink@ucsd.edu
www.adcs.org

Alzheimer's Disease Education and Referral Center (ADEAR)
National Institute on Aging
P.O. Box 8250
Silver Spring, MD 20907
(800) 438-4380
Fax: (301) 495-3334
adear@nia.nih.gov
www.alzheimers.nia.nih.gov

Alzheimer's Disease Research Center
Harvard University
Massachusetts General Hospital
114 16th St. Room 2009
Charlestown, MA 02129
(617) 726-3987
www.madrc.org

Alzheimer's Disease Research Center
Johns Hopkins University
Department of Pathology
Ross 558
720 Rutland Ave.
Baltimore, MD 21205
(410) 502-5164
Fax: (410) 955-9777
edelman1@jhmi.edu

Alzheimer's Disease Research Center
Mount Sinai School of Medicine
One Gustave Levy Place, Box 1230
New York, NY 10029
(212) 241-8329

Alzheimer's Disease Research Center
University of California, Irvine
Gillespie Neuroscience Research Facility, Rm. 1113
Irvine, CA 92697
(949) 824-5847
Fax: (949) 824-2071
www.alz.uci.edu

Alzheimer's Disease Research Center
University of California, Los Angeles
10911 Weyburn Ave. Ste. 200
Los Angeles, CA 90095
(310) 794-3665
www.eastonAD.ucla.edu

Alzheimer's Disease Research Center
University of California, San Diego
Department of Neurosciences
UCSD School of Medicine
9500 Gilman Dr.
La Jolla, CA 92093
(858) 622-5800
www.adrc.ucsd.edu

Alzheimer's Disease Research Center
University of California, San Francisco
350 Parnassus Ave. Suite 905
San Francisco, CA 94143
(415) 476-6880
www.memory.ucsf.edu

Alzheimer's Disease Research Center
University of Michigan
Department of Neurology
2101 Commonwealth, Suite D
Ann Arbor, MI 48105
(734) 936-8281
www.med.umich.edu/alzheimers

Alzheimer's Disease Research Center
University of Pittsburgh
Department of Neurology
3501 Forbes Ave, Suite 830
Pittsburgh, PA 15213
(412) 692-2700
www.adrc.pitt.edu

Alzheimer's Disease Research Center
University of Southern California
Health Consultation Center
1510 San Pablo St. HCC643
Los Angeles, CA 90033
www.usc.edu/dept/gero/ADRC
(323) 442-7600

Alzheimer's Disease Research Center
Washington University School of Medicine
Department of Neurology
4488 Forest Park Ave., Suite 130
St. Louis, MO 63108-2293
(314) 286-2881
www.alzheimer.wustl.edu

Alzheimer's Disease Training for Police
43 Thorndike St., 2nd Floor
Cambridge, MA 02141
(800) 234-0056
Fax: (617) 354-6515
info@apbweb.com
www.apbweb.com/about-apb.html

Alzheimer's Research and Prevention Foundation
6300 E. El Dorado Plaza, Suite 400
Tucson, AZ 85715
(888) 908-5766
Fax: (520) 296-6640

American Academy of Neurology
1080 Montreal Ave.
Saint Paul, MN 55116
(800) 879-1960
Fax: (651) 695-2791
memberservices@aan.com

Arizona Alzheimer's Disease Center/Sun Health Research Institute
Banner Alzheimer's Institute
901 E. Willeta St.
Phoenix, AZ 85006
(602) 239-6500
www.azalz.org

Charles F. and Joanne Knight Alzheimer's Disease Research Center
Washington University School of Medicine
4488 Forest Park
St Louis, MO 63108
(314) 286-2683

Cognitive Neurology and Alzheimer's Disease Center
Feinberg School of Medicine
Northwestern University
675 N St. Claire, Galter 20-100
Chicago, IL 60611
(312) 926-1851
www.brain.northwestern.edu

Columbia University Alzheimer's Disease Center
630 West 168th St. P&S 15-402
New York, NY 10032
(212) 305-2077
www.alzheimercenter.org

Division of Behavioral and Social Research (DBSR)
National Institute on Aging
Gateway Building, Suite 533
7201 Wisconsin Ave., MSC 9205
Bethesda, MD 20892-9205
(301) 496-3131
bsrquery@nia.nih.gov

Division of Geriatrics and Clinical Gerontology (DGCG)
National Institute on Aging
Gateway Building, Suite 3C307
7201 Wisconsin Ave., MSC 9205
Bethesda, MD 20892-9205
(301) 496-6761
gcgquery@nia.nih.gov

Division of Neuroscience (DN)
National Institute on Aging
Gateway Building, Suite 350
7201 Wisconsin Ave., MSC 9205
Bethesda, MD 20892
(301) 496-9350
nnaquery@nia.nih.gov

Fisher Center for Alzheimer's Research Foundation
1 Intrepid Square W. 46th St.
New York, NY 10036
(800) ALZINFO (259-4636)
Fax: (646) 381-5159
info@alzinfo.org

Florida Alzheimer's Disease Research Center
Byrd Alzheimer's Institute
4001 East Fletcher Ave.
Tampa, FL 33613
(866) 700-7773
www.floridaadrc.org

Indiana Alzheimer Disease Center
Department of Pathology and Lab Medicine
Indiana University School of Medicine
635 Barnhill Dr., MS-A-138
Indianapolis, IN 46202
(317) 274-1590
www.iadc.iupui.edu

Joseph and Kathleen Bryan Alzheimer's Disease Research Center
Duke University Medical Center
2200 West Main St.
Suite A-200
Durham, NC 27705
(866) 444-2372
www.adrc.mc.duke.edu

Mayo Clinic Alzheimer's Disease Research Center
4111 Highway 52 North
Rochester, MN 55901
(507) 284-1324

Medifecta Healthcare Training
A Division of Health Care Training Systems, Inc.
1911 United Way
Medford, OR 97504
(888) 846-7008
Fax: (541) 858-6696
info@medifecta.com

National Alzheimer's Coordinating Center
4311 11th Ave. NE, #300
Seattle, WA 98105
(206) 543-8637
Fax: (206) 616-5927
naccmail@u.washington.edu
www.alz.washington.edu

National Cell Repository for Alzheimer's Disease
975 West Walnut St. Room IB-130
Indianapolis, IN 46202-5251
(800) 526-2839
Fax: (317) 274-2387
alzstudy@iupui.edu
www.ncrad.org

National Council of Certified Dementia Practitioners, LLC
103 Valley View Trail
Sparta, NJ 07871
(877) 729-5191
Fax: (973) 860-2244
www.nccdp.org

National Institute on Aging
Building 31, Room 5C27
31 Center Dr., MSC 2292
Bethesda, MD 20892
(800) 222-4225
Fax: (301) 496-1072

Taub Institute for Research in Alzheimer's Disease and the Aging Brain
Columbia University Medical Center
630 West 168th St., P&S Box 16
New York, NY 10032
(212) 305-1818
Fax: (212) 342-2849
tabinstitute@columbia.edu

University of Kentucky Alzheimer's Disease Center
Sanders-Brown Center on Aging, Rm. 101
800 South Limestone St.
Lexington, KY 40536
(859) 323-6040
Fax: (859) 323-2866
www.centeronaging.uky.edu

University of Wisconsin Alzheimer's Disease Center
2500 Overlook Terrace
GRECC 11G
Madison, WI 53705
(866) 636-7764
www.wcmp.wisc.edu

Appendix C:
Alzheimer's Disease Organizations

Alzheimer's Association
225 North Michigan Ave.
Floor 17
Chicago, IL 60601
(800) 272-3900
Fax: (866) 699-1246
info@alz.org
www.alz.org

Alzheimer's Foundation of America
322 Eighth Ave.
7th Floor
New York, NY 10001
(866) AFA-8484
Fax: (646) 638-1546
info@alzfdn.org
www.alzfdn.org

Alzheimer's Care Resource Center, Inc.
2328 10th Ave N #601
Lake Worth, FL 33461
(561) 585-0400

Alzheimer's Disease and Related Disorders Association
1850 York Rd. Suite D
Timonium, MD 21093
(800) 272-3900

Alzheimer's Disease Education and Referral Center (ADEAR)
National Institute on Aging
P.O. Box 8250
Silver Spring, MD 20907
(800) 438-4380
Fax: (301) 495-3334
adear@nia.nih.gov
www.alzheimers.nia.nih.gov

Alzheimer's Disease and Related Disorders Association of Victoria (Australia)
98-104 Riversdale Rd
Hawthorn (Melbourne), Victoria 3122
Australia
(03) 9815 5738
Fax: (03) 9815 7801

Alzheimer's Disease International
64 Great Suffolk St. London
SE1 0BL UK
44 (0) 20 79810880
Fax: 44 (0) 20 79282357
info@alz.co.uk

Alzheimer's Drug Discovery Foundation
57 West 57th St.
Suite 904
New York, NY 10019
(212) 901-8000
Fax: (212) 901-8010
info@alzdiscovery.org
www.alzdiscovery.org

Alzheimer's Family Organization
P.O. Box 1939
New Port Richey, FL 34656
(888) 496-8004

Alzheimer Society of British Columbia
300-828 West 8th Ave.
Vancouver, BC V5Z 1E2

Canada
(800) 667-3742
Fax: (604) 669-6907
info@alzheimerbc.org

Alzheimer Society of Calgary
(403) 290-0110
www.alzheimercalgary.com/alzheimercalgary/research

Alzheimer Society of Canada
20 Eglinton Ave. W. Ste. 1600
Toronto, ON M4R 1K8
(800) 616-8816
Fax: (416) 322-6656
info@alzheimer.ca

Alzheimer Society of Manitoba
10-120 Donald St.
Winnipeg, MB
R3C 4G2
(204) 943-6622
Fax: (204) 942-5408
alzmb@alzheimer.mb.ca

Alzheimer's Society
58 St. Katharine's Way
London E1W 1LB
44 (0) 20 7423 3500
Fax: 44 (020) 7423 3501
enquiries@alzheimers.org.uk
www.alzheimers.org.uk
www.alzfdn.org

Alzheimer's Society, Devon House
58 St. Katharine's Way
London E1W 1LB
44 (0) 20 7423 3500
Fax: 44 (02) 7423 3501
enquiries@alzheimers.org.uk

Alzheimer's Society, London and Middlesex
435 Windermere Rd.
London, ON N5X 2T1
Canada
(888) 495-5855
Fax: (519) 680-2864

American Health Assistance Foundation
22512 Gateway Center Dr.
Clarksburg, MD 20871
(301) 948-3244 / (800) 437-AHAF (2423)
Fax: (301) 258-9454
info@ahaf.org
www.ahaf.org/alzheimers

Association for Frontotemporal Degeneration (AFTD)
Radnor Station Building #2, Suite 320
290 King of Prussia Rd.
Radnor, PA 19087
(866) 507-7222
info@theaftd.org
www.theaftd.org

Family Caregiver Alliance/National Center on Caregiving
180 Montgomery St.
Suite 900
San Francisco, CA 94104
(800) 445-8106
Fax: (415) 434-3508
info@caregiver.org
www.caregiver.org

John Douglas French Alzheimer's Foundation
11620 Wilshire Blvd.
Suite 270
Los Angeles, CA 90025
(310) 445-4650
Fax: (310) 479-0516
www.jdfaf.org

Lewy Body Dementia Association
912 Killian Hill Rd. SW
Lilburn, GA 30047
(800) 539-9767
Fax: (480) 422-5434
lbda@lbda.org
www.lbda.org

National Family Caregivers Association
10400 Connecticut Ave.
Suite 500
Kensington, MD 20895
(800) 896-3650
Fax: (301) 942-2302
info@thefamilycaregiver.org
www.thefamilycaregiver.org

National Hospice and Palliative Care Organization/National Hospice Foundation
1731 King St.
Alexandria, VA 22314
(800) 658-8898
Fax: (703) 837-1233
nhpco_info@nhpco.org
www.nhpco.org

National Institute of Mental Health (NIMH)
National Institutes of Health, DHHS
6001 Executive Blvd., Rm. 8184, MSC 9663
Bethesda, MD 20892
(866) 415-8051
Fax: (301) 443-4279
nimhinfo@nih.gov
www.nimh.nih.gov

National Organization for Rare Disorders (NORD)
P.O. Box 1968
55 Kenosia Ave.
Danbury, CT 06813
(800) 999-NORD (6673)
Fax: (203) 798-2291

orphan@rarediseases.org
www.rarediseases.org

National Respite Network and Resource Center
800 Eastowne Dr.
Suite 105
Chapel Hill, NC 27514
(919) 490-5577 x222
Fax: (919) 490-4905
www.archrespite.org

Well Spouse Association
63 West Main St., Suite H
Freehold, NJ 07728
(800) 838-0879
Fax: (732) 577-8644
info@wellspouse.org
www.wellspouse.org

Appendix D:
Nationally Recognized
Alzheimer's Clinics

Albert Einstein College of Medicine, Department of Neurology
Russo Building, Third Floor
1165 Morris Park Ave.
Bronx, NY 10461
(718) 405-8140
Fax: (718) 430-3851

Alois Alzheimer Center
70 Damon Rd.
Cincinnati, OH 45218
(513) 605-1000

Alzheimer's Disease and Memory Disorders Center
2160 South First Ave.
Maywood, IL 60153
(708) 216-5710

Alzheimer's Disease Assistance Center of Long Island
Health Sciences Center T10
East Loop Rd.
Stony Brook, NY 11794
(516) 444-1365

Alzheimer's Disease Center
CR 131, Oregon Health Sciences University
3181 SW Sam Jackson Park Rd.
Portland, OR 97201
(503) 494-6976

Alzheimer's Disease Center, Center for Aging and Developmental Biology
University of Rochester Medical Center
601 Elmwood Ave.
Box 645
Rochester, NY 14642
(585) 275-2581

Alzheimer's Disease Center, Bedford Veterans Administration Center
200 Springs Rd.
Bedford, MA 01730
(781) 687-2632

Alzheimer's Disease Center, Memory Disorders Clinic
Penn-Ralston Center
3615 Chestnut St.
Philadelphia, PA 19104
(215) 662-7810

Alzheimer's Disease Center, University of Pittsburgh
4-West Montefiore University Hospital
200 Lothrop St.
Pittsburgh, PA 15213
(412) 692-2700

Behavioral Neuroscience and Alzheimer's Clinic
1501 North Campbell Ave.
Room 7319
Tucson, AZ 85724
(520) 626-6524

Cleveland University Alzheimer Center
12220 Fairhill Rd.
Cleveland, OH 44120
(800) 252-5048

Cognitive Neurology and Alzheimer's Disease Center
320 East Superior St.
Chicago, IL 60611
(312) 908-9339
Fax: (312) 908-8789

Columbia Presbyterian Medical Center, Memory Disorders Center
722 West 168th St.
Unit 72, Room 1120
New York, NY 10032
(212) 305-6939

Copper Ridge Clinic
710 Obrecht Rd.
Sykesville, MD 21784
(410) 552-3211

Dean Health System Memory Clinic
700 S. Park St.
Madison, WI 53715
(608) 260-3425

Department of Psychiatry, Memory Disorder Center, Mount Sinai School of Medicine
One Gustave L. Levy Place
New York, NY 10029
(212) 241-9382

Duluth Clinic
Third St. Building
400 East Third St
Duluth, MN
(218) 786-1216
www.duluthclinic.org/otherspecialties/eldercare/eldercare.htm

Fairview Crosstown Clinic, Dementia Assessment Clinic
6545 France Ave.
Edina, MN 55435
(952) 848-5545

Georgia Neurological Institute
4750 Waters Ave.
Savannah, GA 31404
(912) 350-3355

Geriatric Psychiatry Program Memory Clinic
Harvard Institutes of Medicine
77 Louis Pasteur Ave., Room 645
Boston, MA 02115
(617) 726-1276
Fax: (617) 724-1480
jmontana@partners.org

**Geriatric Research and Education Clinic Center Memory Assessment/
Dementia Clinic**
2500 Overlook Terrace
Madison, WI 53705
(608) 280-7000

Guthrie Healthcare System Memory Clinic
One Guthrie Square
Sayre, PA 18840
(570) 882-3107

Hillside Hospital/Long Island Jewish Medical Center
Center for Mental Health Services
Lowenstein Research Building
P.O. Box 38
Glen Oaks, NY 11004
(718) 470-8140

Indiana Alzheimer's Disease Center
Indiana University School of Medicine,
Department of Pathology and Laboratory Medicine,
635 Barnhill Dr. MS-A142
Indianapolis, IN 46202
(317) 278-2030

Institute for Brain Aging and Dementia, Memory Assessment Clinic
Gottschalk Medical Plaza
1100 Medical Plaza Dr. Room 1100
Irvine, CA 92697
(949) 824-2382

Maimonides Medical Center
4802 10th Ave.
Brooklyn, NY 11219
(718) 283-7470
Fax: (718) 283-8836

Marshfield Clinic, Indianhead Center
Marshfield Clinic Lakewoods Family Center
1215 W. Knapp St.
Rice Lake, WI 54868
(866) 333-1996
www.marshfieldclinic.org

Memory and Alzheimer's Treatment Center
Johns Hopkins Bayview Medical Center
5300 Alpha Commons Dr.
Baltimore, MD 21224

Memory Assessment Clinic
Moundview Hospital and Clinic
402 West Lake St.
P.O. Box 41
Friendship, WI 53934
(608) 839-8360

Memory Assessment Clinic and Eldercare Resource Center
2360 Sweeten Creek Rd.
Asheville, NC 28803
(828) 771-2219

Memory Diagnostic Center, Teal Lake Medical Center
Marquette General Hospital
420 West Magnetic St.
Marquette, MI 49855
(800) 562-9753 ext. 3993

Memory Disorder Center, Medical College of Pennsylvania
Department of Neurology
3300 Henry Ave.
Philadelphia, PA 19129
(215) 842-7151

Michigan Alzheimer's Disease Research Center
300 North Ingalls, Room 3D03
Ann Arbor, MI 48109
(734) 764-2190

Milwaukee Health Services
MLK Heritage Health Center
2555 N. Dr. Martin Luther King Jr. Dr.
Milwaukee, WI 53212
(414) 372-8080

Mission Medical Center in Tijuana
4492 Camino de la Plaza, Suite 362
San Ysidro, CA 92173
(619) 662-1578

Montefiore Medical Center
Division of Geriatric Medicine
3400 Bainbridge Ave., 2nd Floor
Bronx, NY 10467
(718) 920-6721

Neuroscience Group of Northeast Wisconsin
1305 W. American Dr.
Neenah, WI 54956
(920) 725-9373

North Broward Memory Disorder Center
201 East Sample Rd.
Pompano Beach, FL 33064
(954) 786-7392

Northeast Rehabilitation Health Network Memory Disorders Clinic
70 Butler St.
Salem, NH 03079
(603) 893-2900, ext. 728
Fax: (603) 893-1628

NYU Langone Medical Center
Center of Excellence on Brain Aging
145 E 32nd St, 5th Floor
New York, NY 10016

(212) 263-8088
www.med.nyu.edu/adc

NYU Silberstein Aging and Dementia Research Center
New York University School of Medicine
550 First Ave., Room 314
New York, NY 10016
(212) 263-8088

Ocala Neurodiagnostic Center
1901 SE 18th Ave., Building 400-A
Ocala, FL 34471
(352) 732-7095

Orlando Neurological Services of Orlando
1111 South Orange Ave.
Suite 300
Orlando, FL 32806
(407) 540-1774

Orlando Regional Memory Disorder Clinic
818 Main Lane
Orlando, FL 32801
(407) 244-3281
Fax: (407) 244-3285

Sanders-Brown Research Center on Aging, University of Kentucky
101 Sanders-Brown Building
Lexington, KY 40536
(859) 323-6040

San Francisco Alzheimer's and Dementia Clinic
909 Hyde St., Suite 322
San Francisco, CA 94109
(415) 673-4600
Fax: (415) 673-9532

Sioux Valley Neuroscience Center, Memory Disorders Clinic
1305 West 18th St.
Sioux Falls, SD 57117
(605) 333-4567

Southern Illinois University Center for Alzheimer's Disease and Related Disorders
P.O. Box 19643
Springfield, IL 62794
(217) 545-8249
Fax: (217) 545-1903

St. Luke's Roosevelt Hospital Center, Division of Geriatric Medicine
1111 Amsterdam Ave.
New York, NY 10025
(212) 523-5934

St. Rita's Medical Center Memory Disorders Clinic
730 West Market St.
Lima, OH 45801
(419) 227-3361

UCSF Memory and Aging Center
350 Parnassus Ave.
Suite 706
San Francisco, CA 94143
(415) 476-6880

University of Florida Memory Disorder Clinic
McKnight Brain Institute
Box 100236
Gainesville, FL 32610
(352) 392-3491

University of Georgia Memory Assessment Clinic
255 East Hancock Ave.
Athens, GA 30602
(706) 542-1173

University of Wisconsin Health Clinics Geriatric Assessment Clinic (East)
5249 E. Terrace Dr.
Madison, WI 53718
(800) 323-8942

University of Wisconsin Health Neurology Memory Disorders Clinic
600 Highland Ave.
Madison, WI 53792
(608) 263-5442

VGH and UBC Hospital Foundation
Vancouver Coastal Health
855 West 12th Ave.
Vancouver, BC V5Z 1M9

Wien Center, Mount Sinai Medical Center
4300 Alton Rd.
Miami Beach, FL 33140
(305) 674-2543

Appendix E:
Selected Studies

Abhorring the Vacuum: Use of Alzheimer's Disease Medications in Fronto-temporal Dementia
Stanford Center for Memory Disorders, Stanford University Medical Center, 300 Pasteur Dr. Room A343, Stanford, CA 94305-5235. kerchner@stanford .edu, May 2011.
www.ncbi.nlm.nih.gov/pubmed/21728274

The Accuracy of the Clock Drawing Test Compared to That of Standard Screening Tests for Alzheimer's Disease: Results from a Study of Brazilian with Heterogeneous Educational Background
Gerontology Division, University of Campinas, São Paulo, Brazil. ivan.apra-hamian@terra.com.br. February 2010.
www.ncbi.nlm.nih.gov/pubmed/19814841

Altered Functional Connectivity in Early Alzheimer's Disease: A Resting-State fMRI Study
National Laboratory of Pattern Recognition, Institute of Automation, Chinese Academy of Sciences, Beijing, People's Republic of China. October 2007.
www.ncbi.nlm.nih.gov/pubmed/17133390

Alzheimer's Diagnostic Guidelines Updated for First Time in Decades
www.nia.nih.gov/Alzheimers/ResearchInformation/NewsReleases/PR-20110419guidelines.htm

Alzheimer's Disease Neuroimaging Initiative Enters Next Phase of Research
www.nia.nih.gov/Alzheimers/ResearchInformation/NewsReleases/PR 20101021ADNI.htm

Amyloid Deposits in Cognitively Normal People May Predict Risk for Alzheimer's Disease
www.nia.nih.gov/Alzheimers/ResearchInformation/NewsReleases

Antidepressant Treatment in Alzheimer's Disease
Brain and Ageing Research Program and Primary Dementia Collaborative Research Centre, School of Psychiatry, Faculty of Medicine, University of New South Wales, NSW 2052, Australia. June 19, 2011.
www.ncbi.nlm.nih.gov/pubmed/21764117

Different Patterns of Brain Activation between Patients of Alzheimer's Disease with and without Depression: A Functional MRI Study during Emotion Stroop Task
Department of Neurology, Xuanwu Hospital, Capital University of Medical Sciences, Beijing 100053, China. April 2007.
www.ncbi.nlm.nih.gov/pubmed/17650397

Divergent Network Connectivity Changes in Behavioral Variant Fronto-temporal Dementia and Alzheimer's Disease
www.ncbi.nlm.nih.gov/pmc/articles/PMC2912696/?tool=pmcentrez

Filling an Unmet Need: A Support Group for Early Stage/Young Onset Alzheimer's Disease and Related Dementias
Alzheimer's Association, West Virginia Chapter. May–June 2011.
www.ncbi.nlm.nih.gov/pubmed/21702419

An FMRI Stroop Task Study of Prefrontal Cortical Function in Normal Aging, Mild Cognitive Impairment, and Alzheimer's Disease
Department of Neurology, Xinqiao Hospital, Third Military Medical University, 400037, China. December 2009.
www.ncbi.nlm.nih.gov/pubmed/19747163

Gene Linked to Alzheimer's Disease Plays Key Role in Cell Survival
www.nia.nih.gov/Alzheimers/ResearchInformation/NewsReleases/PR 20100610presenilin.htm

Higher Levels of HDL Cholesterol Reduce the Risk of Alzheimer's Disease
January 19, 2011
www.naturalnews.com/031046_HDL_cholesterol_Alzheimers.html

Huge New Screening (and Drug Treatment) Push for Alzheimer's Disease
www.naturalnews.com/030900_Alzheimers_screening.html

Impact of Alzheimer's Disease on the Functional Connectivity of Spontaneous Brain Activity

Department of Psychiatry, Klinikum rechts der Isar, Technische Universität München, Ismaninger Strasse 22, 81675 Munich, Germany. c.sorg@lrz.tum.de. December 2009.
www.ncbi.nlm.nih.gov/pubmed/19747154

Impaired Clearance, Not Overproduction of Toxic Proteins, May Underlie Alzheimer's Disease

www.nia.nih.gov/Alzheimers/ResearchInformation/NewsReleases/PR20101209amyloid.htm

Impairment: A Mini Review on fMRI and ERP Studies

Department of Clinical Neurophysiology, Neurological Institute, Graduate School of Medical Sciences, Kyushu University, 3-1-1 Maidashi, Higashi-ku, Fukuoka 812-8582, Japan. July 7, 2011.
www.ncbi.nlm.nih.gov/pubmed/21773027

Large-Scale Functional Brain Network Abnormalities in Alzheimer's Disease: Insights From Functional Neuroimaging

Department of Neurology, Harvard Medical School, Boston. bradd@nmr.mgh.harvard.edu. 2009.
www.ncbi.nlm.nih.gov/pubmed/19847046

Memantine: A Review of Studies into Its Safety and Efficacy in Treating Alzheimer's Disease and Other Dementias

Department of Neurology and Psychiatry, Saint Louis University School of Medicine, St. Louis, MO. October 12, 2009.
www.ncbi.nlm.nih.gov/pubmed/19851512

Mild Cognitive Impairment More Common in Older Men than Older Women

www.nia.nih.gov/Alzheimers/ResearchInformation/NewsReleases/PR20100907MCIgender.htm

Mouse Study Shows Effect of Blood Pressure Drug on Alzheimer's Disease

www.nia.nih.gov/Alzheimers/ResearchInformation/NewsReleases/PR20101115diazoxide.htm

Neurotoxic Effects of Aluminum among Foundry Workers and Alzheimer's Disease
Dipartimento di Medicina del Lavoro dell'Università di Torino, Servizio di Medicina del Lavoro, ASL 8, 10044 Carignano, TO, Torino, Italy. mdl8to@cometacom.it. December 2002.
www.ncbi.nlm.nih.gov/pubmed/12520766

New Study Provides Further Evidence that Apple Juice Can Delay Onset of Alzheimer's Disease
Center for Cellular Neurobiology and Neurodegeneration Research at the University of Massachusetts.
www.physorg.com/news151842200.html

NIH-Supported Study Looks for Earliest Changes in the Brain that May Lead to Alzheimer's Disease
www.nia.nih.gov/Alzheimers/ResearchInformation/NewsReleases

The Predisposing Factors, Biological Markers, Neuroimaging Techniques and Medical Complications Associated with Alzheimer's Disease
West Virginia University School of Medicine. May–June 2011.
www.ncbi.nlm.nih.gov/pubmed/21702411

Recovery Funds Advance Alzheimer's Disease Research
www.nia.nih.gov/Alzheimers/ResearchInformation/NewsReleases/PR20091123ARRA.htm

Scientists Identify Two Gene Variants Associated with Alzheimer's Risk
www.nia.nih.gov/Alzheimers/ResearchInformation/NewsReleases/PR20090908GWAS.htm

Scientists Report Important Step in Biomarker Testing for Alzheimer's Disease
www.nia.nih.gov/Alzheimers/ResearchInformation/NewsReleases/PR20090317biomarkers.htm

Sertaline or Mirtazapine for Depression in Dementia (HTA-SADD): A Randomized, Multicenter, Double-Blind, Placebo-Controlled
Institute of Psychiatry, Health Services and Population Research Department, King's College London, London, UK. July 19, 2011.
www.ncbi.nlm.nih.gov/pubmed/21764118

Studies Find Possible New Genetic Risk Factors for Alzheimer's Disease
www.nia.nih.gov/Alzheimers/ResearchInformation/NewsReleases/PR
20110404GWAS.htm

Study Ties Blood Protein to Alzheimer's Brain Abnormalities
www.nia.nih.gov/Alzheimers/ResearchInformation/NewsReleases/PR-
20101220amyloidtest.htm

Training to Rewire Brain Offers Hope for Alzheimer's
www.psychcentral.com/news/2011/03/24/training-to-rewire-brain-offers-
hope-for-alzheimers/24646.html

Treatment with Vitamin C Dissolves Toxic Protein Aggregates in Alzheimer's Disease
Lund University, Sweden. +46 (0) +46 222 40 77, 46 (0) 70 295 86 22. katrin
.mani@med.lu.se.

Understanding the Pathophysiology of Alzheimer's Disease and Mild Cognitive Validation of the Short Cognitive Battery (B2C): Value in Screening for Alzheimer's Disease and Depressive Disorders in Psychiatric Practice
Centre Mémoire de Ressources et de Recherches, Nice, France. May–June
2003.
www.ncbi.nlm.nih.gov/pubmed/12876552

Notes

PREFACE

1. Han SH, Jung ES, Sohn JH, Hong HJ, Hong HS, Kim JW, Na DL, Kim M, Kim H, Ha HJ, Kim YH, Huh N, Jung MW, Mook-Jung I. Human serum transthyretin levels correlate inversely with Alzheimer's disease. *Journal of Alzheimer's Disease*. 2011 Jan 1;25(1):77–84.

2. Mistur R, Mosconi L, Santi SD, Guzman M, Li Y, Tsui W, de Leon MJ. Current challenges for the early detection of Alzheimer's disease: Brain imaging and CSF studies. *Journal of Clinical Neurology*. 2009 Dec;5(4):153–66.

3. Brookmeyer R, Johnson E, Ziegler-Graham K, Arrighi HM. Forecasting the global burden of Alzheimer's disease. *Alzheimer's and Dementia*. 2007 Jul;3(3):186–91.

4. Sheridan C. *Failure Free Activities for the Alzheimer's Patient*. London: Macmillan; 1992.

5. Mistur et al. Current challenges.

6. Ehrlich LB. Alzheimer's Disease Second Most Feared Health Condition. Harvard Crimson. July 26, 2011. www.thecrimson.com/. Accessed July 28, 2011.

7. Ibid.

8. Ditter SM, Mirra SS. Neuropathologic and clinical features of Parkinson's disease in Alzheimer's disease patients. *Neurology*. 1987 May;37(5):754–60.

9. Han et al. Human serum transthyretin levels.

10. Lambert K. How Sleepwalking Works. www.science.howstuffworks.com/. Accessed January 17, 2012.

11. Vancouver Sun. Brain, Body, and Alzheimer's. July 28, 2011. www.vancouversun.com/. Accessed August 31, 2011.

12. Borland S. How Healthy Lifestyle Can Prevent Half of All Alzheimer's Cases as a Million Expected to Suffer from Disease within a Decade. Mail Online. www.dailymail.co.uk/. Updated July 19, 2011. Accessed July 27, 2011.

13. American Health Assistance Foundation. The Facts on Alzheimer's Disease. June 7, 2011. www.ahaf.org/. Accessed August 31, 2011.

14. Cao C, Wang L, Lin X, Mamcarz M, Zhang C, Bai G, Nong J, Sussman S, Arendash G. Caffeine synergizes with another coffee component to increase plasma GCSF: Linkage to cognitive benefits in Alzheimer's mice. *Journal of Alzheimer's Disease*. 2011 Jan 1;25(2):323–35.

15. Lindsay J. Risk factors for Alzheimer's disease: A prospective analysis from the Canadian study of health and aging. *American Journal of Epidemiological Research*. 2002;156:445–53.

16. Barnes DE, Yaffe K. The projected effect of risk factor reduction on Alzheimer's disease prevalence. *Lancet Neurology*. 2011 Sep;10(9):819–28.

CHAPTER 1

1. Ferney V. The Hierarchy of Mental Illness: Which Diagnosis Is the Least Debilitating? New York City Voices. Winter 2003. www.nycvoices.org/. Accessed August 22, 2011.

2. Heinimaa M. Incomprehensibility: The role of the concept in DSM-IV definition of schizophrenic delusions. *Medicine, Health Care and Philosophy*. 2002;5(3):291–95.

3. Kaplan HI, Sadock BJ. *Kaplan and Sadock's Synopsis of Psychiatry: Behavioral Sciences–Clinical Psychiatry*. 8th ed. Philadelphia: Lippincott Williams and Wilkins; 1998.

4. Hallmann-Mikołajczak A. Ebers Papyrus: The book of medical knowledge of the 16th century B.C. Egyptians [Polish]. *Archiwum Historii I Filozofii Medycyny (Archives of the History and Philosophy of Medicine)*. 2004;67(1):5–14.

5. Okasha A. Mental health in the Middle East: An Egyptian perspective. *Clinical Psychology Reviews*. 1999 Dec;19(8):917–33.

6. Brüne M, Brüne-Cohrs U, McGrew WC, Preuschoft S. Psychopathology in great apes: Concepts, treatment options and possible homologies to human psychiatric disorders. *Neuroscience and Biobehavioral Reviews*. 2006;30(8):1246–59.

7. Allen JP, Manuelian PD, *eds. The Ancient Egyptian Pyramid Texts* (Writings from the Ancient World, No. 23). Boston: Brill Academic Publishers; 2005; Brown RW. Ancient Civilizations to 300 BC—Introduction: The Invention and Diffusion of Civilization. University of North Carolina at Pembroke online lecture. www.uncp.edu/. Accessed January 15, 2012.

8. National Institute of Mental Health. Prevalence of Serious Mental Illness among U.S. Adults by Age, Sex, and Race. www.nimh.gov/. Accessed January 14, 2012.

9. Demyttenaere K, Bruffaerts R, Posada-Villa J, Gasquet I, Kovess V, Lepine JP, Angermeyer MC, Bernert S, de Girolamo G, Morosini P, Polidori G, Kikkawa T, Kawakami N, Ono Y, Takeshima T, Uda H, Karam EG, Fayyad JA, Karam AN, Mneimneh ZN, Medina-Mora ME, Borges G, Lara C, de Graaf R, Ormel J, Gureje O, Shen Y, Huang Y, Zhang M, Alonso J, Haro JM, Vilagut G, Bromet EJ, Gluzman S, Webb C, Kessler RC, Merikangas KR, Anthony JC, Von Korff MR, Wang PS, Brugha TS, Aguilar-Gaxiola S, Lee S, Heeringa S, Pennell BE, Zaslavsky AM, Ustun TB, Chatterji S. WHO World Mental Health Survey Consortium. Prevalence, severity and unmet need for treatment of mental disorders in the World Health Organization world mental health surveys. *Journal of the American Medical Association*. 2004;291(21):2581–90.

10. Magliano L, De Rosa C, Fiorillo A, Malangone C, Maj M. Perception of patients' unpredictability and beliefs on the causes and consequences of schizophrenia: A community survey. *Social Psychiatry and Psychiatric Epidemiology*. 2004 May;39(5):410–16.

11. Crossley N. Contextualizing Contention. In: *Contesting Psychiatry: Social Movements in Mental Health*. 1st ed. New York: Routledge; 2006.

12. Berrios GE. Melancholia and depression during the 19th century. A conceptual history. *British Journal of Psychiatry*. 1988;153:298–304.

13. Tiraboschi P, Hansen LA, Thal LJ, Corey-Bloom J. The importance of neurotic plaques and tangles to the development and evolution of AD. *Neurology*. 62(11):1984–89.

14. Maurer K, Volk S, Gerbaldo H. Auguste D and Alzheimer's disease. *Lancet*. 1997 May 24;349(9064):1546–49.

15. Pederson K. Hippocratic Era Begins. 2005. New Medicine. www.thenewmedicine.org/. Accessed August 8, 2011.

16. Alzheimer A. A new disease of the cortex [German]. *Allgemeine Zeitschrift Fur Psychiatrie.* 1907;64:146–48.

17. Maurer et al. *Lancet.*

18. Alzheimer A. Über eine eigenartige erkrankung der hirnrinde [About a peculiar disease of the cerebral cortex]. *Allgemeine Zeitschrift fur Psychiatrie und Psychisch-Gerichtlich Medizin.* 1907;64(1–2):146–48.

19. Kraepelin E, Diefendorf AR. *Clinical Psychiatry: A Textbook for Students and Physicians.* Whitefish, MT: Kessinger Publishing; 2007; 568.

20. Graeber MB, Kösel S, Egensperger R, Banati RB, Müller U, Bise K, Hoff P, Möller HJ, Fujisawa K, Mehraein P. Rediscovery of the case described by Alois Alzheimer in 1911: Historical, histological and molecular genetic analysis. *Neurogenetics.* 1997;1(1):73–80.

21. Alois Alzheimer. Alzheimer's Disease International. www.alz.co.uk/. Accessed August 1, 2011.

22. Farlex. Nissl. Free Dictionary. http://medical-dictionary.thefreedictionary.com/. Accessed January 2, 2012.

23. Enerson OD. Franz Nissl. 2011. Whonamedit? www.whonamedit.com/. Accessed August 18, 2011.

24. Ibid.

25. Whaley NS. *Senility, Confusion, Debate, Fear: Conceptualizing Alzheimer's Disease and the History of Senile Dementia.* [Thesis]. Drew University, Madison, NJ. 2002.

26. Ibid.; Swerdlow RH. Brain aging, Alzheimer's disease, and mitochondria. *Biochimica et Biophysica Acta.* 2011 Dec;1812(12):1630–9.

27. Desai AK, Grossberg GT. Recognition and management of behavioral disturbances in dementia. *Primary Care Companion to the Journal of Clinical Psychiatry.* 2001 Jun;3(3):93–109.

28. Blacker D, Albert MS, Bassett SS, Go RC, Harrell LE, Folstein MF. Reliability and validity of NINCDS–ADRDA criteria for Alzheimer's disease. National Institute of Mental Health Genetics Initiative. *Archives of Neurology.* 1994 Dec;51(12):1198–204.

29. Jarrott SE. Social aspect of activity stimuli is related to positive affect in persons with Alzheimer's disease. *Evidence Based Nursing.* 2012 Jan;15(1):20–21.

30. Fotenos AF, Mintun MA, Snyder AZ, Morris JC, Buckner RL. Brain volume decline in aging: Evidence for a relation between socioeconomic status, preclinical Alzheimer's disease, and reserve. *Archives in Neurology.* 2008 Jan;65(1):113–20.

31. 10 Disorders Commonly Mistaken for Alzheimer's Disease. In: What Is Alzheimer's Disease? Alzheimer's Research Center. www.alzheimersinfo.org/. Accessed August 1, 2011.

32. World Health Organization International Consortium in Psychiatric Epidemiology. Cross-national comparisons of the prevalences and correlates of mental disorders. *Bulletin of the World Health Organization.* 2000;78(4):413–26.

33. Yu YP, Xu QQ, Zhang Q, Zhang WP, Zhang LH, Wei EQ. Intranasal recombinant human erythropoietin protects rats against focal cerebral ischemia. *Neuroscience Letters.* 2005 Oct 14;387(1):5–10.

CHAPTER 2

1. Merriam-Webster. Anatomy. www.merriam-webster.com/. Accessed January 4, 2012.

2. The Medical Dictionary. Physiology. www.medical-dictionary.com/. Accessed June 8, 2011.

3. Stedman TL, Williams RH, *eds.* Pathology. In: *Stedman's Medical Dictionary.* 28th ed. Philadelphia: Lippincott Williams & Wilkins; 2005.

4. Farlex. Pathology. Free Dictionary. www.medical-dictionary.thefreedictionary.com/. Accessed June 8, 2011; Merriam-Webster. Pathology. http://www.merriam-webster.com/. Accessed January 4, 2012.

5. Burns A, Guthrie E, Marino-Francis F, Busby C, Morris J, Russell E, Margison F, Lennon S, Byrne J. Brief psychotherapy in Alzheimer's disease: Randomised controlled trial. *British Journal of Psychiatry.* 2005 Aug;187:143–47.

6. University of Pennsylvania School of Medicine. Nervous System. www.pennmedicine.org/. Accessed December 13, 2011.

7. Boeree CG. General Psychology: The Cerebrum. Shippensburg University web portal. http://webspace.ship.edu/. Accessed June 9, 2011.

8. Clark BC, Taylor JL. Age-related changes in motor cortical properties and voluntary activation of skeletal muscle. *Current Aging Science.* 2011 Apr 29. Published online ahead of print.

9. Vingerhoets G, Acke F, Alderweireldt AS, Nys J, Vandemaele P, Achten E. Cerebral lateralization of praxis in right- and left-handedness: Same pattern, different strength. *Human Brain Mapping.* 2011 Apr 15. Published online ahead of print.

10. Jensen E. Teaching with the Brain in Mind. In: *Glossary of Brain Terminology.* Alexandria, VA: ASCD (formerly the Association for Supervision and Curriculum Development) Publications; 1998.

11. National Organization for Disorders of the Corpus Callosum. What Is the Corpus Callosum? 2009. www.nodcc.org/. Accessed August 22, 2011.

12. Luders E, Thompson PM, Toga AW. The development of the corpus callosum in the healthy human brain. *Journal of Neuroscience.* 2010 August 18;30(33):10985–90.

13. California Institute of Technology Corpus Callosum Research Program. Information and FAQs: Corpus Callosum. www.emotion.caltech.edu/agcc. Accessed June 9, 2011.

14. American Health Assistance Foundation. Alzheimer's Disease Research. www.ahaf.org. Accessed June 9, 2011; National Institute of Neurological Disorders and Stroke. Brain Basics: Know Your Brain. www.ninds.nih.gov/. Accessed August 16, 2011.

15. California Institute of Technology Corpus Callosum Research Program, Information and FAQs.

16. Chen J, Cohen ML, Lerner AJ, Yang Y, Herrup K. DNA damage and cell cycle events implicate cerebellar dentate nucleus neurons as targets of Alzheimer's disease. *Molecular Neurodegeneration.* 2010 Dec 20;5:60.

17. Jin K, Peel AL, Mao XO, Xie L, Cottrell BA, Henshall DC, Greenberg DA. Increased hippocampal neurogenesis in Alzheimer's disease. *Proceedings of the National Academy of Science USA.* 2004 Jan 6;101(1):343–47.

18. Schuff N, Woerner N, Boreta L, Kornfield T, Shaw LM, Trojanowski JQ, Thompson PM, Jack CR Jr, Weiner MW. MRI of hippocampal volume loss in early Alzheimer's disease in relation to ApoE genotype and biomarkers. *Brain.* 2009 Apr;132(Pt 4):1067–77.

19. MedicineNet.com. Definition of Hippocampus. www.medterms.com/. Accessed June 14, 2011.

20. De Jong LW, van der Hiele K, Veer IM, Houwing JJ, Westendorp RG, Bollen EL, de Bruin PW, Middelkoop HA, van Buchem MA, van der Grond J. Strongly reduced volumes of putamen and thalamus in Alzheimer's disease: An MRI study. *Brain.* 2008 Dec;131(Pt 12):3277–85.

21. Bryn Mawr College. Brain Structures and Their Functions. www.serendip.brynmawr.edu/. Accessed June 11, 2011.

22. MedicineNet.com, Definition of Hippocampus.

23. Baloyannis SI. The hypothalamus in Alzheimer's disease: A study with silver impregnation techniques and electron microscope. *Alzheimer's & Dementia.* 2009 Jul;(5)4[Suppl]:P299.

24. Saper C. Hypothalamus. Scholarpedia [The peer-reviewed online encyclopedia]. www .scholarpedia.org/. Accessed June 11, 2011.

25. Gomez JM, Aguilar M, Soler J. Growth hormone and thyrotropin hormone secretion in Alzheimer's disease. *Journal of Nutrition Health & Aging.* 2000;4(4):229–32.

26. Bowen RA. Functional Anatomy of the Hypothalamus and Pituitary Gland. Vivo (Colorado State University). www.vivo.colostate.edu/. Updated September 4, 2001. Accessed June 13, 2011.

27. Jacobs DH, Adair JC, Williamson DJ, Na DL, Gold M, Foundas AL, Shuren JE, Cibula JE, Heilman KM. Apraxia and motor-skill acquisition in Alzheimer's disease are dissociable. *Neuropsychologia.* 1999 Jun;37(7):875–80.

28. Bryn Mawr College, Brain Structures and Their Functions.

29. Schneider JA, Bienias JL, Gilley DW, Kvarnberg DE, Mufson EJ, Bennett DA. Improved detection of substantia nigra pathology in Alzheimer's disease. *Journal of Histochemistry and Cytochemistry.* 2002 Jan;50(1):99–106; Nelson PT, Schmitt FA, Lin Y, Abner EL, Jicha GA, Patel E, Thomason PC, Neltner JH, Smith CD, Santacruz KS, Sonnen JA, Poon LW, Gearing M, Green RC, Woodard JL, Van Eldik LJ, Kryscio RJ. Hippocampal sclerosis in advanced age: Clinical and pathological features. *Brain.* 2011 May;134(Pt 5):1506–18; Maarouf CL, Daugs ID, Kokjohn TA, Walker DG, Hunter JM, Kruchowsky JC, Woltjer R, Kaye J, Castaño EM, Sabbagh MN, Beach TG, Roher AE. Alzheimer's disease and non-demented high pathology control nonagenarians: Comparing and contrasting the biochemistry of cognitively successful aging. *PLoS One (Public Library of Science).* 2011;6(11):e27291.

30. University of Illinois College of Medicine. Introduction to Pathology. 2011. www.peoria.medicine.uic.edu/. Accessed September 1, 2011.

31. Rank the Universe. Famous Pathologists. www.ranker.com/. Accessed June 14, 2011.

32. Ibid.

33. Farlex. Pathology. Free Dictionary. www.medical-dictionary.thefreedictionary.com/. Accessed June 8, 2011.

34. Crutch S. The Brain and Behavior. Alzheimer's Society. www.alzheimers.org.uk/. Accessed June 15, 2011.

35. Mori E, Hirono N, Yamashita H, Imamura T, Ikejiri Y, Ikeda M, Kitagaki H, Shimomura T, Yoneda Y. Premorbid brain size as a determinant of reserve capacity against intellectual decline in Alzheimer's disease. *American Journal of Psychiatry.* 1997 Jan;154(1):18–24; Oprica M, Hjorth E, Spulber S, Popescu BO, Ankarcrona M, Winblad B, Schultzberg M. Studies on brain volume, Alzheimer-related proteins and cytokines in mice with chronic overexpression of IL-1 receptor antagonist. *Journal of Cellular and Molecular Medicine.* 2007 Jul–Aug;11(4):810–25.

36. American Health Assistance Foundation, Alzheimer's Disease Research.

37. Hoozemans JJ, Veerhuis R, Rozemuller JM, Eikelenboom P. Neuroinflammation and regeneration in the early stages of Alzheimer's disease pathology. *International Journal of Developmental Neuroscience.* 2006 Apr–May;24(2–3):157–65.

38. Waters CE, French G, Burt M. Difficulty in brainstem death testing in the presence of high spinal cord injury. *British Journal of Anaesthesia.* 2004;92(5):760–64.

CHAPTER 3

1. Zubenko GS, Winwood E, Jacobs B, Teply I, Stiffler JS, Hughes HB 3rd, Huff FJ, Sunderland T, Martinez AJ. Prospective study of risk factors for Alzheimer's disease: Results at 7.5 years. *American Journal of Psychiatry.* 1999 Jan;156(1):50–57.

2. Baum LW. Sex, hormones, and Alzheimer's disease. *Journals of Gerontology. Series A, Biological Sciences and Medical Sciences.* 2005 Jun;60(6):736–43; Peri A, Serio M. Estrogen receptor-mediated neuroprotection: The role of the Alzheimer's disease-related gene seladin-1. *Journal of Neuropsychiatric Disease and Treatment.* 2008 Aug;4(4):817–24.

3. Kawas C, Resnick S, Morrison A, Brookmeyer R, Corrada M, Zonderman A, Bacal C, Lingle DD, Metter E. A prospective study of estrogen replacement therapy and the risk of developing Alzheimer's disease: The Baltimore Longitudinal Study of Aging. *Neurology.* 1997 Jun;48(6):1517–21.

4. Barford A, Dorling D, Davey Smith G, Shaw M. Life expectancy: Women now on top everywhere. *British Medical Journal.* 2006 Apr 8;332(7545):808.

5. Harman D. Alzheimer's disease: A hypothesis on pathogenesis. *AGE: Journal of the American Aging Association.* 2000 Jul;23(3):147–61.

6. Rocchi A, Orsucci D, Tognoni G, Ceravolo R, Siciliano G. The role of vascular factors in late-onset sporadic Alzheimer's disease: Genetic and molecular aspects. *Current Alzheimer Research.* 2009 Jun;6(3):224–37.

7. Bird TD. Early-Onset Familial Alzheimer Disease. In: Pagon RA, Bird TD, Dolan CR, Stephens K, *eds.* Seattle: University of Washington; 1993–1999.

8. Ibid.

9. Cupples LA, Farrer LA, Sadovnick AD, Relkin N, Whitehouse P, Green RC. Estimating risk curves for first-degree relatives of patients with Alzheimer's disease: The REVEAL study. *Genetics in Medicine.* 2004 Jul–Aug;6(4):192–96; Lautenschlager NT, Cupples LA, Rao VS, Auerbach SA, Becker R, Burke J, Chui H, Duara R, Foley EJ, Glatt SL, Green RC, Jones R, Karlinsky H, Kukull WA, Kurz A, Larson EB, Martelli K, Sadovnick AD, Volicer L, Waring SC, Growdon JH, Farrer LA. Risk of dementia among relatives of Alzheimer's disease patients in the MIRAGE study: What is in store for the oldest old? *Neurology.* 1996 Mar;46(3):641–50.

10. Mueller SG, Weiner MW. Selective effect of age, Apo e4, and Alzheimer's disease on hippocampal subfields. *Hippocampus.* 2009 Jun;19(6):558–64.

11. Ibid.; Taylor DH Jr, Cook-Deegan RM, Hiraki S, Roberts JS, Blazer DG, Green RC. Genetic testing for Alzheimer's and long-term care insurance. *Health Affairs (Millwood).* 2010 Jan–Feb;29(1):102–8; Hall K, Murrell J, Ogunniyi A, Deeg M, Baiyewu O, Gao S, Gureje O, Dickens J, Evans R, Smith-Gamble V, Unverzagt FW, Shen J, Hendrie H. Cholesterol, APOE genotype, and Alzheimer disease: An epidemiologic study of Nigerian Yoruba. *Neurology.* 2006 Jan 24;66(2):223–27.

12. Raux G, Guyant-Maréchal L, Martin C, Bou J, Penet C, Brice A, Hannequin D, Frebourg T, Campion D. Molecular diagnosis of autosomal dominant early onset Alzheimer's disease: an update. *Journal of Medical Genetics.* 2005 Oct;42(10):793–5.

13. Zetzsche T, Rujescu D, Hardy J, Hampel H. Advances and perspectives from genetic research: Development of biological markers in Alzheimer's disease. *Expert Review of Molecular Diagnostics.* 2010 Jul;10(5):667–90.

14. Ibid.

15. Bekris LM, Yu CE, Bird TD, Tsuang DW. Genetics of Alzheimer's disease. *Journal of Geriatric Psychiatry and Neurology.* 2010 Dec;23(4):213–27.

16. Pope SK, Shue VM, Beck C. Will a healthy lifestyle help prevent Alzheimer's disease? *Annual Review of Public Health.* 2003;24:111–32.

17. Vadstrup ES, Frølich A, Perrild H, Borg E, Røder M. Lifestyle intervention for type 2 diabetes patients: Trial protocol of the Copenhagen Type 2 Diabetes Rehabilitation Project. *BioMed Central (BMC) Public Health.* 2009 May 29;9:166.

18. Sima AA, Li ZG. Diabetes and Alzheimer's disease: Is there a connection? *Review of Diabetic Studies.* 2006 Winter;3(4):161–68.

19. Mielke MM, Rosenberg PB, Tschanz J, Cook L, Corcoran C, Hayden KM, Norton M, Rabins PV, Green RC, Welsh-Bohmer KA, Breitner JC, Munger R, Lyketsos CG. Vascular factors predict rate of progression in Alzheimer disease. *Neurology.* 2007;69:1850–58.

20. Gatz M, Svedberg P, Pedersen NL, Mortimer JA, Berg S, Johansson B. Education and the risk of Alzheimer's disease: Findings from the study of dementia in Swedish twins. *Journals of Gerontology. Series B, Psychological Sciences and Social Sciences.* 2001 Sep;56(5):P292–300.

21. Perneczky R, Wagenpfeil S, Lunetta KL, Cupples LA, Green RC, DeCarli C, Farrer LA, Kurz A. Education attenuates the effect of medial temporal lobe atrophy on cognitive function in Alzheimer's disease: The MIRAGE study. *Journal of Alzheimer's Disease.* 2009;17(4):855–62.

22. Ibid.

23. Ibid.

24. Perl DP, Good PF. Aluminum and the neurofibrillary tangle: Results of tissue microprobe studies. *Ciba Foundation Symposium.* 1992;169:227–36.

25. Morgan TE, Davis DA, Iwata N, Tanner JA, Snyder D, Ning Z, Kam W, Hsu YT, Winkler JW, Chen JC, Petasis NA, Baudry M, Sioutas C, Finch CE. Glutamatergic neurons in rodent models respond to nanoscale particulat urban air pollutants in vivo and in vitro. *Environmental Health Perspectives.* 2011 Jul;119(7):1003–9.

26. Sloane JA, Hinman JD, Lubonia M, Hollander W, Abraham CR. Age-dependent myelin degeneration and proteolysis of oligodendrocyte proteins is associated with the activation of calpain-1 in the rhesus monkey. *Journal of Neurochemistry.* 2003 Jan;84(1):157–68.

27. Choi JH, Berger JD, Mazzella MJ, Morales-Corraliza J, Cataldo AM, Nixon RA, Ginsberg SD, Levy E, Mathews PM. Age-dependent dysregulation of brain amyloid precursor protein in the Ts65Dn Down syndrome mouse model. *Journal of Neurochemistry.* 2009 Sep;110(6):1818–27.

28. Braak H, Braak E, Yilmazer D, de Vos RA, Jansen EN, Bohl J. Neurofibrillary tangles and neuropil threads as a cause of dementia in Parkinson's disease. *Journal of Neural Transmission.* 1997;51:49–55.

29. Reitz C, Brayne C, Mayeux R. Epidemiology of Alzheimer's disease. *Nature Reviews Neurology.* 2011 Mar;7(3):137–52.

30. Takahashi M, Tsujioka Y, Yamada T, Tsuboi Y, Okada H, Yamamoto T, Liposits Z. Glycosylation of microtubule-associated protein tau in Alzheimer's disease brain. *Acta Neuropathologica.* 1999 Jun;97(6):635–41.

31. Ehrenstein G, Galdzicki Z, Lange GD. The choline-leakage hypothesis for the loss of acetylcholine in Alzheimer's disease. *Biophysical Journal.* 1997 Sep;73(3):1276–80.

32. Tabet N. Acetylcholinesterase inhibitors for Alzheimer's disease: Anti-inflammatories in acetylcholine clothing! *Age and Ageing.* 2006 Jul;35(4):336–38.

33. Hefti F, Weiner WJ. Nerve growth factor and Alzheimer's disease. *Annals of Neurology.* 1986 Sep;20(3):275–81.

34. Fischer W, Sirevaag A, Wiegand SJ, Lindsay RM, Björklund A. Reversal of spatial memory impairments in aged rats by nerve growth factor and neurotrophins 3 and 4/5 but not by brain-derived neurotrophic factor. *Proceedings of the National Academy of Science USA.* 1994 Aug 30;91(18):8607–11.

35. Szutowicz A. Aluminum, NO, and nerve growth factor neurotoxicity in cholinergic neurons. *Journal of Neuroscience Research.* 2001 Dec 1;66(5):1009–18.

36. Hardy J, Selkoe DJ. The amyloid hypothesis of Alzheimer's disease: Progress and problems on the road to therapeutics. *Science.* 2002 Jul 19;297(5580):353–56.

37. Struble RG, Ala T, Patrylo PR, Brewer GJ, Yan XX. Is brain amyloid production a cause or a result of dementia of the Alzheimer's type? *Journal of Alzheimer's Disease.* 2010;22(2):393–99.

38. Winters HV. Relationship of amyloid to Alzheimer's disease. *Western Journal of Medicine.* 1991 Jan;154(1):94–35.

39. Hu D, Qin Z, Xue B, Fink AL, Uversky VN. Effect of methionine oxidation on the structural properties, conformational stability, and aggregation of immunoglobulin light chain LEN. *Biochemistry.* 2008 Aug 19;47(33):8665–77.

40. Ouchi E, Nomura N, Watabe S, Seiji K, Sato J. Clinical significance of Congo red test. *Tohoku Journal of Experimental Medicine.* 1976;118 Suppl:191–98.

41. Ando Y, Haraoka K, Terazaki H, Tanoue Y, Ishikawa K, Katsuragi S, Nakamura M, Sun X, Nakagawa K, Sasamoto K, Takesako K, Ishizaki T, Sasaki Y, Doh-ura K. A novel tool for detecting amyloid deposits in systemic amyloidosis in vitro and in vivo. *Laboratory Investigation: A Journal of Technical Methods and Pathology.* 2003 Dec;83(12):1751–59.

42. University of Maryland Medical Center. Amyloidosis. 2011. www.umm.edu/. Accessed August 17, 2011.

43. Tuppo EE, Arias HR. The role of inflammation in Alzheimer's disease. *International Journal of Biochemistry & Cell Biology.* 2005 Feb;37(2):289–305.

44. Ibid.; Kiyota T, Okuyama S, Swan RJ, Jacobsen MT, Gendelman HE, Ikezu T. CNS expression of anti-inflammatory cytokine interleukin-4 attenuates Alzheimer's disease-like pathogenesis in APP+PS1 bigenic mice. *Federation of American Societies for Experimental Biology (FASEB) Journal.* 2010 Aug;24(8):3093–102.

45. Akiyama H, Barger S, Barnum S, Bradt B, Bauer J, Cole GM, Cooper NR, Eikelenboom P, Emmerling M, Fiebich BL, Finch CE, Frautschy S, Griffin WS, Hampel H, Hull M, Landreth G, Lue L, Mrak R, Mackenzie IR, McGeer PL, O'Banion MK, Pachter J, Pasinetti G, Plata-Salaman C, Rogers J, Rydel R, Shen Y, Streit W, Strohmeyer R, Tooyoma I, Van Muiswinkel FL, Veerhuis R, Walker D, Webster S, Wegrzyniak B, Wenk G, Wyss-Coray T. Inflammation and Alzheimer's disease. *Neurobiology of Aging.* 2000 May–June;(21)3:383–421.

46. Dringen R. Metabolism and functions of glutathione in brain. *Progress in Neurobiology.* 2000 Dec;62(6):649–71.

47. Brunet-Rossinni AK. Reduced free-radical production and extreme longevity in the little brown bat (Myotis lucifugus) versus two non-flying mammals. *Mechanisms of Ageing and Development.* 2004 Jan;125(1):11–20.

48. Pogocki D. Alzheimer's beta-amyloid peptide as a source of neurotoxic free radicals: The role of structural effects. *Acta Neurobiologiae Experimentalis (Warsaw).* 2003;63(2):131–45.

49. Perl, Good, Aluminum and the neurofibrillary tangle, 227–36.

CHAPTER 4

1. Prabhat. Difference between Signs and Symptoms. Differencebetween.net. www.differencebetween.net/. Updated October 6, 2009. Accessed June 8, 2001.

2. University of Maryland Medical Center. Alzheimer's Disease-Symptoms. 2011. www.umm.edu/. Accessed June 8, 2011.

3. Healthgrades. Retrograde Amnesia. www.wrongdiagnosis.pubs.righthealth.com/. Accessed June 13, 2011.

4. Ibid.

5. Long CJ. Brain Lesions & Amnesia. University of Memphis. http://neuro.psyc.memphis.edu/neuropsyc/np-ugp-memory.htm#lesion. Accessed January 5, 2012; de Guise E. Amnesia. University of Buffalo Center for International Rehabilitation Research Information & Exchange (CIRRIE). www.cirrie.buffalo.edu/. Accessed January 5, 2012.

6. Warrington EK. Studies of retrograde memory: A long-term view. *Proceedings of the National Academy of Sciences USA.* 1996 Nov 26;93(24):13523–26.

7. Mayes AR, Daum I, Markowisch HJ, Sauter B. The relationship between retrograde and anterograde amnesia in patients with typical global amnesia. *Cortex.* 1997 Jun;33(2):197–217.

8. Bright P, Buckman J, Fradera A, Yoshimasu H, Colchester AC, Kopelman MD. Retrograde amnesia in patients with hippocampal, medial temporal, temporal lobe, or frontal pathology. *Learning & Memory.* 2006 Sep–Oct;13(5):545–57.

9. Markowitsch HJ, Calabrese P, Neufeld H, Gehlen W, Durwen HF. Retrograde amnesia for world knowledge and preserved memory for autobiographic events: A case report. *Cortex.* 1999 Apr;35(2):243–52.

10. Healthgrades. Anterograde Amnesia. www.wrongdiagnosis.pubs.righthealth.com/. Accessed June 13, 2011.

11. Kirshner HS. Approaches to intellectual and memory impairments. In: Gradley WG, Daroff RB, Fenichel GM, Jankovic J, eds. *Neurology in Clinical Practice.* 5th ed. Philadelphia: Butterworth-Heinemann; 2008:chap 6.

12. Bartsch T, Deuschl G. Transient global amnesia: Functional anatomy and clinical implications. *Lancet Neurology.* 2010 Feb;9(2):205–14.

13. Milner B. The medial temporal-lobe amnesic syndrome. *Psychiatric Clinics of North America.* 2005 Sep;28(3):599–611, 609; Stracciari A, Guarino M, Pazzaglia P. Transient procedural amnesia. *Italian Journal of Neurological Sciences.* 1997 Feb;18(1):35–36.

14. Healthwise. Dementia: Topic overview. WebMD. www.webmd.com/. Updated June 17, 2009. Accessed June 13, 2011.

15. Scazufca M, Menezes PR, Vallada HP, Crepaldi AL, Pastor-Valero M, Coutinho LM, Di Rienzo VD, Almeida OP. High prevalence of dementia among older adults from poor socioeconomic backgrounds in São Paulo, Brazil. *International Psychogeriatric Association.* 2008 Apr;20(2):394–405.

16. Nordqvist C. What Is Dementia? What Causes Dementia? Symptoms of Dementia. March 13, 2009. www.medicalnewstoday.com/. Accessed June 15, 2011.

17. Cleveland Clinic. Diseases & Conditions: Types of Dementia. www.my.clevelandclinic .org/. Accessed June 15, 2011.

18. Reeves AG, Swenson RS. *Disorders of the Nervous System* (online e-book). Dartmouth Medical School. www.dartmouth.edu/. Accessed June 13, 2011.

19. Bartsch, Deuschl, Transient global amnesia.

20. eMedTV. Alzheimer's Articles. http://alzheimers.emedtv.com/. Accessed June 15, 2011.

21. Reeves, Swenson, *Disorders of the Nervous System.*

22. Mason DJ. Diseases. *The Memory Dr.* 2006. www.memorydr.com/. Accessed July 25, 2011.

23. Alzheimer's Society. Types of Dementia. www.alzheimers.org.uk/. Accessed June 13, 2011.

24. Alzheimer's Society. Vascular Dementia. www.alzheimers.org.uk/. Accessed June 13, 2011.

25. Hale A, *reviewer.* Am I at Risk of Developing Dementia? Alzheimer's Society. www .alzheimers.org.uk/. Updated December 2010. Accessed August 23, 2011.

26. Honig LS, Tang MX, Albert S, Costa R, Luchsinger J, Manly J, Stern Y, Mayeux R. Stroke and the risk of Alzheimer's disease. *Archives of Neurology.* 2003;60(12):1707–12.

27. Förstl H, Howard R, Levy R. Binswanger's clinical and neuropathological criteria for "Binswanger's disease." *Journal of Neurology, Neurosurgery, and Psychiatry.* 1991 Dec;54(12):1122–23.

28. National Institute of Neurological Disorders and Stroke (NINDS). Binswanger's Disease Information Page. www.ninds.nih.gov/. Updated November 19, 2010. Accessed August 23, 2011.

29. Alzheimer's Society. What Is Dementia with Lewy Bodies? www.alzheimers.org.uk/. Accessed June 13, 2011.

30. O'Brien JT. Role of imaging techniques in the diagnosis of dementia. *British Journal of Radiology.* 2007 Dec;80[Special](2):S74.

31. Nelson PT, Kryscio RJ, Jicha GA, Abner EL, Schmitt FA, Xu LO, Cooper G, Smith CD, Markesbery WR. Relative preservation of MMSE scores in autopsy-proven dementia with Lewy bodies. *Neurology.* 2009 Oct 6;73(14):1127–33.

32. McKeith I, Mintzer J, Aarsland D, Burn D, Chiu H, Cohen-Mansfield J, Dickson D, Dubois B, Duda JE, Feldman H, Gauthier S, Halliday G, Lawlor B, Lippa C, Lopez OL, Carlos Machado J, O'Brien J, Playfer J, Reid W. Dementia with Lewy bodies. *Lancet Neurology.* 2004 Jan;3:19.

33. Ferman TJ, Boeve BF. Dementia with Lewy bodies. *Neurologic Clinics.* 2007 Aug;25(3):741–60, vii.

34. dbS Productions. Alzheimer's Disease and Related Disorders SAR Research. www.dbs-sar.com/. Accessed June 15, 2011.

35. Pineda P, Gould DJ. The neuroanatomical relationship of dementia pugilistica and Alzheimer's disease. *Neuroanatomy.* 2010;9(1):5–7.

36. Alzheimer's Society. What Is Fronto-Temporal Dementia (Including Pick's Disease)? www.alzheimers.org.uk/. Accessed June 13, 2011.

37. Snowden JS, Bathgate D, Varma A, Blackshaw A, Gibbons ZC, Neary D. Distinct behavioural profiles in frontotemporal dementia and semantic dementia. *Journal of Neurology, Neurosurgery, and Psychiatry.* 2001;70:329.

38. Mourik JC, Rosso SM, Niermeijer MF, Duivenvoorden HJ, Van Swieten JC, Tibben A. Frontotemporal dementia: Behavioral symptoms and caregiver distress. *Dementia and Geriatric Cognitive Disorders.* 2004;18(3–4):299–306.

39. Thompson SA, Patterson K, Hodges JR. Left/right asymmetry of atrophy in semantic dementia: Behavioral-cognitive implications. *Neurology.* 2003 Nov 11;61(9):1196–203.

40. Sabbagh MN, Sandhu SS, Farlow MR, Vedders L, Shill HA, Caviness JN, Connor DJ, Sue L, Adler CH, Beach TG. Correlation of clinical features with argyrophilic grains at autopsy. *Alzheimer Disease & Associated Disorders.* 2009 Jul–Sep;23(3):229–33.

41. Braak H, Braak E. Argyrophilic grain disease: Frequency of occurrence in different age categories and neuropathological diagnostic criteria. *Journal of Neural Transmission.* 1998;105(8–9):801–19; Soma K, Fu YJ, Wakabayashi K, Onodera O, Kakita A, Takahashi H. Co-occurrence of argyrophilic grain disease in sporadic amyotrophic lateral sclerosis. *Neuropathology and Applied Neurobiology.* 2011 Mar 28. Published online ahead of print.

42. Hampton J. The Physical Effects of Alzheimer's Disease. www.livestrong.com/. Accessed June 14, 2011.

43. Davidson HA, Borrie MJ, Crilly RG. Copy task performance and urinary incontinence in Alzheimer's disease. *Journal of the American Geriatric Society.* 1991 May;39(5):467–71; Sugiyama T, Hashimoto K, Kiwamoto H, Ohnishi N, Esa A, Park YC, Kurita T. Urinary incontinence in senile dementia of the Alzheimer type (SDAT). *International Journal of Urology.* 1994 Dec;1(4):337–40; Lancioni GE, Singh NN, O'Reilly MF, Sigafoos J, Bosco A, Zonno N, Badagliacca F. Persons with mild or moderate Alzheimer's disease learn to use urine alarms and prompts to avoid large urinary accidents. *Research in Developmental Disabilities.* 2011 Sep–Oct;32(5):1998–2004.

44. Gerstner E, Lazar RM, Keller C, Honig LS, Lazar GS, Marshall RS. A case of progressive apraxia of speech in pathologically verified Alzheimer disease. *Cognitive and Behavioral Neurology.* 2007 Mar;20(1):15–20.

45. Gregory GC, Macdonald V, Schofield PR, Kril JJ, Halliday GM. Differences in regional brain atrophy in genetic forms of Alzheimer's disease. *Neurobiology of Aging.* 2006 Mar;27(3):387–93.

46. Burns JM, Cronk BB, Anderson HS, Donnelly JE, Thomas GP, Harsha A, Brooks WM, Swerdlow RH. Cardiorespiratory fitness and brain atrophy in early Alzheimer disease. *Neurology.* 2008 Jul 15;71(3):210–16.

47. Yu F, Savik K, Wyman JF, Bronas UG. Maintaining physical fitness and function in Alzheimer's disease: A pilot study. *American Journal of Alzheimer's Disease and Other Dementias.* 2011 Aug;26(5):406–12.

48. Gregory et al., Differences in regional brain atrophy.

49. Petersen R. Alzheimer's Research Must Be Accelerated. CNN Opinion. www.cnn .com/. Accessed June 15, 2011.

50. Huether SE, McCance KL, *eds. Understanding Pathophysiology.* 2nd ed. St. Louis: Mosby; 2000:407–8.

51. Petersen, Alzheimer's Research.

52. *New York Times* (About.com). Importance of Early Diagnosis in Alzheimer's Disease. www.alzheimers.about.com/. June 15, 2011.

CHAPTER 5

1. Elias MF, Beiser A, Wolf PA, Au R, White RF, D'Agostino RB. The preclinical phase of Alzheimer's disease: A 22-year prospective study of the Framingham cohort. *Archives of Neurology.* 2000;57:808–13; Kawas CH, Corrada MM, Brookmeyer R, Morrison A, Resnick SM, Zonderman AB, Arenberg D. Visual memory predicts Alzheimer's disease more than a decade before diagnosis. *Neurology.* 2003;60:1089–93; LaRue A, Jarvik LF. Cognitive function and prediction of dementia in old age. *International Journal of Aging and Human Development.* 1987;25:79–89.

2. DeNoon DJ. New Alzheimer's Guidelines Stress Early Diagnosis. WebMD Health News. www.webmd.com/. Updated April 19, 2011. Accessed May 24, 2011.

3. Sweetwood J. Alzheimer's Disease Overview. Better Medicine. www.bettermedicine .com/. Updated July 16, 2009. Accessed May 25, 2011.

4. Glass J. Making the Diagnosis of Alzheimer's Disease. WebMD. www.webmd.com/. Updated June 16, 2009. Accessed May 26, 2011.

5. McKhann G, Drachman D, Folstein M, Katzman R, Price D, Stadlan EM. Clinical diagnosis of Alzheimer's disease: Report of the NINCDS-ADRDA Work Group under the auspices of Department of Health and Human Services Task Force on Alzheimer's Disease. *Neurology.* 1984 Jul;34(7):939–44.

6. Jack CR Jr, Albert MS, Knopman DS, McKhann GM, Sperling RA, Carrillo MC, Thies B, Phelps CH. Introduction to the recommendations from the National Institute on Aging–Alzheimer's Association workgroups on diagnostic guidelines for Alzheimer's disease. *Alzheimer's and Dementia.* 2011 May;7(3):257–62.

7. National Institutes of Health. Alzheimer's Diagnostic Guidelines Updated for First Time in Decades. April 19, 2011. www.nih.gov/news. Updated May 27, 2011. Accessed May 30, 2011.

8. Hampel H, Bürger K, Teipel SJ, Bokde AL, Zetterberg H, Blennow K. Core candidate neurochemical and imaging biomarkers of Alzheimer's disease. *Alzheimer's & Dementia.* 2008 Jan;4(1):38–48.

9. Alzheimer's Association. Genetic Testing. www.sitesearch.alz.org. Updated November 2008. Accessed May 30, 2011; Mrak RE, Griffin WS. Potential inflammatory biomarkers in Alzheimer's disease. *Journal of Alzheimer's Disease.* 2005 Mar;8(4):369–75.

10. National Institutes on Health, Alzheimer's Diagnostic Guidelines Updated.

11. Cosentino S. Biomarkers' Could Spot Alzheimer's Disease Early, Studies Suggest. www .wrongdiagnosis.com/. Accessed May 30, 2011.

12. Alzheimer's Association. Diagnosing Alzheimer's. www.alz.org/. Updated May 18, 2011. Accessed May 24, 2011.

13. National Institute of Aging. Diagnosis. www.nia.nih.gov/. Updated January 10, 2011. Accessed May 29, 2011.

14. Alzheimer's Association, Diagnosing Alzheimer's.

15. Alzheimer's Association. Why Get Checked. www.alz.org.com/. Updated March 29, 2011. Accessed May 24, 2011.

16. Glass, Making the Diagnosis of Alzheimer's.

17. Alzheimer's Association, Diagnosing Alzheimer's.

18. National Institute of Aging, Diagnosis.

19. Alzheimer's Association, Diagnosing Alzheimer's.

20. Alzheimer's Association. Medical Evaluation. www.alz.org/. Updated May 18, 2011. Accessed May 26, 2011.

21. Alzheimer's Association, Diagnosing Alzheimer's.

22. Glass, Making the Diagnosis of Alzheimer's.

23. Alzheimer's Association, Diagnosing Alzheimer's.

24. National Institute of Aging, Diagnosis.

25. Alzheimer's Association, Diagnosing Alzheimer's.

26. National Institute of Aging, Diagnosis.

27. Alzheimer's Association, Diagnosing Alzheimer's.

28. Marieb EN. *Essentials of Anatomy & Physiology.* 7th ed. Jurong, Singapore: Pearson Education South Asia; 2004.

29. *Mosby's Pocket Dictionary of Medicine, Nursing & Allied Health.* 4th ed. Philippines: Elsevier Singapore; 2002.

30. Alzheimer's Association, Diagnosing Alzheimer's.

31. *Mosby's Pocket Dictionary.*

32. National Institute of Aging, Diagnosis.

33. Alzheimer's Association, Diagnosing Alzheimer's.

34. Better Medicine. Diagnosing Alzheimer's Disease. www.bettermedicine.com/. Updated February 1, 2009. Accessed May 25, 2011.

35. Alzheimer's Association, Medical Evaluation.

36. Better Medicine, Diagnosing Alzheimer's Disease.

37. Ibid.

38. Alzheimer's Association, Diagnosing Alzheimer's.

39. Better Medicine, Diagnosing Alzheimer's Disease.

40. National Institute of Aging, Diagnosis.

41. Better Medicine, Diagnosing Alzheimer's Disease.

42. Alzheimer's Association, Diagnosing Alzheimer's.

43. Marieb, *Essentials of Anatomy & Physiology.*

44. Alzheimer's Association. Diagnostic Overview. www.alz.org/. Updated April 17, 2009. Accessed May 28, 2011.

45. *Mosby's Pocket Dictionary.*

46. Alzheimer's Association, Diagnosing Alzheimer's.

47. Nettina SM, *ed. The Lippincott Manual of Nursing Practice.* 7th ed. Philadelphia: Lippincott-Raven Publishers; 2001.

48. Alzheimer's Association, Medical Evaluation.

49. Alzheimer's Association, Diagnosing Alzheimer's.

50. Nettina, *Lippincott Manual.*

51. Glass, Making the Diagnosis of Alzheimer's.

52. Alzheimer's Association, Medical Evaluation.

53. Better Medicine, Diagnosing Alzheimer's Disease.

54. Glass, Making the Diagnosis of Alzheimer's.

55. Better Medicine, Diagnosing Alzheimer's Disease.

56. Alzheimer's Association, Diagnosing Alzheimer's.

57. Phillips JR, Carroll J, Ehsanullah M. Screening for acute myocardial infarction in elderly patients with collapse, confusion and falls. *International Journal of Clinical Practice.* 1999 Mar;53(2):93–95.

58. Better Medicine, Diagnosing Alzheimer's Disease.

59. Silvestri LA. *Saunders Comprehensive Review for the NCLEX-RN Examination.* 4th ed. St. Louis, MO: Elsevier; 2008.

60. Nettina, *Lippincott Manual.*

61. Better Medicine, Diagnosing Alzheimer's Disease.

62. Hu YY, He SS, Wang X, Duan QH, Grundke-Iqbal I, Iqbal K, Wang J. Levels of non-phosphorylated and phosphorylated tau in cerebrospinal fluid of Alzheimer's disease patients: An ultrasensitive bienzyme-substrate-recycle enzyme-linked immunosorbent assay. *American Journal of Pathology.* 2002;160(4):1269–78; Maddalena A, Papassotiropoulos A, Müller-Tillmanns B, Jung HH, Hegi T, Nitsch RM, Hock C. Biochemical diagnosis of Alzheimer disease by measuring the cerebrospinal fluid ratio of phosphorylated tau protein to beta-amyloid peptide42. *Archives of Neurology.* 2003 Sep;60(9):1202–6.

63. Nettina, *Lippincott Manual.*

64. Glass, Making the Diagnosis of Alzheimer's.

65. Alzheimer's Association, Medical Evaluation.

66. Better Medicine, Diagnosing Alzheimer's Disease.

67. Ibid.

68. Marieb, *Essentials of Anatomy & Physiology.*

69. Nettina, *Lippincott Manual.*

70. *Mosby's Pocket Dictionary.*

71. Silvestri, *Saunders Comprehensive Review.*

72. *Mosby's Pocket Dictionary.*

73. Glass, Making the Diagnosis of Alzheimer's.

74. Sekhar M. Anaemia and lead toxicity. *Chemical Hazards and Poisons Report.* 2006 Nov;8:12–13.

75. Whitfield CL, Ch'ien LT, Whitehead JD. Lead encephalopathy in adults. *American Journal of Medicine.* 1972 Mar;52(3):289–98.

76. Healthwise. Thyroid-Stimulating Hormone (TSH). WebMD. www.webmd.com/. Updated April 21, 2010. Accessed August 18, 2011.

77. Ibid.

78. *Mosby's Pocket Dictionary.*

79. Muir JL. Acetylcholine, aging, and Alzheimer's disease. *Pharmacology, Biochemistry, and Behavior.* 1997 Apr;56(4):687–96.

80. [No author listed]. Emerging therapeutic strategies for treating Alzheimer's disease in primary care. *Primary Care Companion to the Journal of Clinical Psychiatry.* 2003 Dec;5(6):268–75.

81. Glass, Making the Diagnosis of Alzheimer's.

82. Tietz NW ed. *Clinical Guide to Laboratory Tests.* 3rd ed. Philadelphia: W. B. Saunders; 1995.

83. Powell AL, Coyne AC, Jen L. A retrospective study of syphilis seropositivity in a cohort of demented patients. *Alzheimer Disease and Associated Disorders.* 1993 Spring;7(1):33–38.

84. Kennard J. Signs and Symptoms of Syphilis. *New York Times* (About.com). www.meanshealth.about.com/. Updated March 5, 2010. Accessed May 30, 2011.

85. Brown DL, Frank JE. Diagnosis and management of syphilis. *American Family Physician.* 2003 Jul 15;68(2):283–90.

86. Nettina, *Lippincott Manual.*

87. National Aids Trust. *Home Testing for HIV.* London: National Aids Trust; September 2008:1–9.

88. AVERT (formerly known as the AIDS Education and Research Trust). Getting Tested for HIV. www.avert.org/. Accessed July 19, 2011.

89. *Mosby's Pocket Dictionary.*

90. Glass, Making the Diagnosis of Alzheimer's.

91. Dixit NK, Vazquez LD, Cross NJ, Kuhl EA, Serber ER, Kovacs A, Dede DE, Conti JB, Sears SF. Cardiac resynchronization therapy: A pilot study examining cognitive change in patients before and after treatment. *Clinical Cardiology.* 2010 Feb;33(2):84–88.

92. Hammond CJ, Hallock LR, Howanski RJ, Appelt DM, Little CS, Balin BJ. Immunohistological detection of Chlamydia pneumoniae in the Alzheimer's disease brain. *BMC (BioMed Central) Neuroscience.* 2010 Sep 23;11:121.

93. Glass, Making the Diagnosis of Alzheimer's.

94. Nettina, *Lippincott Manual.*

95. Glass, Making the Diagnosis of Alzheimer's.

96. Silvestri, *Saunders Comprehensive Review.*

97. Better Medicine, Diagnosing Alzheimer's Disease.

98. Glass, Making the Diagnosis of Alzheimer's.

99. Nettina, *Lippincott Manual.*

100. *Mosby's Pocket Dictionary.*

101. Glass, Making the Diagnosis of Alzheimer's.

102. *Mosby's Pocket Dictionary.*

103. Tan G, Thornby J, Hammond DC, Strehl U, Canady B, Arnemann K, Kaiser DA. Meta-analysis of EEG biofeedback in treating epilepsy. *Clinical EEG & Neuroscience.* 2009 Jul;40(3):173–79; Cortez MA, McKerlie C, Snead OC III. A model of atypical absence seizures: EEG, pharmacology, and developmental characterization. *Neurology.* 2001 Feb 13;56(3):341–49.

104. Kowalski JW, Gawel M, Pfeffer A, Barcikowska M. The diagnostic value of EEG in Alzheimer disease: Correlation with the severity of mental impairment. *Journal of Clinical Neurophysiology.* 2001 Nov;18(6):570–75; Dauwels J, Vialatte F, Cichocki A. Diagnosis of Alzheimer's disease from EEG signals: Where are we standing? *Current Alzheimer Research.* 2010 Sep;7(6):487–505.

105. Polich J. EEG and ERP assessment of normal aging. *Electroencephalography and Clinical Neurophysiology.* 1997 May;104(3):244–56.

106. Silvestri, *Saunders Comprehensive Review.*

107. *Mosby's Pocket Dictionary.*

108. Glass, Making the Diagnosis of Alzheimer's.

109. Alzheimer's Association, Genetic Testing.

110. Alzheimer's Association. Diagnostic Disclosure. www.alz.org/. Updated January 6, 2007. Accessed May 30, 2011.

CHAPTER 6

1. Galluzzi KE, Appelt DM, Balin BJ. Modern care for patients with Alzheimer disease: Rationale for early intervention. *Journal of the American Osteopathic Association.* 2010 Sep;110(9 Suppl 8):S37–42.

2. Wilson GT, O'Leary KD, Nathan PE. *Abnormal Psychology.* Upper Saddle River, NJ: Prentice Hall; 1992:406.

3. Associated Press. No Cure Yet for Mind-Robbing Alzheimer's. MSNBC.com. 2004. www.msnbc.msn.com/. Accessed July 13, 2011.

4. Kennard C. Importance of Early Diagnosis in Alzheimer's Disease. *New York Times* (About .com). www.alzheimers.about.com/. Updated November 7, 2006. Accessed July 13, 2011.

5. Alzheimer's Association. What We Know Today about Alzheimer's Disease. www.alz .org/. Accessed July 14, 2011.

6. Dalmau J, Gleichman AJ, Hughes EG, Rossi JE, Peng X, Lai M, Dessain SK, Rosenfeld MR, Balice-Gordon R, Lynch DR. Anti-NMDA-receptor encephalitis: Case series and analysis of the effects of antibodies. *Lancet Neurology*. 2008 Dec;7(12):1091–98.

7. National Institute for Aging. Alzheimer's Disease Medication Fact Sheet. www.nia.nih .gov/. Accessed July 14, 2011.

8. MedicineNet.com. Memantine: Oral, Namenda. www.medicinenet.com/. Accessed July 14, 2011.

9. Babington PW, Spiegel DR. Treatment of catatonia with olanzapine and amantadine. *Psychosomatics*. 2007;48(6):534–36.

10. MedicineNet.com. Memantine (Namenda). www.medicinenet.com/. Accessed July 7, 2011.

11. MedicineNet.com, Memantine (Namenda); Forest Laboratories. Namenda. www .namenda.com/. Accessed July 4, 2011.

12. Erkulwater S, Pillai R. Amantadine and the end-stage dementia of Alzheimer's type. *Southern Medical Journal*. 1989 May;82(5):550–54.

13. Meythaler JM, Brunner RC, Johnson A, Novack TA. Amantadine to improve neurorecovery in traumatic brain injury-associated diffuse axonal injury: A pilot double-blind randomized trial. *Journal of Head Trauma Rehabilitation*. 2002 Aug;17(4):300–313.

14. National Institutes of Health. Amantadine. September 1, 2008. www.nlm.nih.gov/. Accessed July 4, 2011.

15. British Columbia Ministry of Health. Cholinesterase Inhibitors. www.health.gov.bc.ca/. Accessed July 4, 2011.

16. Drugs.com. Razadyne. www.drugs.com/. Accessed July 4, 2011.

17. Drugs.com. Razadyne ER Side Effects. www.drugs.com/. Accessed July 14, 2011.

18. Ibid.; WebMD. Razadyne Oral. www.webmd.com/. Accessed July 14, 2011.

19. Epocrates. Galantamine. https://online.epocrates.com/. Accessed July 14, 2011; MedicineNet.com. Galantamine (Razadyne, Razadyne ER—formerly known as Reminyl). www .medicinenet.com/. Accessed July 4, 2011.

20. Clinaero. Rivastigmine. www.senior-health.emedtv.com/. Accessed July 13, 2011.

21. Drugsite Trust. Rivastigmine Side Effects. www.drugs.com/. Accessed July 14, 2011.

22. Clinaero, Rivastigmine.

23. MedicineNet.com. Rivastigmine (Exelon). www.medicinenet.com/. Accessed July 4, 2011.

24. Clinaero. Exelon Overdose. www.alzheimers.emedtv.com/. Accessed July 5, 2011; Dhillon S. Rivastigmine transdermal patch: A review of its use in the management of dementia of the Alzheimer's type. *Drugs*. 2011 Jun 18;71(9):1209–31.

25. MedicineNet.com. Donepezil, Aricept, Aricept ODT. www.medicinenet.com/. Accessed July 7, 2011.

26. Clinaero. Donepezil Side Effects. www.drugs.emedtv.com/. Accessed July 13, 2011.

27. Vlad SC, Miller DR, Kowall NW, Felson DT. Protective effects of NSAIDs on the development of Alzheimer disease. *Neurology*. 2008 May 6;70(19):1672–77.

28. Drugsite Trust. Cognex. www.drugs.com/. Accessed July 8, 2011.

29. Davis KL, Thal LJ, Gamzu ER, Davis CS, Woolson RF, Gracon SI, Drachman DA, Schneider LS, Whitehouse PJ, Hoover TM. A double-blind, placebo-controlled multicenter study of tacrine for Alzheimer's disease. The Tacrine Collaborative Study Group. *New England Journal of Medicine*. 1992 Oct 29;327(18):1253–59.

30. MedicineNet.com. Tacrine. www.medicinenet.com. Last reviewed November 19, 2003. Accessed July 4, 2011.

31. National Institute for Aging. Alzheimer's Disease.

32. Panza F, Frisardi V, Imbimbo BP, D'Onofrio G, Pietrarossa G, Seripa D, Pilotto A, Solfrizzi V. Bapineuzumab: Anti-ß-amyloid monoclonal antibodies for the treatment of Alzheimer's disease. *Immunotherapy.* 2010 Nov;2(6):767–82.

33. Alzheimer's Research Forums. Drugs in Clinical Trials. www.alzforum.org/. Accessed July 18, 2011.

34. Medivation. Dimebon: Overview. www.medivation.com/. Accessed July 14, 2011.

35. DeNoon D. Dimebon Shines as Alzheimer's Therapy. WebMD. www.webmd.com/. Accessed July 14, 2011.

36. Dimebon Dimebolin Information Availability. www.dimebonalzheimers.com/. Accessed July 15, 2011.

37. BuyDimebon.com. Dimebon Side Effects. www.buydimebon.com/. Accessed July 14, 2011; Layton D, Wilton L, Boshier A, Cornelius V, Harris S, Shakir SA. Comparison of the risk of drowsiness and sedation between levocetirizine and desloratadine: A prescription-event monitoring study in England. *Drug Safety.* 2006;29(10):897–909.

38. Doody RS, Gavrilova SI, Sano M, Thomas RG, Aisen PS, Bachurin SO, Seely L, Hung D, Dimebon investigators. Effect of Dimebon on cognition, activities of daily living, behaviour, and global function in patients with mild-to-moderate Alzheimer's disease: A randomised, double-blind, placebo-controlled study. *Lancet.* 2008 Jul 19;372(9634):207–15.

39. BusinessWire. Pfizer and Medivation Announce Results from Two Phase 3 Studies in Dimebon (latrepirdine) Alzheimer's Disease Clinical Development Program. March 3, 2010. http://investors.medivation.com/. Accessed January 6, 2012; USA Today, Gannett Corp. Pfizer Alzheimer's drug fails in study. March 3, 2010. www.usatoday.com. Accessed January 6, 2012.

40. Bezprozvanny I. The rise and fall of Dimebon. *Drug News and Perspectives.* 2010 Oct;23(8):518–23.

41. Jeffrey S. Phase 2a Trial of PBT2 in AD Supports Further Investigation. www.medscape.com/. Accessed July 14, 2011.

42. Alzheimer Research Forum. Drugs in Clinical Trials: PBT2. www.alzforum.org/drg/drc/detail.asp?id=110. Accessed July 13, 2011.

43. Francis YI, Fà M, Ashraf H, Zhang H, Staniszewski A, Latchman DS, Arancio O. Dysregulation of histone acetylation in the APP/PS1 mouse model of Alzheimer's disease. *Journal of Alzheimer's Disease.* 2009;18(1):131–39.

44. Rubin A, Rubin H, *eds.* Possible New Drugs for Alzheimer's Disease Treatment: Part V. www.therubins.com/. Accessed July 14, 2011.

45. Francis et al. Dysregulation of histone acetylation.

46. Li G, Larson EB, Sonnen JA, Shofer JB, Petrie EC, Schantz A, Peskind ER, Raskind MA, Breitner JC, Montine TJ. Statin therapy is associated with reduced neuropathologic changes of Alzheimer disease. *Neurology.* 2007 Aug 28;69(9):878–85.

47. Ibid.

48. University of Rochester. Epilepsy Drug Useful to Treat Alzheimer's, Studies Find. www.rochester.edu/. Accessed July 14, 2011.

49. Ibid.

50. Roman MW. Axona (Accera, Inc.): A new medical food therapy for persons with Alzheimer's disease. *Issues in Mental Health Nursing.* 2010 Jun;31(6):435–36.

51. Rubin and Rubin, Possible New Drugs.

CHAPTER 7

1. Grill JD, Cummings JL. Current therapeutic targets for the treatment of Alzheimer's disease. *Expert Review of Neurotherapeutics.* 2010 May;10(5):711–28.

2. Press D, Alexander M. Cholinesterase Inhibitors in the Treatment of Dementia. 2011. www.uptodate.com/. Accessed April 23 2009.

3. Newson W. Natural Cures for Alzheimer's Disease. www.about-alzheimers.com/. Accessed July 9, 2011.

4. Alzheimer's Association. Natural Cures for Alzheimer's Disease. www.alz.org/. Accessed July 9, 2011.

5. Healthline Networks. Caprylic Acid. http://healthline.com/. Accessed July 14, 2011.

6. Birks J, Grimley Evans J. Ginkgo biloba for cognitive impairment and dementia. *Cochrane Database of Systematic Reviews.* 2009 Jan 21;(1):CD003120.

7. Newson W. Alzheimer's Prevention: How to Keep Your Brain in Tip-Top Shape. www.about-alzheimers.com/. Accessed July 9, 2011.

8. Monson K. Gingko Biloba Side Effects. www.alzheimers.emedtv.com/. Accessed July 14, 2011.

9. Wang R, Tang XC. Neuroprotective effects of huperzine A: A natural cholinesterase inhibitor for the treatment of Alzheimer's disease. *Neurosignals.* 2005;14(1–2):71–82.

10. Wang BS, Wang H, Wei ZH, Song YY, Zhang L, Chen HZ. Efficacy and safety of natural acetylcholinesterase inhibitor huperzine A in the treatment of Alzheimer's disease: An updated meta-analysis. *Journal of Neural Transmission.* 2009 Apr;116(4):457–65.

11. Bai DL, Tang XC, He XC. Huperzine A: A potential therapeutic agent for treatment of Alzheimer's disease. *Current Medicinal Chemistry.* 2000 Mar;7(3):355–74.

12. Gold Medal Nutraceuticals. Huperzine Side Effects. www.huperzine.net/. Accessed September 8, 2011.

13. Aisen P, Gauthier S, Ferris S, Garceau D, Samier D, Duong A, Sampalis J. A Phase III, placebo-controlled, double-blind randomized trial of tramiprosate in the clinical management of patients with mild-to-moderate Alzheimer's disease (the Alphase Study). *Neurology.* 2009;72(Suppl 3):A271.

14. Schwarcz, J. It's Natural, so It's Marketable. Montreal Gazette. www.montrealgazette.com/. November 16, 2008.

15. Santa-Maria I, Hernández F, Del Rio J, Moreno FJ, Avila J. Tramiprosate, a drug of potential interest for the treatment of Alzheimer's disease, promotes an abnormal aggregation of tau. *Molecular Neurodegeneration.* 2007 Sep 6;2:17.

16. Giugliano D, Ceriello A, Esposito K. The effects of diet on inflammation: Emphasis on the metabolic syndrome. *Journal of the American College of Cardiology.* 2006 Aug 15;48(4):677–85.

17. Ma QL, Teter B, Ubeda OJ, Morihara T, Dhoot D, Nyby MD, Tuck ML, Frautschy SA, Cole GM. Omega-3 fatty acid docosahexaenoic acid increases SorLA/LR11, a sorting protein with reduced expression in sporadic Alzheimer's disease (AD): Relevance to AD prevention. *Journal of Neuroscience.* 2007 Dec 26;27(52):14299–307.

18. Monson K. Side Effects of Omega-3 Fatty Acids. www.stroke.emedtv.com/. Accessed July 14, 2011.

19. Kato-Kataoka A, Sakai M, Ebina R, Nonaka C, Asano T, Miyamori T. Soybean-derived phosphatidylserine improves memory function of the elderly Japanese subjects with memory complaints. *Journal of Clinical Biochemistry and Nutrition.* 2010 Nov;47(3):246–55.

20. Richter Y, Herzog Y, Cohen T, Steinhart Y. The effect of phosphatidylserine-containing omega-3 fatty acids on memory abilities in subjects with subjective memory complaints: A pilot study. *Clinical Interventions in Aging.* 2010 Nov 2;5:313–16.

21. Crook T, Petrie W, Wells C, Massari DC. Effects of phosphatidylserine in Alzheimer's disease. *Psychopharmacol Bull.* 1992;28(1):61–66.

22. Aguilaniu H, Durieux J, Dillin A. Metabolism, ubiquinone synthesis, and longevity. *Genes & Development.* 2005;19(20):2399–406.

23. Mayo Clinic. Coenzyme Q10. http://mayoclinic.com/. Accessed July 9, 2011.

24. U.S. National Library of Medicine. Coenzyme Q-10: Are There Safety Concerns? Natural Medicines Comprehensive Database. www.nlm.nih.gov/. Last reviewed July 12, 2011. Accessed July 14, 2011.

25. Escott-Stump S, *ed. Nutrition and Diagnosis-Related Care.* 6th ed. Philadelphia: Lippincott Williams & Wilkins; 2008.

26. Office of Dietary Supplements, National Institutes of Health. Dietary Supplement Fact Sheet: Vitamin E. www.ods.od.nih.gov/. Accessed September 8, 2011.

27. Rauscher M. Vitamin E May Slow Alzheimer's Disease. May 4, 2009. www.reuters.com/. Accessed July 14, 2011.

28. Royal College of Psychiatrists. Drug Treatments in Alzheimer's. www.rcpsych.ac.uk/. Updated March 2011.

29. Escott-Stump, Nutrition and Diagnosis.

30. Bodenstein CJ. Intravenous vitamin E and deaths in the intensive care unit. *Pediatrics.* 1984 May;73(5):733.

31. Monson, K. Vitamin E Side Effects. www.alzheimers.emedtv.com/. Accessed July 14, 2011.

32. Freedom Home Care. Alzheimer's Care. www.freedomhomecare.net/. Accessed July 9, 2011.

33. Kalmijn S, Launer LJ, Ott A, Witteman JC, Hofman A, Breteler MM. Dietary fat intake and the risk of incident dementia in the Rotterdam Study. *Annals of Neurology.* 1997 Nov;42(5):776–82; Granholm AC, Bimonte-Nelson HA, Moore AB, Nelson ME, Freeman LR, Sambamurti K. Effects of a saturated fat and high cholesterol diet on memory and hippocampal morphology in the middle-aged rat. *Journal of Alzheimer's Disease.* 2008 Jun;14(2):133–45.

34. Fisher Center for Alzheimer's Research Foundation. Diet, Exercise & Health: How Can Overall Health and Well-Being Be Maintained in a Person Suffering from Alzheimer's Disease? www.alzinfo.org/. Accessed July 10, 2011.

35. Russell D, de Benedictis T, Saisan J. Dementia and Alzheimer's Care: Planning and Preparing for the Road Ahead. March 2011. www.helpguide.org/. July 11, 2011.

36. Covinsky KE, Newcomer R, Fox P, Wood J, Sands L, Dane K, Yaffe K. Patient and caregiver characteristics associated with depression in caregivers of patients with dementia. *Journal of General Internal Medicine.* 2003;18(12):1006–14.

37. Epstein DK, Connor JR. Dementia in the elderly: An overview, *Generations.* 1999 Fall;23(3):9–16.

38. Ibid.

39. Hodon S. Caring for Our Parents and Grandparents: Alzheimer's and Kids. GRAND Magazine. 2009. www.grandmagazine.com/. Accessed September 8, 2011.

40. Ibid.

41. De Nazelle A, Nieuwenhuijsen MJ, Antó JM, Brauer M, Briggs D, Braun-Fahrlander C, Cavill N, Cooper AR, Desqueyroux H, Fruin S, Hoek G, Panis LI, Janssen N, Jerrett M, Joffe M, Andersen ZJ, van Kempen E, Kingham S, Kubesch N, Leyden KM, Marshall JD, Matamala J, Mellios G, Mendez M, Nassif H, Ogilvie D, Peiró R, Pérez K, Rabl A, Ragettli M, Rodríguez D, Rojas D, Ruiz P, Sallis JF, Terwoert J, Toussaint JF, Tuomisto J, Zuurbier M, Lebret E. Improving health through policies that promote active travel: A review of evidence to support integrated health impact assessment. *Environmental International.* 2011 May;37(4):766–77.

42. Richards KC, Beck C, O'Sullivan PS, Shue VM. Effect of individualized social activity on sleep in nursing home residents with dementia. *Journal of the American Geriatric Society.* 2005 Sep;53(9):1510–17; Schreiner AS, Yamamoto E, Shiotani H. Positive affect among nursing

home residents with Alzheimer's dementia: The effect of recreational activity. *Aging and Mental Health.* 2005 Mar;9(2):129–34.

43. Farina E, Mantovani F, Fioravanti R, Rotella G, Villanelli F, Imbornone E, Olivotto F, Tincani M, Alberoni M, Petrone E, Nemni R, Postiglione A. Efficacy of recreational and occupational activities associated to psychologic support in mild to moderate Alzheimer disease: A multicenter controlled study. *Alzheimer Disease & Associated Disorders.* 2006 Oct–Dec;20(4):275–82.

44. Fisher Center for Alzheimer's Research Foundation. Alzheimer's Therapeutic Activities. www.alzinfo.org/. Accessed June 21, 2010.

45. Wilson RS, Krueger KR, Arnold SE, Schneider JA, Kelly JF, Barnes LL, Tang Y, Bennett DA. Loneliness and risk of Alzheimer disease. *Archives of General Psychiatry.* 2007 Feb;64(2):234–40.

46. Jayson S. Power of a Super Attitude. USA Today. October 12, 2004. www.usatoday.com/. Accessed September 8, 2011.

47. Fisher Center, Diet, Exercise & Health.

48. American Academy of Family Physicians. Mind/Body Connection: How Your Emotions Affect Your Health: What Is Good Emotional Health [Audio file]. www.familydoctor.org/. Accessed September 8, 2011. Reviewed December 2010.

49. Richeson NE. Effects of animal-assisted therapy on agitated behaviors and social interactions of older adults with dementia. *American Journal of Alzheimer's Disease and Other Dementias.* 2003 Nov–Dec;18(6):353–58.

50. Lite J, Vann M. Animal Rx: 11 Ways Pets Make You Healthy. www.everydayhealth.com/. Last updated July 15 2011. Accessed July 14, 2011.

51. Reyner A, Pelkauskas L, Martin L, O'Mansky A. *Successful Craft and Game Ideas for Alzheimer's Activities.* Colchester, CT: S & S Worldwide; 2006:3–11.

52. Fritsch T, Smyth KA, Debanne SM, Petot GJ, Friedland RP. Participation in novelty-seeking leisure activities and Alzheimer's disease. *Journal of Geriatric Psychiatry and Neurology.* 2005 Sep;18(3):134–41.

53. Aldridge D. Music and Alzheimer's disease—Assessment and therapy: Discussion paper. *Journal of the Royal Society of Medicine.* 1993 Feb;86(2):93–95.

54. Assist Guide Information Services (AGIS) Network. Top Ten Reasons Why Alzheimer's Patients Need Activities. 2008. www.agis.com/. Accessed July 14, 2011.

55. Kiyosaki R. Alzheimer's Games in All Flavors. www.best-alzheimers-products.com/. Accessed July 14, 2011.

56. Pevtzow L. Laughter Is the Test Medicine: Alzheimer's Patients Try Improv as Researchers Study Its Effects on Memory, Mood. July 13, 2011. Chicago Tribune. www.chicagotribune.com/. Accessed July 14, 2011.

57. American Association of Retired Persons (AARP). Activities for People with Alzheimer's Disease. www.assets.aarp.org/. Accessed July 15, 2011.

58. Beck C, Zgola J, Shue V. Activities of daily living: An essential component of programming for persons with Alzheimer's disease. *Alzheimer's Care Quarterly.* 2000 Spring;1(2):46–55.

59. Kemp G, Robinson L, Segal J, *contributors.* Dietary Supplements: The Smart and Safe Use of Vitamins and Supplements. www.helpguide.org/. Accessed September 8, 2011.

60. Gustafson T. Flower Power: The Pros and Cons of Taking Herbal Supplements. October 2010. www.timigustafson.com/. Accessed July 14, 2011.

61. Grunnet J. Advantages and Disadvantages of Herbal Medicine. www.herbs.lovetoknow.com/. Accessed July 14, 2011.

62. Ibid.

CHAPTER 8

1. American Health Assistance Foundation. www.ahaf.org/. Updated June 10, 2011. Accessed June 29, 2011.

2. Wischik C. Alzheimer's Scotland: Action on Dementia. www.alzscot.org/. Accessed June 29, 2011.

3. ICNF World. Interviews with Scientists. www.icn-frankfurt.de/. Accessed June 29, 2011.

4. Dementia Care Central. Stages of Dementia. www.dementiacarecentral.com/. Accessed June 29, 2011.

5. McKhann GM, Knopman DS, Chertkow H, Hyman BT, Jack CR Jr, Kawas CH, Klunk WE, Koroshetz WJ, Manly JJ, Mayeux R, Mohs RC, Morris JC, Rossor MN, Scheltens P, Carrillo MC, Thies B, Weintraub S, Phelps CH. The diagnosis of dementia due to Alzheimer's disease: Recommendations from the National Institute on Aging–Alzheimer's Association workgroups on diagnostic guidelines for Alzheimer's disease. *Alzheimer's & Dementia*. 2011;7,3:263–69.

6. American Geriatrics Society. What's New in Clinical Medicine. AGS News Week in Review. May 6, 2011. www.americangeriatrics.org/. Accessed June 29, 2011.

7. McKhann et al., Diagnosis of dementia.

8. Alzheimer's Association. New Diagnostic Criteria and Guidelines for Alzheimer's Disease. www.alz.org/. Accessed June 29, 2011.

9. Alzheimer's Association. Stages of Alzheimer's Disease. www.alz.org/. Updated October 2003. Accessed June 29, 2011.

10. Archer T, Kostrzewa RM. Staging Neurological Disorders: Expressions of Cognitive and Motor Disorder. *Neurotoxicity Research*. 2010 August;18:107–11.

11. Park M. 3 Stages of Alzheimer's Disease Introduced. CNN. www.edition.cnn.com/. Updated April 19, 2011. Accessed June 29, 2011.

12. Robinson L, Saisan J, and Segal J. Stages of Alzheimer's Disease. www.helpguide.org/. Updated June 2011. Accessed July 3, 2011.

13. Sperling RA, Aisen PS, Beckett LA, Bennett DA, Craft S, Fagan AM, Iwatsubo T, Jack CR Jr, Kaye J, Montine TJ, Park DC, Reiman EM, Rowe CC, Siemers E, Stern Y, Yaffe K, Carrillo MC, Thies B, Morrison-Bogorad M, Wagster MV, Phelps CH. Toward defining the preclinical stages of Alzheimer's disease: Recommendations from the National Institute on Aging–Alzheimer's Association workgroups on diagnostic guidelines for Alzheimer's disease. *Alzheimer's & Dementia*. 2011;7(3):280–92.

14. Robinson, Saisan, and Segal, Stages of Alzheimer's.

15. Fisher Center for Alzheimer's Research Foundation. Genetic Risk Factors. www.alz-info.org/. Accessed July 3, 2011.

16. Alzheimer's Association, Stages of Alzheimer's.

17. Sperling et al., Toward defining the preclinical stages.

18. Robinson, Saisan, and Segal, Stages of Alzheimer's.

19. Sergeant N, Bombois S, Ghestem A, Drobecq H, Kostanjevecki V, Missiaen C, Wattez A, David JP, Vanmechelen E, Sergheraert C, Delacourte A. Truncated beta-amyloid peptide species in pre-clinical Alzheimer's disease as new targets for the vaccination approach. *Journal of Neurochemistry*. 2003 Jun;85(6):1581–91.

20. Berger P, *ed*. New Guidelines to Detect MCI, Alzheimer's, Dementia. *Dementia & Alzheimer's Weekly*. 2011 April 24–May 1.

21. Sperling et al., Toward defining the preclinical stages.

22. Shaw LM, Vanderstichele H, Knapik-Czajka M, Clark CM, Aisen PS, Petersen RC, Blennow K, Soares H, Simon A, Lewczuk P, Dean R, Siemers E, Potter W, Lee VM, Trojanowski JQ. Cerebrospinal fluid biomarker signature in Alzheimer's disease neuroimaging initiative subjects. *Annals of Neurology*. 2009;65:403–13.

23. Ibid.

24. Fagan AM, Mintun MA, Mach RH, Lee SY, Dence CS, Shah AR, LaRossa GN, Spinner ML, Klunk WE, Mathis CA, DeKosky ST, Morris JC, Holtzman DM. Inverse relation between in vivo amyloid imaging load and cerebrospinal fluid Abeta42 in humans. *Annals of Neurology.* 2006;59:512–19.

25. Sperling et al., Toward defining the preclinical stages.

26. Ibid.

27. Ibid.

28. Campbell N, Ayub A, Boustani MA, Fox C, Farlow M, Maidment I, Howards R. Impact of cholinesterase inhibitors on behavioral and psychological symptoms of Alzheimer's disease: A meta-analysis. *Journal of Clinical Interventions in Aging.* 2008;3(4):719–28.

29. Vivacare. Alzheimer's Disease Medications. www.fromyourdoctor.com/. Updated April 4, 2011. Accessed July 3, 2011.

30. Robinson, Saisan, and Segal, Stages of Alzheimer's.

31. Ibid.

32. Ibid.

33. Albert MS, DeKosky ST, Dickson D, Dubois B, Feldman HH, Fox NC, Gamst A, Holtzman DM, Jagust WJ, Petersen RC, Snyder PJ, Carrillo MC, Thies B, Phelps CH. The diagnosis of mild cognitive impairment due to Alzheimer's disease: Recommendations from the National Institute on Aging–Alzheimer's Association workgroups on diagnostic guidelines for Alzheimer's disease. *Alzheimer's & Dementia.* 2011;7(3):270–79.

34. Ibid.

35. Ibid.

36. Ibid.

37. Bupa's Health Information Team. Alzheimer's Disease. February 2011. www.bupa .co.uk/. Accessed July 3, 2011.

38. Vivacare. Alzheimer's Disease Medications.

39. Austrom MG, Lu Y. Long term caregiving: Helping families of persons with mild cognitive impairment cope. *Current Alzheimer Research.* 2009;6(4):392–98.

40. Robinson, Saisan, and Segal, Stages of Alzheimer's.

41. Ibid.

42. Alzheimer's Association, Stages of Alzheimer's.

43. Robinson, Saisan, and Segal, Stages of Alzheimer's.

44. McKhann et al., Diagnosis of dementia.

45. Ibid.

46. Ibid.

47. Brickman AM, Muraskin J, Zimmerman ME. Structural neuroimaging in Alzheimer's disease: Do white matter hyperintensities matter? *Dialogues in Clinical Neuroscience.* 2009;11(2):181–90.

48. McKhann et al., Diagnosis of dementia.

49. Ibid.

50. Vivacare. Alzheimer's Disease Medications.

51. Ibid.

52. Ibid.

53. Ibid.

54. Fisher Center for Alzheimer's Research Foundation. Alzheimer's Research on Caregiving. www.alzinfo.org/. Accessed July 3, 2011.

55. Robinson, Saisan, and Segal, Stages of Alzheimer's.

56. Fisher Center for Alzheimer's Research Foundation. Clinical Stages of Alzheimer's. www.alzinfo.org/. Accessed July 3, 2011.

57. Berger, New Guidelines to Detect MCI.

58. Ibid.

59. Khachaturian ZS. Revised criteria for diagnosis of Alzheimer's disease: Recommendations from the National Institute on Aging–Alzheimer's Association workgroups on diagnostic guidelines for Alzheimer's disease. *Alzheimer's & Dementia.* 2011;7,3:253–56.

60. Ibid.

CHAPTER 9

1. Goethe Institute of Frankfurt. Eva Braak homepage. www.med.uni-frankfurt.de/. Updated November 20, 2006. Accessed July 15, 2011.

2. Braak H, Braak E. Neuropathological staging of Alzheimer's-related changes. *Acta Neuropathologica.* 1991;82(4):239–59.

3. Interdisciplinary Center for Neuroscience Frankfurt (ICNF). Interview with Prof. Dr. Heiko Braak: A Pioneer of Brain Research Reports. www.icn-frankfurt.de/. Updated May 14, 2009. Accessed July 13, 2011.

4. Braak H. Das ependym der hirnventrikel von chimaera monstrosa (mit besonderer berücksichtigung des organon vasculare praeopticum) [German]. *Zeitschrift für Zellforschung und Mikroskopische Anatomie.* 1963;60:582–608.

5. Braak H. Biogene amine im gehirn vom frosch (Rana esculenta) [German]. *Zeitschrift für Zellforschung und Mikroskopische Anatomie.*1970;106(2):269–308.

6. Michael J. Fox Foundation for Parkinson's Research. Researcher Bio: Heiko Braak, MD. www.michaeljfox.org/. Updated July 13, 2011. Accessed July 13, 2011.

7. Ibid.

8. Goethe Institute of Frankfurt, Eva Braak home page.

9. Ibid.

10. Braak H, Del Tredici K. The pathological process underlying Alzheimer's disease in individuals under thirty. *Acta Neuropathologica.* 2011;121:171–81.

11. TauRX Therapeutics. Tau Tangles in Alzheimer's Disease. www.tau-rx.com/. Updated July 30, 2008. Accessed July 14, 2011.

12. TheRibbon.com. The Three Stages of Alzheimer's Disease. www.theribbon.com/. Updated July 17, 2011. Accessed July 17, 2011.

13. Alzheimer Gesellschaft Berlin (Alzheimer's Association of Berlin). *Stationen der Alzheimer-Krankheit (Stages of Alzheimer's Disease).* Freiburg, Germany: Verlag Herder; 2000:52–55.

14. Ibid.

15. Braak and Braak, Neuropathological staging.

16. Braak H, Braak E. Evolution of Alzheimer's Disease Related Intraneuronal Changes. www.alzforum.org/. Updated July 17, 2011. Accessed July 17, 2011.

17. University of Washington. BrainInfo. www.braininfo.org/. Updated July 5, 2011. Accessed July 15, 2011.

18. Finck O. *Verstehende Diagnostik als Chance zur rehistorisierenden Diagnostik für und mit chronisch verwirrten Menschen zur Bewahrung der biographischen Integrität.* Munich, Germany: Grin Verlag; 2007:40–44.

19. TauRX, Tau Tangles.

20. Ibid.

21. Ibid.

22. Finck, *Verstehende Diagnostik.*

23. University of Washington. BrainInfo.

24. Rajmohan V, Mohandas E. The limbic system. *Indian Journal of Psychiatry.* 2007 Apr;49(2):132–39.

25. TauRX, Tau Tangles.

26. Ibid.

27. Finck, *Verstehende Diagnostik.*

28. TauRX, Tau Tangles.

29. Manaye KF, McIntire DD, Mann DM, German DC. Locus coeruleus cell loss in the aging human brain: A non-random process. *Journal of Comparative Neurology.* 1995 Jul 17;358(1):79–87.

30. Finck, *Verstehende Diagnostik.*

31. Braak and Braak, Neuropathological staging.

32. Braak and Del Tredici, Pathological process underlying Alzheimer's.

33. Rauch J. Alzheimer Beginnt Schon in der Kindheit. www.wissenschaft.de/. Updated July 14, 2011. Accessed July 14, 2011.

CHAPTER 10

1. Hamdy RC. The Clinical Stages. 1992. www.zarcrom.com/. Accessed July 2, 2011.

2. Alzheimer's Association. Stages of Alzheimer's. www.alz.org/. Accessed June 28 2011.

3. Alzheimer Gesellschaft Berlin (Alzheimer's Association of Berlin). *Stationen der Alzheimer-Krankheit (Stages of Alzheimer's Disease).* Freiburg, Germany: Verlag Herder; 2000: 52–55.

4. New York University Langone Medical Center. Barry Reisberg, MD. www .med.nyu.edu/. Accessed January 8, 2012.

5. International Psychogeriatric Association. IPA Profiles: Barry Reisberg, MD. www.ipa-online.org/. Accessed June 28, 2011.

6. Ibid.

7. Alzheimer's Association. Stages of Alzheimer's.

8. Memory Study. The 7 Stages of Alzheimer's. www.memorystudy.org/. Accessed June 28 2011.

9. Robinson L, Saisan J, Segal J. Alzheimer's Disease: Symptoms, Stages and Coping with Alzheimer's Disease. www.helpguide.org/. Updated August 2011. Accessed September 15, 2011.

10. Nordqvist C. What Is Alzheimer's Disease? What Causes Alzheimer's Disease? July 31, 2009. www.medicalnewstoday.com/. Accessed September 15, 2011.

11. Mania I, Evcimen H, Mathews M. Citalopram treatment for inappropriate sexual behavior in a cognitively impaired patient. *Primary Care Companion to the Journal of Clinical Psychiatry.* 2006;8(2):106.

12. Memory Study, 7 Stages.

13. Wormald T. The Complete Guide to Treating and Coping with Alzheimer's Disease. 2006. www.health-directories.com/. Accessed April 26, 2012.

14. The Fisher Center for Alzheimer's Research Foundation. The Clinical Stages of Alzheimer's. www.alzinfo.org/. Accessed June 28 2011.

CHAPTER 11

1. Demyttenaere K, Bruffaerts R, Posada-Villa J, Gasquet I, Kovess V, Lepine JP, Angermeyer MC, Bernert S, de Girolamo G, Morosini P, Polidori G, Kikkawa T, Kawakami N, Ono Y, Takeshima T, Uda H, Karam EG, Fayyad JA, Karam AN, Mneimneh ZN, Medina-Mora ME, Borges G, Lara C, de Graaf R, Ormel J, Gureje O, Shen Y, Huang Y, Zhang M, Alonso J,

Haro JM, Vilagut G, Bromet EJ, Gluzman S, Webb C, Kessler RC, Merikangas KR, Anthony JC, Von Korff MR, Wang PS, Brugha TS, Aguilar-Gaxiola S, Lee S, Heeringa S, Pennell BE, Zaslavsky AM, Ustun TB, Chatterji S. Prevalence, severity, and unmet need for treatment of mental disorders in the World Health Organization World Mental Health Surveys. *Journal of the American Medical Association*. 2004 Jun 2;291(21):2581–90.

2. Holmes L. Mental Disorders Common throughout the World. www.mentalhealth .about.com/. Updated November 5, 2005. Accessed May 28, 2011.

3. Demyttenaere et al., Prevalence, severity, and unmet need.

4. Holmes, Mental Disorders.

5. Cherry K. What Is Cognition? www.psychology.about.com/. Accessed June 1, 2011.

6. U.S. National Library of Medicine. Multi-infarct Dementia. Reviewed March 22, 2010. www.ncbi.nlm.nih.gov/. Accessed January 14, 2012.

7. Boyles S. Depression Linked to Alzheimer's Disease: Study Shows Depression in Elderly Doubles Dementia Risk. WebMD. www.webmd.com/. Accessed May 30, 2011.

8. Nordqvist C. Depression. Medical News Today. June 1, 2004. www.medicalnewstoday .com/. Updated April 7, 2009. Accessed May 30, 2011.

9. Egede LE. Major depression in individuals with chronic medical disorders: Prevalence, correlates and association with health resource utilization, lost productivity and functional disability. *General Hospital Psychiatry*. 2007 Sep–Oct;29(5):409–16.

10. National Alliance on Mental Illness. What Is Depression? www.nami.org/. Accessed June 2, 2011.

11. Cannon-Spoor HE, Levy JA, Zubenko GS, Zubenko WW, Cohen RM, Mirza N, Putnam K, Sunderland T. Effects of previous major depressive illness on cognition in Alzheimer disease patients. *American Journal of Geriatric Psychiatry*. 2005 Apr;13(4):312–18.

12. Migliorelli R, Tesón A, Sabe L, Petracchi M, Leiguarda R, Starkstein SE. Prevalence and correlates of dysthymia and major depression among patients with Alzheimer's disease. *American Journal of Psychiatry*. 1995 Jan;152(1):37–44.

13. Whitley KP. Mood and anxiety disorders in women. *Psychiatric Services* 2007 Sep;58:1234.

14. Saczynski JS, Beiser A, Seshadri S, Auerbach S, Wolf PA, Au R. Depressive symptoms and risk of dementia: The Framingham Heart Study. *Neurology*. 2010 Jul 6;75(1):35–41.

15. Ibid.

16. O'Leary D, Jyringi D, Sedler M. Childhood conduct problems, stages of Alzheimer's disease, and physical aggression against caregivers. *International Journal of Geriatric Psychiatry*. 2005 May;20(5):401–5.

17. Alzheimer's Association. 10 Signs of Alzheimer's. www.alz.org/. Updated August 23, 2011. Accessed September 16, 2011; Alzheimer's Association. Stages of Alzheimer's. www .alz.org/. Updated June 1, 2011. Accessed September 16, 2011; Forest Laboratories. Stages of Alzheimer's Disease. www.namenda.com/. Accessed September 16, 2011.

18. Seignourel PJ, Kunik ME, Snow L, Wilson N, Stanley M. Anxiety in dementia: A critical review. *Clinical Psychology Review*. 2008 Oct;28(7):1071–82; Cooper C, Katona C, Orrell M, Livingston G. Coping strategies and anxiety in caregivers of people with Alzheimer's disease: The LASER-AD study. *Journal of Affective Disorders*. 2006 Jan;90(1):15–20; Chemerinski E, Petracca G, Manes F, Leiguarda R, Starkstein SE. Prevalence and correlates of anxiety in Alzheimer's disease. *Depression and Anxiety*. 1998;7(4):166–70.

19. Nordqvist C, ed. What Is Anxiety? What Causes Anxiety? What to Do About It. Medical News Today. April 23, 2004. www.medicalnewstoday.com/. Updated February 10, 2009. Accessed May 30, 2011.

20. MedicineNet.com. Generalized Anxiety Disorder. www.medicinenet.com/. Accessed June 2, 2011.

21. Chakraburtty A, *reviewer*. Anxiety Disorders. WebMD. February 9, 2009. www.web md.com/. Accessed May 31, 2011.

22. Branan N. Anxiety and Alzheimer's: A lifetime of stress could lead to memory problems and disease. Scientific American. October 2007. www.scientificamerican.com/. Accessed May 31, 2011.

23. Silverstien N, Salmons T. Wandering Behavior in Community-Residing Persons with Alzheimer's Disease Registered in Safe Return. Boston: Gerontology Institute; 1996.

24. Synder LH, Rupprecht P, Pyrek J, Brekhus S, Moss T. Wandering. *Gerontologist.* 1978;18(3):272–80.

25. Hussain RA, Davis RL. Responsive care. In: Behavior Interventions with Elderly Persons. Champaign, IL: Research Press; 1985.

26. Butler J, Barnett C. Window of wandering. *Geriatric Nursing.* 1991;Sep/Oct: 226–27.

27. National Center for Health Statistics. The National Nursing Home Survey, series 13, no. 97. Hyattsville, MD: DDHS, USPHS; 1989:89–1758.

28. O'Boyle R. Managing Agitation Behavior in Alzheimer's Patients. Healing Well. www .healingwell.com/. Accessed June 2, 2011.

29. Watson Institute. Repetitive or Unusual Behaviors. www.thewatsoninstitute.org/. Accessed May 31, 2011.

30. Alexander G, Hanna A, Serna V, Younkin L, Younkin S, Janus C. Increased aggression in males in transgenic Tg2576 mouse model of Alzheimer's disease. *Behavioural Brain Research.* 2011 Jan 1;216(1):77–83.

31. Eustace A, Kidd N, Greene E, Fallon C, Bhrain SN, Cunningham C, Coen R, Walsh JB, Coakley D, Lawlor BA. Verbal aggression in Alzheimer's disease: Clinical, functional and neuropsychological correlates. *International Journal of Geriatric Psychiatry.* 2001 Sep;16(9):858–61.

32. Alzheimer's Association. Aggression. www.alz.org/. Accessed June 3, 2011.

33. National Center for Health Statistics, National Nursing Home Survey.

34. Hwang JP, Tsai SJ, Yang CH, Liu KM, Lirng JF. Hoarding behavior in dementia: A preliminary report. *American Journal of Geriatric Psychiatry.* 1998 Fall;6(4):285–89; Bakker R. Hoarding and Alzheimer's Disease (AD): One Daughter's Story [Presentation]. Weill Cornell Center for Aging Research and Clinical Care. n.d.:1–11.

35. Mayo Clinic. Hoarding. www.mayoclinic/. Accessed May 31, 2011.

36. Ibid.

37. Brink TL. Paranoia in Alzheimer's patients: Prevalence and impact on caretakers. *International Journal of Behavioral Geriatrics.* 1983 Winter;1(4):53–55.

38. Fauci AS, Braunwald E, Kasper DL, Hauser SL, Longo DL, Jameson JL, Loscalzo J. Harrison's Principles of Internal Medicine. 17th ed. New York: McGraw-Hill Professional; 2008.

39. Ibid.

40. DepressionGuide.com. Paranoia. www.depression-guide.com/. Accessed May 31, 2011.

41. Wilson RS, Gilley DW, Bennett DA, Beckett LA, Evans DA. Hallucinations, delusions, and cognitive decline in Alzheimer's disease. *Journal of Neurology, Neurosurgery & Psychiatry.* 2000 Aug;69(2):172–77; Bassiony MM, Steinberg MS, Warren A, Rosenblatt A, Baker AS, Lyketsos CG. Delusions and hallucinations in Alzheimer's disease: Prevalence and clinical correlates. *International Journal of Geriatric Psychiatry.* 2000 Feb;15(2):99–107.

42. Iaria G, Fox CJ, Scheel M, Stowe RM, Barton JJ. A case of persistent visual hallucinations of faces following LSD abuse: A functional Magnetic Resonance Imaging study. *Neurocase.* 2010 Apr;16(2):106–18.

43. Ballas C, reviewer. Hallucinations. New York Times Health Guide. www.health.nytimes .com/. Accessed May 31, 2011.

44. Skovdahl K, Sörlie V, Kihlgren M. Tactile stimulation associated with nursing care to individuals with dementia showing aggressive or restless tendencies: An intervention study in dementia care. *International Journal of Older People Nursing.* 2007 Sep;2(3):162–70.

45. Agüera-Ortiz L, Perez MI, Osorio RS, Sacks H, Palomo T. Prevalence and clinical correlates of restless legs syndrome among psychogeriatric patients. *International Journal of*

Geriatric Psychiatry. 2011 Dec;26(12):1252–59; Bliwise DL. Restless Legs Syndrome: Manifestations in Aging and Dementia. In: Geriatric Sleep Medicine. 1st ed. New York: Informa Plc (Health); September 2008:280.

46. HealthGrades. Restlessness. www.wrongdiagnosis.com/. Accessed June 1, 2011.

47. Sokol DK, Maloney B, Long JM, Ray B, Lahiri DK. Autism, Alzheimer disease, and fragile X: APP, FMRP, and mGluR5 are molecular links. *Neurology*. 2011 Apr 12;76(15):1344–52.

48. Nordqvist C. What Is Autism? What Causes Autism? www.medicalnewstoday.com/. Accessed June 2, 2011.

49. National Institute of Mental Health. Treatment Research in Mental Illness: Improving the Nation's Public Mental Health Care through NIMH Funded Interventions Research. January 2005. www.nimh.nih.gov/. Accessed June 2, 2011.

CHAPTER 12

1. Arvanitakis Z, Wilson RS, Bienias JL, Evans DA, Bennett DA. Diabetes mellitus and risk of Alzheimer disease and decline in cognitive function. *Archives of Neurology*. 2004 May;61(5):661–66; Li ZG, Zhang W, Sima AA. Increased beta-amyloid and phospho-tau in diabetic encephalopathy. *Diabetes*. 2006;55:A190.

2. Tan ZS, Vasan RS. Thyroid function and Alzheimer's disease. *Journal of Alzheimer's Disease*. 2009;16(3):503–7.

3. Kugler M. Niemann-Pick Disease. www.rarediseases.about.com/. Updated March 3, 2009. Accessed June 4, 2011.

4. Office of Communications and Public Liaison. National Institute of Neurological Disorders and Stroke (NINDS) Niemann-Pick Disease Information Page. www.ninds.nih.gov/. Updated June 10, 2011. Accessed June 11, 2011.

5. Jan MM, Camfield PR. Nova Scotia Niemann-Pick disease (type D): Clinical study of 20 cases. *Journal of Child Neurology*. 1998 Feb;13(2):75–78.

6. Lott IT, Head E. Down syndrome and Alzheimer's disease: A link between development and aging. *Mental Retardation and Developmental Disabilities Research Reviews*. 2001;7(3):172–78.

7. Nemours Foundation. Down Syndrome. August 2008. www.kidshealth.org/. Accessed June 6, 2011.

8. National Institute of Neurological Disorders and Stroke (NINDS). Creutzfeldt-Jakob Disease Fact Sheet. www.ninds.nih.gov/. Accessed September 16, 2011.

9. Ibid.

10. Korenberg JR, Bradley C, Disteche C. Down syndrome: Molecular mapping of the congenital heart disease and duodenal stenosis. *American Journal of Human Genetics*. 1992;50:294–302.

11. WebMD. Down Syndrome and Alzheimer's Disease Risk. www.webmd.com/. Updated June 16, 2009. Accessed June 6, 2011.

12. Debatin L, Streffer J, Geissen M, Matschke J, Aguzzi A, Glatzel M. Association between deposition of beta-amyloid and pathological prion protein in sporadic Creutzfeldt-Jakob disease. *Neurodegenerative Diseases*. 2008;5(6):347–54.

13. Talbott SD, Plato BM, Sattenberg RJ, Parker J, Heidenreich JO. Cortical restricted diffusion as the predominant MRI finding in sporadic Creutzfeldt-Jakob disease. *Acta Radiologica*. 2011 Apr 1;52(3):336–39.

14. NINDS, Creutzfeldt-Jakob Disease.

15. Will RG. Acquired prion disease: Iatrogenic CJD, variant CJD, kuru. *British Medical Bulletin.* 2003;66:255–65.

16. National Institute of Neurological Disorders and Stroke. Disorder Index. http://www .ninds.nih.gov/. Accessed June 15, 2011.

17. North Dakota State University Department of Psychology. Introduction to Creutzfeldt Jakob Disease. www.psych.ndsu.nodak.edu/. Accessed September 20, 2011.

18. NINDS, Creutzfeldt-Jakob Disease.

19. Ibid.

20. Selkoe DJ. Cell biology of protein misfolding: the examples of Alzheimer's and Parkinson's diseases. *Nature Cell Biology.* 2004 Nov;6(11):1054–61.

21. Knopman DS. Alzheimer's disease and other dementias. In: Goldman L, Ausiello D, eds. *Cecil Medicine.* 23rd ed. Philadelphia: Saunders Elsevier; 2007:chap. 425.

22. Tan, E. The Basic Neurobiology of Huntington's Disease. HOPES Huntington's Outreach Project for Education at Stanford. www.hopes.stanford.edu/. Accessed June 15, 2011.

23. Nance MA, Myers RH. Juvenile onset Huntington's disease: Clinical and research perspectives. *Mental Retardation and Developmental Disabilities Research Reviews.* 2001;7(3):153–57; Smith JA, Brewer HM, Eatough V, Stanley CA, Glendinning NW, Quarrell OW. The personal experience of juvenile Huntington's disease: An interpretative phenomenological analysis of parents' accounts of the primary features of a rare genetic condition. *Clinical Genetics.* 2006 Jun;69(6):486–96.

24. Novak MJ, Tabrizi SJ. Huntington's disease. *British Medical Journal.* 2010;340:c3109.

25. Ibid.

26. Nussbaum RL, Ellis CE. Alzheimer's disease and Parkinson's disease. *New England Journal of Medicine.* 2003;348:1356–64.

27. Houghton PJ, Howes MJ. Natural products and derivatives affecting neurotransmission relevant to Alzheimer's and Parkinson's disease. *Neurosignals.* 2005;14(1–2):6–22.

28. Peppard RF, Martin WR, Clark CM, Carr GD, McGeer PL, Calne DB. Cortical glucose metabolism in Parkinson's and Alzheimer's disease. *Journal of Neuroscience Research.* 1990 Dec;27(4):561–68; Farkas E, De Jong GI, Apró E, De Vos RA, Steur EN, Luiten PG. Similar ultrastructural breakdown of cerebrocortical capillaries in Alzheimer's disease, Parkinson's disease, and experimental hypertension: What is the functional link? *Annals of the New York Academy of Sciences.* 2000 Apr;903:72–82.

29. Lolekha P, Phanthumchinda K, Bhidayasiri R. Prevalence and risk factors of Parkinson's disease in retired Thai traditional boxers. *Movement Disorders.* 2010 Sep 15;25(12):1895–901.

30. Schapira AH. Etiology and pathogenesis of Parkinson disease. *Neurology Clinics.* 2009;27:583.

31. Burton RR. Parkinson's disease without tremor masquerading as mechanical back pain: A case report. *Journal of the Canadian Chiropractic Association.* 2008 Aug;52(3):185–92.

32. Kamin J, Manwani S, Hughes D. Emergency psychiatry: Extrapyramidal side effects in the psychiatric emergency service. *Psychiatric Services.* 2000 Mar;51(3):287–89.

33. Berardelli A, Rothwell JC, Thompson PD, Hallett M. Pathophysiology of bradykinesia in Parkinson's disease. *Brain.* 2001 Nov;124(Pt 11):2131–46; Hill C. What is Alzheimer's Disease? *New York Times* (About.com). www.alzheimers.about.com/. Updated November 22, 2010. Accessed August 22, 2011.

34. Tyrrell PJ, Sawle GV, Ibanez V, Bloomfield PM, Leenders KL, Frackowiak RS, Rossor MN. Clinical and positron emission tomographic studies in the "extrapyramidal syndrome" of dementia of the Alzheimer type. *Archives of Neurology.* 1990 Dec;47(12):1318–23.

35. Flanagan M. *The Downside of Upright Posture: The Anatomical Causes of Alzheimer's, Parkinson's and Multiple Sclerosis.* Minneapolis: Two Harbors Press; 2010.

36. Asgari M, Shafran I. Predicting severity of Parkinson's disease from speech: Conference proceedings. *Annual International Conference of the IEEE Engineering in Medicine and Biology Society.* 2010;2010:5201–4.

37. Buter TC, van den Hout A, Matthews FE, Larsen JP, Brayne C, Aarsland D. Dementia and survival in Parkinson disease: A 12-year population study. *Neurology.* 2008 Mar 25;70(13):1017–22.

38. National Institute of Neurological Disorders and Stroke, Disorder Index.

39. dbS Productions. Alzheimer's Disease and Related Disorders SAR Research. www.dbs-sar.com/. Accessed June 15, 2011.

40. Clinaero. Alzheimers Articles. http://alzheimers.emedtv.com/. Accessed June 15, 2011.

41. Weller RO, Nicoll JA. Cerebral amyloid angiopathy: Pathogenesis and effects on the ageing and Alzheimer brain. *Neurological Research.* 2003 Sep;25(6):611–16.

42. Savolainen S, Paljärvi L, Vapalahti M. Prevalence of Alzheimer's disease in patients investigated for presumed normal pressure hydrocephalus: A clinical and neuropathological study. *Acta Neurochirurgica.* 1999;141(8):849–53.

43. National Institute of Neurological Disorders and Stroke. Hydrocephalus Fact Sheet. www.ninds.nih.gov/. Accessed January 11, 2012.

44. Eide PK, Sorteberg W. Changes in intracranial pulse pressure amplitudes after shunt implantation and adjustment of shunt valve opening pressure in normal pressure hydrocephalus. *Acta Neurochirurgica.* 2008 Nov;150(11):1141–47.

45. Zarrouf F, Griffith J, Jesse J. Cognitive dysfunction in normal pressure hydrocephalus (NPH): A case report and review of the literature. *West Virginia Medical Journal.* 2009 Mar–Apr;105(2):22, 24–26.

46. Lott and Head, Down syndrome and Alzheimer's disease.

47. DBS Productions. Alzheimer's Disease and Related Disorders: SAR Research. www .dbs-sar.com/. Accessed June 15, 2011.

48. Fishman, MA. Hydrocephalus. In: Eliasson, SG, Prensky, AL, Hardin, WB *eds. Neurological Pathophysiology.* New York: Oxford University Press; 1978.

49. Fishman, Hydrocephalus; Carey, CM, Tullous, MW, Walker, ML. Hydrocephalus: Etiology, Pathologic Effects, Diagnosis, and Natural History. In: Cheek, WR, *ed. Pediatric Neurosurgery,* 3rd ed. Philadelphia: WB Saunders Company; 1994.

50. Fishman, Hydrocephalus; Carey, Tullous, and Walker, Hydrocephalus.

51. Thomas FP. Dementia Due to HIV Infection. eMedicine. www.emedicinehealth.com/. Accessed June 15, 2011.

52. Hill, What Is Alzheimer's?

CHAPTER 13

1. Merskey H, Bogduk N. *Classification of Chronic Pain: Descriptions of Chronic Pain Syndromes and Definition of Pain Terms.* 2nd ed. Seattle: IASP Press; 1994.

2. Kopf A, Patel NB, *eds.* Guide to Pain Management in Low-Resource Settings. www .iasp-pain.org/. Accessed July 27, 2011; Vasudevan S. Physical rehabilitation in managing pain. *Pain Clinical Updates.* 1997;5(3):1–4.

3. Ganong WF. *Review of Medical Physiology.* 20th ed. New York: McGraw-Hill; 2001.

4. Braun D. Alzheimer Disease and Pain Control. www.natural-holistic-health.com/. Accessed July 22, 2011.

5. Scherder E, Bouma A, Slaets J, Ooms M, Ribbe M, Blok A, Sergeant J. Repeated pain assessment in Alzheimer's disease. *Dementia and Geriatric Cognitive Disorders.* 2001;12(6):400–

407; Rainero I, Vighetti S, Bergamasco B, Pinessi L, Benedetti F. Autonomic responses and pain perception in Alzheimer's disease. *European Journal of Pain.* 2001;4(3):267–74.

6. Gibson SJ, Voukelatos X, Ames D, Flicker L, Helme RD. An examination of pain perception and cerebral event-related potentials following carbon dioxide laser stimulation in patients with Alzheimer's disease and age-matched control volunteers. *Pain Research & Management.* 2001 Fall;6(3):126–32; Rainero et al., Autonomic responses; Benedetti F, Vighetti S, Ricco C, Lagna E, Bergamasco B, Pinessi L, Rainero I. Pain threshold and tolerance in Alzheimer's disease. *Pain.* 1999 Mar;80(1–2):377–82.

7. Cole LJ, Farrell MJ, Duff EP, Barber JB, Egan GF, Gibson SJ. Pain sensitivity and fMRI pain-related brain activity in Alzheimer's disease. *Brain.* 2006 Nov;129 (Pt 11):2957–65.

8. Ganong, *Review of Medical Physiology.*

9. Dartmouth-Hitchcock Medical Center. Annual Report 2004. www.dhmc.org/. Accessed July 27, 2011.

10. Ganong, *Review of Medical Physiology.*

11. Kopf and Patel, Guide to Pain Management.

12. Kansas Department on Aging. Medications for Treating Dementia Symptoms. www.agingkansas.org/. Accessed July 28, 2011.

13. Dias MB, Nucci TB, Branco LG, Gargaglioni LH. Opioid μ-receptors in the rostral medullary raphe modulate hypoxia-induced hyperpnea in unanesthetized rats. *Acta Physiologica (Oxford).* 2011 Aug 9. Published online ahead of print.

14. National Institute on Drug Abuse. Research Report Series: Prescription Drugs; Abuse and Addiction. www.nida.nih.gov/. Accessed August 2, 2011; Davidson S, Macleod J, eds. *The Principles and Practice of Medicine.* 10th ed. Edinburgh, UK: Livingstone; 1971.

15. Bell JS, Laitinen ML, Lavikainen P, Lönnroos E, Uosukainen H, Hartikainen S. Use of strong opioids among community-dwelling persons with and without Alzheimer's disease in Finland. *Pain.* 2011;152(3):543–47.

16. Collins KM, Plantevin OM. Use of alfentanil in short anaesthetic procedures. *Journal of the Royal Society of Medicine.* 1985 Jun;78(6):456–58.

17. Ganong, *Review of Medical Physiology;* National Institute on Drug Abuse, Research Report Series; Davidson and Macleod, *Principles and Practice of Medicine.*

18. Wood R. Healing with Food. www.rwood.com/. Accessed August 2, 2011.

19. Watzl B. Anti-inflammatory effects of plant-based foods and of their constituents. *International Journal for Vitamin and Nutrition Research.* 2008 Dec;78(6):293–98; Gertsch J. Anti-inflammatory cannabinoids in diet: Towards a better understanding of CB(2) receptor action? *Communicative & Integrative Biology.* 2008;1(1):26–28; Lin WC, Lin JY. Five bitter compounds display different anti-inflammatory effects through modulating cytokine secretion using mouse primary splenocytes in vitro. *Journal of Agriculture and Food Chemistry.* 2011 Jan 12;59(1):184–92.

20. MetabolismAdvice.com. Food to Fight Pain: Pain Management Diet for Arthritis and Other Pain. www.metabolismadvice.com/. Accessed July 22, 2011.

21. Ibid.

22. Ringman JM, Frautschy SA, Cole GM, Masterman DL, Cummings JL. A potential role of the curry spice curcumin in Alzheimer's disease. *Current Alzheimer Research.* 2005 Apr;2(2):131–36; Yang F, Lim GP, Begum AN, Ubeda OJ, Simmons MR, Ambegaokar SS, Chen PP, Kayed R, Glabe CG, Frautschy SA, Cole GM. Curcumin inhibits formation of amyloid beta oligomers and fibrils, binds plaques, and reduces amyloid in vivo. *Journal of Biological Chemistry.* 2005 Feb 18;280(7):5892–901.

23. Moldofsky H, Warsh JJ. Plasma tryptophan and musculoskeletal pain in non-articular rheumatism ("fibrositis syndrome"). *Pain.* 1978 Jun;5(1):65–71; Seltzer S, Dewart D, Pollack RL, Jackson E. The effects of dietary tryptophan on chronic maxillofacial pain and experimental pain

tolerance. *Journal of Psychiatric Research.* 1982–1983;17(2):181–86; Seltzer S, Stoch R, Marcus R, Jackson E. Alteration of human pain thresholds by nutritional manipulation and L-tryptophan supplementation. *Pain.* 1982 Aug;13(4):385–93.

24. Dattner AM. From medical herbalism to phytotherapy in dermatology: Back to the future. *Dermatologic Therapy.* 2003;16(2):106–13.

25. Halperin AK. Acupuncture in pain management. *Northeast Florida Medicine.* 2005 Summer;56(3):1–30.

26. Mjöberg B, Hellquist E, Mallmin H, Lindh U. Aluminum, Alzheimer's disease and bone fragility. *Acta Orthopaedica Scandinavica.* 1997 Dec;68(6):511–14; Loskutova N, Honea RA, Vidoni ED, Brooks WM, Burns JM. Bone density and brain atrophy in early Alzheimer's disease. *Journal of Alzheimer's Disease.* 2009;18(4):777–85.

27. Wong C. Herbs for Pain Management. www.altmedicine.about.com/. Updated April, 2009. Accessed July 23, 2011.

28. Boecker H, Sprenger T, Spilker ME, Henriksen G, Koppenhoefer M, Wagner KJ, Valet M, Berthele A, Tolle TR. The runner's high: Opioidergic mechanisms in the human brain. *Cerebral Cortex.* 2008 Nov;18(11):2523–31.

29. Mahajan N, Dhawan V, Sharma G, Jain S, Kaul D. Induction of inflammatory gene expression by THP-1 macrophages cultured in normocholesterolaemic hypertensive sera and modulatory effects of green tea polyphenols. *Journal of Human Hypertension.* 2008 Feb;22(2):141–43; Ho MCT, Leung TM, Fung ML, Liong EC, Tipoe GL, Nanji AA, Lau THY. Green tea polyphenols ameliorated pathological changes, oxidative stress and proinflammatory markers in an animal model of non-alcoholic fatty liver disease (NAFLD) animal model. *Hepatology.* 2010;44(4):160A–1063.

30. Beer A, Wegener T. Willow bark extract (Salicis cortex) for gonarthrosis and coxarthrosis: Results of a cohort study with a control group. *Phytomedicine.* 2008 Sep 22. Published online ahead of print.

31. Zollinger PE. Daily vitamin C prevented development of complex regional pain syndrome in adults with wrist fractures. *Evidence Based Medicine.* 2008;13:48; Zollinger PE, Tuinebreijer WE, Breederveld RS, Kreis RW. Can vitamin C prevent complex regional pain syndrome in patients with wrist fractures? A randomized, controlled, multicenter dose-response study. *Journal of Bone and Joint Surgery.* 2007 Jul;89(7):1424–31.

32. Boecker et al., The runner's high.

33. Wang H, Nair MG, Strasburg GM, Chang YC, Booren AM, Gray JI, DeWitt DL. Antioxidant and antiinflammatory activities of anthocyanins and their aglycon, cyanidin, from tart cherries. *Journal of Natural Products.* 1999 Feb;62(2):294–96.

34. Kozicz T. Met-enkephalin immunoreactive neurons recruited by acute stress are innervated by axon terminals immunopositive for tyrosine hydroxylase and dopamine-alpha-hydroxylase in the anterolateral division of bed nuclei of the stria terminalis in the rat. *European Journal of Neuroscience.* 2002 Sep;16(5):823–35; Nabeshima T, Katoh A, Kameyama T. Inhibition of enkephalin degradation attenuated stress-induced motor suppression (conditioned suppression of motility). *Journal of Pharmacology and Experimental Therapeutics.* 1988 Jan;244(1):303–9; Mansi JA, Laforest S, Drolet G. Effect of stress exposure on the activation pattern of enkephalin-containing perikarya in the rat ventral medulla. *Journal of Neurochemistry.* 2000 Jun;74(6):2568–75.

35. Demand Media, Inc. Alzheimer's Guidelines. www.livestrong.com/. Accessed August 2, 2011.

36. National Center for Complementary and Alternative Medicine. Acupuncture for Pain. http://nccam.nih.gov/. Accessed August 2, 2011; AcupunctureforAmerica.com. Acupuncture for Alzheimer's Disease. www.acupunctureamerica.com/. Accessed August 3, 2011.

37. Lee MS, Shin BC, Ernst E. Acupuncture for Alzheimer's disease: A systematic review. *International Journal of Clinical Practice.* 2009 Jun;63(6):874–79; Peng XW, Dong KL. Clinical observation on acupuncture combined with Yizhi Jiannao granules for treatment of

Alzheimer's disease [Chinese]. *Zhongguo Zhen Jiu (Chinese Acupuncture & Moxibustion)*. 2009 Apr;29(4):269–71.

38. Tse MMY, Wan VTC, Ho SSK. Physical exercise: Does it help in relieving pain and increasing mobility among older adults with chronic pain? *Journal of Clinical Nursing*. 2011; 20:5–6.

39. Pulugurtha S. Vitamins to Relieve Pain. www.livestrong.com/. Updated November 24, 2010. Accessed July 23, 2011.

CHAPTER 14

1. Organisation for Economic Co-operation and Development (OECD). Old age social spending. *Social Issues: Key Tables from OECD. 2011;(3)*:table 3. www.oecd-ilibrary.org/. Accessed August 1, 2011.

2. Social Security Administration. The Budget for Fiscal Year 2011. 2011:139–41. http://www.gpoaccess.gov/. Accessed July 25, 2011.

3. Ibid.

4. Ibid.

5. President's Budget for Fiscal Year 2012. http://www.whitehouse.gov/. Accessed July 25, 2011.

6. OECD, Old age social spending.

7. The Next Phase of Canada's Economic Action Plan: A Low Tax Plan for Jobs and Growth. http://www.budget.gc.ca/. Accessed July 25, 2011.

8. Crawford T, Stewart M. Budget 2011: Deficit Slaying Remains the Top Priority. Conference Board of Canada. http://www.conferenceboard.ca/. Accessed July 25, 2011.

9. Access Economics. *The Dementia Epidemic: Economic Impact and Positive Solutions for Australia*. Canberra, Australia: Alzheimer's Australia; 2003:36–39.

10. Australia's Final Budget Outcome. http://www.budget.gov.au/. Accessed August 2, 2011.

11. OECD, Old age social spending.

12. AtGuardianAngel. The Financial Impact of Alzheimer's Disease. http://www.issueswithalzheimers.com/. Accessed July 29, 2011.

13. Alzheimer's Association, Thies W, Bleiler L. 2011 Alzheimer's disease facts and figures. *Alzheimer's & Dementia*. 2011 Mar;7(2):208–44.

14. Ibid.

15. Alzheimer's Association. Alzheimer's Disease Facts and Figures 2007. www.alz.org/. Accessed July 29, 2011.

16. MetLife Mature Market Institute. *Market Survey of Long-Term Care Costs: The 2009 MetLife Market Survey of Nursing Home, Assisted Living, Adult Day Services and Home Care Costs*, October 2009.

17. Alzheimer's Association, Thies, Bleiler, 2011 Alzheimer's disease facts.

18. Ibid.

19. Ibid.

20. Alzheimer's Association, Alzheimer's Disease Facts 2007.

21. Alzheimer's Association, Thies, Bleiler, 2011 Alzheimer's disease facts.

22. Alzheimer's Disease Research. The Facts on Alzheimer's Disease. http://www.ahaf.org/. Updated June 7, 2011. Accessed July 29, 2011.

23. Belluck, P. Giving Alzheimer's Patients Their Way, Even Chocolate. New York Times. December 31, 2010. www.nytimes.com/. Accessed August 1, 2010.

24. Langa KM, Chernew ME, Kabeto MU, Herzog AR, Ofstedal MB, Willis RJ, Wallace RB, Mucha LM, Straus WL, Fendrick AM. National estimates of the quantity and cost of

informal caregiving for the elderly with dementia. *Journal of General Internal Medicine.* 2001; 16(11): 770–78.

25. Arno PS, Levine C, Memmot MM. The economic value of informal care. *Health Affairs.*1999;18(2):182–88.

26. Alzheimer's Association, Thies, Bleiler, 2011 Alzheimer's disease facts.

27. Alzheimer's Association, Alzheimer's Disease Facts 2007.

28. 2004 Task Force on Aging Research Funding. Meeting the Needs of the 21st Century. http://www.semeg.es/. Accessed August 1, 2011.

29. Alzheimer's Disease Research, Facts on Alzheimer's Disease.

30. Ibid.

31. Alzheimer's Association, Thies, Bleiler, 2011 Alzheimer's disease facts.

32. Ibid.

33. Steenhuysen J. Alzheimer's in U.S. Claims $202 Billion in Unpaid Care. March 15, 2011. www.reuters.com/. Accessed September 25, 2011.

34. Alzheimer's Association. 2009 Alzheimer's Disease Facts and Figures. *Alzheimer's & Dementia.* 2009;5(3):47–48.

35. Alzheimer's Association, Thies, Bleiler, 2011 Alzheimer's disease facts.

36. Gingrich N, Egge R. Let's Pay Up for Alzheimer's. Bloomberg Businessweek. December 11, 2006. http://www.businessweek.com/. Accessed July 25, 2011.

37. Alzheimer's Association, Alzheimer's Disease Facts 2007.

38. Alzheimer's Association, Thies, Bleiler, 2011 Alzheimer's disease facts.

39. Ibid.

40. Access Economics, *Dementia Epidemic.*

41. EurekAlert. Medicare claims for Alzheimer's disease skyrocket 250 percent. http://www.eurekalert.org/. Updated July 19, 2004. Accessed July 29, 2011.

42. Personal Social Services Research Unit (PSSRU), *preparer.* Dementia UK: Full Report. 2007:95–97.

43. Tucker ME. Rising Alzheimer's Rates, Costs Expected to "Overwhelm" U.S. Health Care System. *Clinical Psychiatry News.* October 2004. www.findarticles.com/. Accessed January 2, 2012.

44. Barford A, Dorling D, Davey Smith G, Shaw M. Life expectancy: Women now on top everywhere. *British Medical Journal.* 2006 Apr 8;332(7545):808.

45. EurekAlert, Medicare claims.

46. Desai AK, Grossberg GT. Diagnosis and treatment of Alzheimer's disease. *Neurology.* 2005 Jun 28;64(12 Suppl 3):S34–39.

47. Leon J, Cheng CK, Neumann PJ. Alzheimer's disease care: Costs and potential savings. *Health Affairs.* 1998;17(6):206–16.

48. Ibid.

49. Ibid.

50. Harvey R, Rossor M, Skelton-Robinson M, Garralda E. Young Onset Dementia: Epidemiology, clinical symptoms, family burden, support and outcome. 1998. http://home.kosha.net/. Accessed August 4, 2011.

51. Maslow K, *preparer.* Early Onset Dementia: A National Challenge, a Future in Crisis. Alzheimer's Association. June 2006. www.alz.org/. Accessed December 7, 2011.

52. McDaniel S. The costs of early-onset Alzheimer's disease and the federal benefits dilemma. *West Virginia Law Review.* 2010;113:140–49.

53. Maslow, Early Onset Dementia.

54. Alzheimer's Association, Thies, Bleiler, 2011 Alzheimer's disease facts.

55. Access Economics, *Dementia Epidemic.*

56. Access Economics. The dementia epidemic: Economic impact and positive solutions for Australia. *Report for Alzheimer's Australia.* 2003.

57. Access Economics, *Dementia Epidemic.*

58. PSSRU, Dementia.

59. X-Rates.com. http://www.x-rates.com/. Accessed July 29, 2011.

60. Søgaard R, Sørensen J, Waldorff FB, Eckermann A, Buss DV, Waldemar G. Private costs almost equal health care costs when intervening in mild Alzheimer's: A cohort study alongside the DAISY trial. *BMC (BioMed Central) Health Services Research.* 2009 Nov 25;9:215.

61. Access Economics, *Dementia Epidemic.*

62. PSSRU, Dementia.

63. Access Economics, *Dementia Epidemic.*

64. Tanna S. Priority Medicines for Europe and the World: "A Public Health Approach to Innovation." *Alzheimer's Disease "Opportunities to Address Pharmaceutical Gaps."* 2004:15.

65. Alzheimer's Australia. Dementia Facts & Statistics 2008. http://203.17.29.161/upload/StatisticsMar08.pdf. Updated March 2008. Accessed July 29, 2011.

66. Access Economics, *Dementia Epidemic.*

67. RiskAnalytica. Rising Tide: The Impact of Dementia on Canadian Society. Canada: Alzheimer's Society; 2010.

68. Alzheimer's Society. Advocating for Change: National Strategy. www.alzheimer.ca/. Updated September 2007. Accessed July 29, 2011.

69. Access Economics, *Dementia Epidemic.*

70. PSSRU, Dementia.

71. Better Business Bureau. Alzheimer's Association. http://www.bbb.org/. Updated January 2011. Accessed August 1, 2011.

72. Better Business Bureau. American Health Assistance Foundation. www.bbb.org/. Updated November 2009. Accessed August 1, 2011.

73. Ibid.

74. Alzheimer's Society. Annual Report and Financial Statements 2009/10. http://alzheimers.org.uk/. Accessed August 1, 2011.

75. Alzheimer's Society of Canada. http://www.alzheimer.ca/. Accessed August 1, 2011.

76. Alzheimer's Disease International. Financial Report. http://www.alz.co.uk/. Accessed August 1, 2011.

77. Alzheimer's Australia. 2009/2010 Annual Report. http://www.alzheimers.org.au/. Accessed August 1, 2011.

78. Wimo A, Winblad B, Jönsson L. An estimate of the total worldwide societal costs of dementia in 2005. *Alzheimer's & Dementia.* 2007 Apr;3(2):81–91.

79. Tanna, Priority Medicines.

CHAPTER 15

1. Alzheimer's Association. Alzheimer's Disease Facts and Figures 2008. www.alz.org/.

2. Ibid.

3. Jack CR Jr, Albert MS, Knopman DS, McKhann GM, Sperling RA, Carrillo MC, Thies B, Phelps CH. Introduction to the recommendations from the National Institute on Aging and the Alzheimer's Association Workgroups on Diagnostic Guidelines for Alzheimer's Disease. *Alzheimer's & Dementia.* 2011:1–6.

4. Jack CR Jr, Albert MS, Knopman DS, McKhann GM, Sperling RA, Carrillo MC, Thies B, Phelps CH. The diagnosis of dementia due to Alzheimer's disease: Recommendations from the National Institute on Aging and the Alzheimer's Association Workgroup. *Alzheimer's & Dementia.* 2011:1–7.

5. De Rosa R, Garcia AA, Braschi C, Capsoni S, Maffei L, Berardi N, Cattaneo A. Normal MRI appearance and motion-related phenomena of CSF. *American Journal of Roentgenology.* 2007 Mar;188(3):716–25.

6. Mattsson N, Zetterberg H, Blennow K. Lessons from multicenter studies on CSF biomarkers for Alzheimer's disease. *International Journal of Alzheimer's Disease.* 2010 Jul 8;2010. pii: 610613.

7. De Meyer G, Shapiro F, Vanderstichele H, Vanmechelen E, Engelborghs S, De Deyn PP, Coart E, Hansson O, Minthon L, Zetterberg H, Blennow K, Shaw L, Trojanowski JQ. Diagnosis-independent Alzheimer disease biomarker signature in cognitively normal elderly people. *Archives of Neurology.* 2010 Aug;67(8):949–56.

8. Ibid.

9. Dotti CG, De Strooper B. Alzheimer's dementia by circulation disorders: When trees hide the forest. *Nature Cell Biology.* 2009 Feb;11(2):114–16; Buerger K, Ernst A, Ewers M, Uspenskaya O, Omerovic M, Morgenthaler NG, Knauer K, Bergmann A, Hampel H. Blood-based microcirculation markers in Alzheimer's disease-diagnostic value of midregional pro-atrial natriuretic peptide/C-terminal endothelin-1 precursor fragment ratio. *Biological Psychiatry.* 2009 Jun 1;65(11):979–84; De la Torre JC, Mussivand T. Can disturbed brain microcirculation cause Alzheimer's disease? *Neurological Research.* 1993 Jun;15(3):146–53.

10. Shipton OA, Leitz JR, Dworzak J, Acton CE, Tunbridge EM, Denk F, Dawson HN, Vitek MP, Wade-Martins R, Paulsen O, Vargas-Caballero M. Tau protein is required for amyloid {beta}-induced impairment of hippocampal long-term potentiation. *Journal of Neuroscience.* 2011 Feb 2;31(5):1688–92; Ittner LM, Götz J. Amyloid-β and tau: A toxic pas de deux in Alzheimer's disease. *Nature Reviews Neuroscience.* 2011 Feb;12(2):65–72.

11. Oz M, Lorke DE, Petroianu GA. Methylene blue and Alzheimer's disease. *Biochemistry & Pharmacology.* 2009 Oct 15;78(8):927–32.

12. Jorenby DE, Hays JT, Rigotti NA, Azoulay S, Watsky EJ, Williams KE, Billing CB, Gong J, Reeves KR. Efficacy of varenicline, an alpha4beta2 nicotinic acetylcholine receptor partial agonist, vs placebo or sustained-release bupropion for smoking cessation: A randomized controlled trial. *Journal of the American Medical Association.* 2006 Jul 5;296(1):56–63; Hays JT, Ebbert JO, Sood A. Efficacy and safety of varenicline for smoking cessation. *American Journal of Medicine.* 2008 Apr;121(4 Suppl 1):S32–42.

13. Pfizer. Evaluation of the Efficacy of Varenicline on Cognition, Safety, Tolerability and Pharmacokinetics in Subjects with Mild-to-Moderate Alzheimer's Disease. www.clinicaltrials .gov/. Updated December 17, 2010. Accessed May 26, 2011.

14. Mendiondo MS, Ashford JW, Kryscio RJ, Schmitt FA. Modelling mini mental state examination changes in Alzheimer's disease. *Statistical Methods.* 2000 Jun 15–30;19(11–12): 1607–16.

15. Kolata G. Doubt on Tactic in Alzheimer's Battle. New York Times. www.nytimes .com/. Updated August 18, 2010. Accessed May 26, 2011.

16. Ibid.

17. Eli Lilly and Company. [Main Page]. www.lilly.com/. Accessed October 1, 2011.

18. Wilson D. Lilly Stops Alzheimer's Drug Trials. August 17, 2010. New York Times. www.nytimes.com/. Accessed October 1, 2011.

19. Yu YP, Xu QQ, Zhang Q, Zhang WP, Zhang LH, Wei EQ. Intranasal recombinant human erythropoietin protects rats against focal cerebral ischemia. *Neuroscience Letters.* 2005 Oct 14;387(1):5–10.

20. Craft S. Insulin resistance and Alzheimer's disease pathogenesis: Potential mechanisms and implications for treatment. *Current Alzheimer Research.* 2007 Apr;4(2):147–52; Watson GS, Craft S. The role of insulin resistance in the pathogenesis of Alzheimer's disease: Implications for treatment. *Central Nervous System (CNS) Drugs.* 2003;17(1):27–45.

21. Zhongling Feng, Gang Zhao, Lei Yu. Neural stem cells and Alzheimer's disease: Challenges and hope. *American Journal of Alzheimer's Disease and Other Dementias.* 2009

Feb–Mar;24(1):52–57; Taupin P. Adult neurogenesis, neural stem cells and Alzheimer's disease: Developments, limitations, problems and promises. *Current Alzheimer Research.* 2009 Dec;6(6):461–70; Abdel-Salam OM. Stem cell therapy for Alzheimer's disease. *CNS & Neurological Disorders: Drug Targets.* 2011 Jun;10(4):459–85.

22. Kolata G. Stem Cells. New York Times. www.topics.nytimes.com/. Updated May 2, 2011. Accessed May 25, 2011.

23. Arizona Board of Regents. Dickey-Wicker Amendment. www.embryo.asu.edu/. Accessed January 12, 2012.

24. White House. George W. Bush. www.whitehouse.gov/. Accessed October 1, 2011.

25. Ibid.

26. Alzheimer's Research Center. Adult Stem Cell Research. www.alzheimersinfo.org/. Accessed August 1, 2011.

27. O'Keeffe FE, Scott SA, Tyers P, O'Keeffe GW, Dalley JW, Zufferey R, Caldwell MA. Induction of A9 dopaminergic neurons from neural stem cells improves motor function in an animal model of Parkinson's disease. *Brain.* 2008 Mar;131(Pt 3):630–41.

28. Bjornson CR, Rietze RL, Reynolds BA, Magli MC, Vescovi AL. Turning brain into blood: A hematopoietic fate adopted by adult neural stem cells in vivo. *Science.* 1999 Jan 22;283(5401):534–37.

29. Alzheimer's Research Center, Adult Stem Cell Research.

30. Alzheimer's Research Center. Intranasal Nerve Growth Factor Research. www.alzheimersinfo.org/. Accessed August 1, 2011.

31. Ibid.

32. Alzheimer's Research Center. [Main Page]. www.alzheimersinfo.org/. Accessed October 1, 2011.

33. Yu et al., Intranasal recombinant human erythropoietin; Yu YP, Xu QQ, Zhang Q, Zhang WP, Zhang LH, Wei EQ. Cerebral neurogenesis is induced by intranasal administration of growth factors. *Annals of Neurology.* 2003 Mar;53(3):405–9; De Rosa R, Garcia AA, Braschi C, Capsoni S, Maffei L, Berardi N, Cattaneo A. Intranasal administration of nerve growth factor (NGF) rescues recognition memory deficits in AD11 anti-NGF transgenic mice. *Proceedings of the National Academy of Sciences USA.* 2005 Mar 8;102(10):3811–16.

34. Alzheimer's Research Center, Adult Stem Cell Research.

35. Kennard C. Volunteering for Alzheimer's Research. www.alzheimers.about.com/. Updated December 10, 2005. Accessed October 2. 2011.

36. Ibid.

37. Fackelmann K. A Dose of Hope vs. Alzheimer's. USA Today. July 27, 2003. www.usatoday.com/. Updated July 27, 2003. Accessed October 2, 2011.

38. Massachusetts General Hospital. Unforgettable Breakthroughs in Alzheimer's. www.massgeneralmag.org/. Accessed August 1, 2011.

CHAPTER 16

1. Merriam-Webster. Diet. www.merriam-webster.com/. Accessed July 26, 2011.

2. Weir K. Food for thought. *Current Health 2.* 2006 Feb;32(6):23–25.

3. Ibid.

4. Alzheimer's Association. Maintain Your Brain. www.alz.org/. Accessed July 26, 2011.

5. Sacks F. Ask the Expert: Omega-3 Fatty Acids. Harvard School of Public Health Nutrition Source. www.hsph.harvard.edu/. Accessed July 26, 2011.

6. Alzheimer's Association, Maintain Your Brain.

7. Tsang G. Antioxidants 101. www.healthcastle.com/. Updated March 1, 2011. Accessed July 26, 2011.

8. Health.com. Black Superfoods: Black Is the New Green. March 20, 2011. Huffington Post. www.huffingtonpost.com/. Updated March 23, 2011. Accessed October 11, 2011.

9. Alzheimer's Association, Maintain Your Brain.

10. Healthy J. Bad Fats Break Down Your Brain. www.myhealingkitchen.com/. Accessed July 26, 2011.

11. Ibid.

12. Neville K. Memory boost: 33 Foods that can help. 4 supplements you might consider. *Environmental Nutrition.* 2006 Oct;29(10):1–6.

13. Macrobiotic Guide. Sugar: Its effects on the boy and mind. www.macrobiotics.co.uk/. Accessed July 28, 2011.

14. Ibid.

15. Mulrooney M. Foods with Refined Sugars. www.livestrong.com/. Updated March 30, 2011. Accessed July 28, 2011.

16. Rizzo M, Anderson SW, Dawson J, Nawrot M. Vision and cognition in Alzheimer's disease. *Neuropsychologia.* 2000;38(8):1157–69; Cacace AT. Aging, Alzheimer's disease, and hearing impairment: Highlighting relevant issues and calling for additional research. *American Journal of Audiology.* 2007 Jun;16(1):2–3; Hoffmann I, Nemeth D, Dye CD, Pákáski M, Irinyi T, Kálmán J. Temporal parameters of spontaneous speech in Alzheimer's disease. *International Journal of Speech-Language Pathology.* 2010 Feb;12(1):29–34.

17. Lasik Directory. Nutrition for Better Vision. www.the-lasik-directory.com/. Accessed July 28, 2011.

18. Ibid.

19. Ibid.

20. Ibid.

21. National Institutes of Health: Office of Dietary Supplements. Dietary Supplement Fact Sheet: Vitamin D. http://ods.od.nih.gov/. Accessed August 28, 2011.

22. Hemat RA. *Principles of Orthomolecularism.* Urotext Publications (ebook): 2009; 54.

23. National Institutes of Health. Taking Care of Your Voice. www.nidcd.nih.gov/. Accessed July 29, 2011.

24. Rao J, Oz G, Seaquist ER. Regulation of cerebral glucose metabolism. *Minerva Endocrinologica.* 2006 Jun;31(2):149–58.

25. Walton P, Rhodes EC. Glycaemic index and optimal performance. *Sports Medicine.* 1997 Mar;23(3):164–72; Ludwig DS, Majzoub JA, Al-Zahrani A, Dallal GE, Blanco I, Roberts SB. High glycemic index foods, overeating, and obesity. *Pediatrics.* 1999 Mar;103(3):E26.

26. Hitti M. High Sugar Foods May Affect Eyesight. www.webmd.com/. Updated July 13, 2007. Accessed July 30, 2011.

27. Aspartame, A. Bitter Sweetener. www.naturodoc.com/. Accessed July 30, 2011.

28. Keate B. Food-Borne Neurotoxins and Tinnitus Part 2: Monosodium Glutamate. www.tinnitusformula.com/. Updated 2010. Accessed July 30, 2011.

29. Keate B. Diet and Tinnitus, What to Eat . . . and What Not to Eat. www.tinnitusformula.com/. Updated 2010. Accessed July 30, 2011.

30. Evans WJ. Protein nutrition, exercise and aging. *Journal of the American College of Nutrition.* 2004 Dec;23(suppl. 6):601S–609S.

31. Warner J. Mediterranean Diet May Keep Aging Mind Sharp. www.webmd.com/. Updated January 7, 2011. Accessed August 1, 2011.

32. BMJ. Modified Mediterranean diet and survival: EPIC-elderly prospective. www.bmj.com/. Accessed August 2, 2011.

33. Karuppagounder SS, Pinto JT, Xu H, Chen HL, Beal MF, Gibson GE. Dietary supplementation with resveratrol reduces plaque pathology in a transgenic model of Alzheimer's disease. *Neurochemistry International.* 2009 Feb;54(2):111–18.

34. BMJ, Modified Mediterranean diet.

35. Albert SG, Nakra BR, Grossberg GT, Caminal ER. Drinking behavior and vasopressin responses to hyperosmolality in Alzheimer's disease. *International Psychogeriatric Association.* 1994 Spring;6(1):79–86; Norbiato G, Bevilacqua M, Carella F, Chebat E, Raggi U, Bertora P, Grassi MP, Mangoni A. Alterations in vasopressin regulation in Alzheimer's disease. *Journal of Neurology, Neurosurgery & Psychiatry.* 1988 Jul;51(7):903–8.

36. Rohmann R. Balanced Diet for the Elderly. www.livestrong.com/. Updated 2010. Accessed August 2, 2011; Williams RJ, Spencer JP. Flavonoids, cognition, and dementia: Actions, mechanisms, and potential therapeutic utility for Alzheimer disease. *Free Radical Biology and Medicine.* 2011 Sep 17.

37. Tapsell LC, Hemphill I, Cobiac L, Patch CS, Sullivan DR, Fenech M, Roodenrys S, Keogh JB, Clifton PM, Williams PG, Fazio VA, Inge KE. Health benefits of herbs and spices: The past, the present, the future. *Medical Journal of Australia.* 2006;185[*Suppl*](4):s1–s23.

38. Wylde B. 10 Worst Foods for Aging. Readers Digest Canada. www.readersdigest.ca/. Accessed August 2, 2011.

39. Ibid.

40. Mayo Clinic. Added Sugar: Don't Get Sabotaged by Sweeteners. www.mayoclinic .com/. Updated April 5, 2011. Accessed August 3, 2011.

41. Bad Effects of Carbonated Drinks. www.drinkhealthydrinks.com/. Updated 2011. Accessed August 3, 2011.

42. Wylde, 10 Worst Foods.

43. Boehlke J. High Sugar Diets Effects on the Elderly. www.livestrong.com/. Updated April 26, 2011. Accessed August 3, 2011.

44. Perrig WJ, Perrig P, Stähelin HB. The relation between antioxidants and memory performance in the old and very old. *Journal of the American Geriatric Society.* 1997 Jun;45(6):718–24.

45. Medletter Associates. Preventing Dementia. *Memory.* 2008 Jan:7–24.

46. Golub C. B Vitamins: Focus on fab three for a healthy heart, mighty memory. *Environmental Nutrition.* 2004 Feb;27(2):1–4.

47. The Battle for Your Brain. *Tufts University Health & Nutrition Letter* [serial online]. October 2010;28(8):1–4. Health Source, Consumer Edition, Ipswich, MA. http://www.tufts-healthletter.com/. Accessed July 30, 2011.

48. Hooshmand B, Solomon A, Kåreholt I, Leiviskä J, Rusanen M, Ahtiluoto S, Winblad B, Laatikainen T, Soininen H, Kivipelto M. Homocysteine and holotranscobalamin and the risk of Alzheimer disease: A longitudinal study. *Neurology.* 2010 Oct 19;75(16):1408–14.

49. Lockrow J, Prakasam A, Huang P, Bimonte-Nelson H, Sambamurti K, Granholm AC. Cholinergic degeneration and memory loss delayed by vitamin E in a Down syndrome mouse model. *Experimental Neurology.* 2009 Apr;216(2):278–89.

50. FCA Publishing. Nature's Prescriptions for Memory Loss. www.fca.com/. Accessed August 3, 2011.

51. Medletter Associates, Preventing Dementia.

52. Perreira KM, Sloan FA. Excess alcohol consumption and health outcomes: A 6-year follow-up of men over age 50 from the health and retirement study. *Addiction.* 2002 Mar;97(3):301–10.

53. White A. What Happened? Alcohol, Memory Blackouts, and the Brain. www.pubs .niaaa.nih.gov/. Updated July 2004. Accessed August 3, 2011.

54. Harvard School of Public Health Nutrition Source. Fats and Cholesterol: Out with the Bad, In with the Good. www.hsph.harvard.edu/. Accessed August 3, 2011.

55. Neville, Memory boost.

56. Pistell PJ, Morrison CD, Gupta S, Knight AG, Keller JN, Ingram DK, Bruce-Keller AJ. Cognitive impairment following high fat diet consumption is associated with brain inflammation. *Journal of Neuroimmunology.* 2010 Feb 26;219(1–2):25–32.

57. Tremblay L. Vitamins that Enhance Cognitive Function. www.livestrong .com/. Updated December 2010. Accessed August 3, 2011.

58. Sears B, Sears M. Best Brain Foods: 11 Ways Food Can Help You Think. www.askdr-sears.com/. Accessed August 4, 2011.

59. Ibid.

60. Pearson O. How Bad Nutrition Can Affect a Person's Life. www.livestrong.com/. Updated June 25, 2011.

61. Ibid.

62. Harvard School of Public Health Nutrition Source. Carbohydrates: Good Carbs Guide the Way. www.hsph.harvard.edu/. Accessed August 4, 2011.

63. Harvard School of Public Health Nutrition Source. Shining the Spotlight on Trans Fats. www.hsph.harvard.edu/. Accessed August 4, 2011.

64. Hooshmand et al., Homocysteine and holotranscobalamin.

65. Dean L. *Blood Groups and Red Cell Antigens.* Chapter 1: Blood and The Cells It Contains. Bethesda, MD: National Center for Biotechnology Information; 2005.

66. Micha R, Wallace SK, Mozaffarian D. Red and processed meat consumption and risk of incident coronary heart disease, stroke, and diabetes mellitus: A systematic review and meta-analysis. *Circulation.* 2010 Jun 1;121(21):2271–83.

67. Ho L, Chen LH, Wang J, Zhao W, Talcott ST, Ono K, Teplow D, Humala N, Cheng A, Percival SS, Ferruzzi M, Janle E, Dickstein DL, Pasinetti GM. Heterogeneity in red wine polyphenolic contents differentially influences Alzheimer's disease-type neuropathology and cognitive deterioration. *Journal of Alzheimer's Disease.* 2009;16(1):59–72.

68. Anekonda TS. Resveratrol: A boon for treating Alzheimer's disease? *Brain Research Reviews.* 2006 Sep;52(2):316–26.

CHAPTER 17

1. National Library of Medicine. Exercise and Physical Fitness. February 25, 2009. www.nlm.nih.gov/medlineplus. Updated October 17, 2011. Accessed October 17, 2011; Franklin Institute. About Physical Exercise. 2004. www.fi.edu/. Accessed October 19, 2011.

2. Alfaro MF, Putney L, Tarkington BK, Hatch GE, Hyde DM, Schelegle ES. Effect of rapid shallow breathing on the distribution of 18O-labeled ozone reaction product in the respiratory tract of the rat. *Inhalation Toxicology.* 2004 Feb;16(2):77–85.

3. Nieman P. Psychosocial aspects of physical activity. *Paediatrics & Child Health.* 2002 May;7(5):309–12.

4. Duman RS. Neurotrophic factors and regulation of mood: Role of exercise, diet and metabolism. *Neurobiology of Aging.* 2005 Dec;26 Suppl 1:88–93.

5. Van de Hinkel A, Feys H, De Weert W. Cognitive and behavioral effects of music-based exercises in patients with dementia. *Clinical Rehabilitation.* 2004 May;18(3):253–60.

6. Van Gelder LH, Bartz SD. The effect of acute stretching on agility performance. *Journal of Strength & Conditioning Research.* 2011 Sep 13. Published online ahead of print.

7. Kennedy JF. The soft American. *Sports Illustrated.* 1960;13:15–17.

8. Ndubuizu O, LaManna JC. Brain tissue oxygen concentration measurements. *Antioxidants & Redox Signaling.* 2007 Aug;9(8):1207–19.

9. Satoh T, Sakurai I, Miyagi K, Hohshaku Y. Walking exercise and improved neuropsychological functioning in elderly patients with cardiac disease. *Journal of Internal Medicine.* 1995 Nov;238(5):423–28.

10. Larson EB, Wang L, Bowen JD, McCormick WC, Teri L, Crane P, Kukull W. Exercise is associated with reduced risk for incident dementia among persons 65 years of age and older. *Annals of Internal Medicine.* 2006 Jan 17;144(2):73–81.

11. Graff-Radford NR. Can aerobic exercise protect against dementia? *Alzheimer's Research & Therapy.* 2011 Feb 28;3(1):6; Mayor S. Regular exercise reduces risk of dementia and Alzheimer's disease. *British Medical Journal.* 2006 Jan;332(7534):137.

12. Segura-García C, Ammendolia A, Procopio L, Papaianni MC, Sinopoli F, Bianco C, De Fazio P, Capranica L. Body uneasiness, eating disorders, and muscle dysmorphia in individuals who overexercise. *Journal of Strength & Conditioning Research.* 2010 Nov;24(11):3098–104.

13. Westerterp KR. Daily physical activity and ageing. *Current Opinion in Clinical Nutrition & Metabolic Care.* 2000 Nov;3(6):485–88.

14. Yu F, Kolanowski AM, Strumpf NE, Eslinger PJ. Improving cognition and function through exercise intervention in Alzheimer's disease. *Journal of Nursing Scholarship.* 2006; 38(4):358–65.

15. Colcombe SJ, Kramer AF, Erickson KI, Scalf P, McAuley E, Cohen NJ, Webb A, Jerome GJ, Marquez DX, Elavsky S. Cardiovascular fitness, cortical plasticity, and aging. *Proceedings of the National Academy of Sciences USA.* 2004 Mar 2;101(9):3316–21.

16. Lane AM, Wilson MG, Whyte GP, Shave R. Physiological correlates of emotion-regulation during prolonged cycling performance. *Applied Psychophysiology and Biofeedback.* 2011 Sep;36(3):181–84.

17. Rogers CD. The Health Effects of Heart-Rate Exercise. March 28, 2011. www.livestrong.com/. Accessed October 19, 2011.

18. Cassilhas RC, Viana VA, Grassmann V, Santos RT, Santos RF, Tufik S, Mello MT. The impact of resistance exercise on the cognitive function of the elderly. *Medicine and Science in Sports and Exercise.* 2007 Aug;39(8):1401–7.

19. Van de Hinkel, Feys, De Weert, Cognitive and behavioral effects.

20. Padilla R. Effectiveness of environment-based interventions for people with Alzheimer's disease and related dementias. *American Journal of Occupational Therapy (AJOT).* 2011 Sep/Oct;65(5):514–22.

21. Elgar K, Campbell R. Annotation: The cognitive neuroscience of face recognition; Implications for developmental disorders. *Journal of Child Psychology and Psychiatry.* 2001 Sep;42(6):705–17.

22. Sahay A, Scobie KN, Hill AS, O'Carroll CM, Kheirbek MA, Burghardt NS, Fenton AA, Dranovsky A, Hen R. Increasing adult hippocampal neurogenesis is sufficient to improve pattern separation. *Nature.* 2011 Apr 28;472(7344):466–70.

23. Sobel BP. Bingo vs. physical intervention in stimulating short-term cognition in Alzheimer's disease patients. *American Journal of Alzheimer's Disease and Other Dementias.* 2001 Mar–Apr;16(2):115–20.

24. Rogers MA, Langa KM. Untreated poor vision: A contributing factor in late-life dementia. *American Journal of Epidemiology.* 2010 Mar 15;171(6):728–35.

25. Peretz C, Korczyn AD, Shatil E, Aharonson V, Birnboim S, Giladi N. Computer-based, personalized cognitive training versus classical computer games: A randomized double-blind prospective trial of cognitive stimulation. *Neuroepidemiology.* 2011;36(2):91–99.

26. Wilson RS, Krueger KR, Arnold SE, Schneider JA, Kelly JF, Barnes LL, Tang Y, Bennett DA. Loneliness and risk of Alzheimer disease. *Archives of General Psychiatry.* 2007 Feb;64(2):234–40.

27. Sugiyama T, Hashimoto K, Kiwamoto H, Ohnishi N, Esa A, Park YC, Kurita T. Urinary incontinence in senile dementia of the Alzheimer type (SDAT). *International Journal of Urology.* 1994 Dec;1(4):337–40.

28. Aslan E, Komurcu N, Beji NK, Yalcin O. Bladder training and Kegel exercises for women with urinary complaints living in a rest home. *Gerontology.* 2008;54(4):224–31.

29. Humbert IA, McLaren DG, Kosmatka K, Fitzgerald M, Johnson S, Porcaro E, Kays S, Umoh EO, Robbins J. Early deficits in cortical control of swallowing in Alzheimer's disease. *Journal of Alzheimer's Disease.* 2010;19(4):1185–97; Correia Sde M, Morillo LS, Jacob

Filho W, Mansur LL. Swallowing in moderate and severe phases of Alzheimer's disease. *Arquivos de Neuro-Psiquiatria.* 2010. Dec;68(6):855–61.

30. National Institute of Neurological Disorders and Stroke (NINDS). NINDS Swallowing Disorders Information Page. www.ninds.nih.gov/. Updated December 22, 2010. Accessed October 23, 2011.

31. Wada H, Nakajoh K, Satoh-Nakagawa T, Suzuki T, Ohrui T, Arai H, Sasaki H. Risk factors of aspiration pneumonia in Alzheimer's disease patients. *Gerontology.* 2001 Sep–Oct;47(5):271–76.

32. Conde M, Lawrence V. Postoperative Pulmonary Infections: Preoperative Care. September 29, 2008. www.clinicalevidence.bmj.com/. Accessed October 23, 2011.

33. Monacelli AM, Cushman LA, Kavcic V, Duffy CJ. Spatial disorientation in Alzheimer's disease: The remembrance of things passed. *Neurology.* 2003 Dec 9;61(11):1491–97.

34. Leandri M, Cammisuli S, Cammarata S, Baratto L, Campbell J, Simonini M, Tabaton M. Balance features in Alzheimer's disease and amnestic mild cognitive impairment. *Journal of Alzheimer's Disease.* 2009;16(1):113–20.

35. Allan LM, Ballard CG, Burn DJ, Kenny RA. Prevalence and severity of gait disorders in Alzheimer's and non-Alzheimer's dementias. *Journal of the American Geriatric Society.* 2005 Oct;53(10):1681–87; Muir SW, Speechley M, Wells J, Borrie M, Gopaul K, Montero-Odasso M. Gait assessment in mild cognitive impairment and Alzheimer's disease: The effect of dual-task challenges across the cognitive spectrum. *Gait Posture.* 2011 Sep 20. Published online ahead of print.

36. Erickson KI, Kramer AF. In reality, according to a strict medical definition, exercise is any form of physical activity that is practiced repetitively in order to improve and maintain both the health and fitness of one's body. *British Journal of Sports Medicine.* 2009 Jan;43(1):22–24.

37. Viña J, Lloret A. Why women have more Alzheimer's disease than men: Gender and mitochondrial toxicity of amyloid-beta peptide. *Journal of Alzheimer's Disease.* 2010;20 Suppl 2:S527–33.

38. Rizzo M, Anderson SW, Dawson J, Nawrot M. Vision and cognition in Alzheimer's disease. *Neuropsychologia.* 2000;38(8):1157–69.

39. Williams PT. Prospective study of incident age-related macular degeneration in relation to vigorous physical activity during a 7-year follow-up. *Investigative Ophthalmology & Visual Science.* 2009 Jan;50(1):101–6.

40. Rogers, Langa, Untreated poor vision.

41. Uhlmann RF, Larson EB, Rees TS, Koepsell TD, Duckert LG. Relationship of hearing impairment to dementia and cognitive dysfunction in older adults. *Journal of the American Medical Association.* 1989 Apr 7;261(13):1916–19.

42. Ibid.

43. Ibid.

44. García-Mesa Y, López-Ramos JC, Giménez-Llort L, Revilla S, Guerra R, Gruart A, Laferla FM, Cristòfol R, Delgado-García JM, Sanfeliu C. Physical exercise protects against Alzheimer's disease in 3xTg-AD mice. *Journal of Alzheimer's Disease.* 2011;24(3):421–54.

CHAPTER 18

1. Robert PH, Darcourt G, Koulibaly MP, Clairet S, Benoit M, Garcia R, Dechaux O, Darcourt J. Lack of initiative and interest in Alzheimer's disease: A single photon emission computed tomography study. *European Journal of Neurology.* 2006 Jul;13(7):729–35.

2. Barak Y, Aizenberg D. Suicide amongst Alzheimer's disease patients: A 10-year survey. *Dementia and Geriatric Cognitive Disorders.* 2002;14(2):101–3.

3. Wimo A, Prince M. *World Alzheimer Report 2010*. London, UK: Alzheimer's Disease International; 2010:4.

4. Kamer AR, Dasanayake AP, Craig RG, Glodzik-Sobanska L, Bry M, de Leon MJ. Alzheimer's disease and peripheral infections: The possible contribution from periodontal infections, model and hypothesis. *Journal of Alzheimer's Disease*. 2008 May;13(4):437–49.

5. Center for Disease Control and Prevention. What is the Burden of Alzheimer's Disease in the United States? www.cdc.gov/. Updated September 10, 2010. Accessed July 20, 2011.

6. Stevenson JP. Family stress related to home care of Alzheimer's disease patients and implications for support. *Journal of Neuroscience Nursing*. 1990 Jun;22(3):179–88.

7. Winslow BW. Effects of formal supports on stress outcomes in family caregivers of Alzheimer's patients. *Research in Nursing and Health*. 1997 Feb;20(1):27–37.

8. Smith AP, Beattie BL. Disclosing a diagnosis of Alzheimer's disease: Patient and family experiences. *Canadian Journal of Neurological Sciences (CJNS)*. 2001 Feb;28 Suppl 1:S67–71.

9. Bahro M, Silber E, Sunderland T. How do patients with Alzheimer's disease cope with their illness? A clinical experience report. *Journal of the American Geriatrics Society*. 1995;43:416.

10. Duncan LR, Hall CR, Wilson PM, Jenny O. Exercise motivation: A cross-sectional analysis examining its relationships with frequency, intensity, and duration of exercise. *International Journal of Behavioral Nutrition and Physical Activity*. 2010 Jan 26;7:7.

11. Nied RJ, Franklin B. Promoting and prescribing exercise for the elderly. *American Family Physician*. 2002 Feb 1;65(3):419–427.

12. Ibid.

13. World Health Organization. Physical Activity and Older Adults. 2011. www.who.int/. Accessed August 20, 2011.

14. Arkin S. Introduction to Alzheimer's Disease and Exercise. University of Illinois at Chicago. Department of Disability and Human Development and the National Center on Physical Activity and Disability. www.ncpad.org/. Updated January 8, 2008. Accessed August 20, 2011.

15. Grant WB, Campbell A, Itzhaki RF, Savory J. The significance of environmental factors in the etiology of Alzheimer's disease. *Journal of Alzheimer's Disease*. 2002 Jun;4(3):179–89.

16. Hurley AC, Gauthier MA, Horvath KJ, Harvey R, Smith SJ, Trudeau S, Cipolloni PB, Hendricks A, Duffy M. Promoting safer home environments for persons with Alzheimer's disease: The Home Safety/Injury Model. *Journal of Gerontological Nursing*. 2004 Jun;30(6):43–51.

17. Ibid.

18. Hickey T, Douglass RL. Mistreatment of the elderly in the domestic setting: An exploratory study. *American Journal of Public Health*. 1981 May;71(5):500–507; Hardin E, Khan-Hudson A. Elder abuse: "society's dilemma." *Journal of the National Medical Association*. 2005 Jan;97(1):91–94; Cohen M, Levin SH, Gagin R, Friedman G. Elder abuse: Disparities between older people's disclosure of abuse, evident signs of abuse, and high risk of abuse. *Journal of the American Geriatric Society*. 2007 Aug;55(8):1224–30; Cooper C, Selwood A, Livingston G. The prevalence of elder abuse and neglect: A systematic review. *Age & Ageing*. 2008 Mar;37(2):151–60.

19. Kennedy RD. Elder abuse and neglect: The experience, knowledge, and attitudes of primary care physicians. *Family Medicine*. 2005 Jul–Aug;37(7):481–85.

20. Levine JM. Elder neglect and abuse: A primer for primary care physicians. *Geriatrics*. 2003 Oct;58(10):37–40, 42–44.

21. Vandeweerd C, Paveza GJ, Fulmer T. Abuse and neglect in older adults with Alzheimer's disease. *Nursing Clinics of North America*. 2006 Mar;41(1):43–55, v–vi.

22. Millán-Calenti JC, Gandoy-Crego M, Antelo-Martelo M, López-Martinez M, Riveiro-López MP, Mayán-Santos JM. Helping the family carers of Alzheimer's patients: From theory . . . to practice; A preliminary study. *Archives of Gerontology and Geriatrics*. 2000 Mar–Apr;30(2):131–38.

23. Bright-Long L. Alzheimer's treatment in nursing homes: Room for improvement. *Journal of the American Medical Directors Association*. 2006 Feb;7(2):90–95.

24. Gogia PP, Rastogi N. *Clinical Alzheimer's Rehabilitation*. New York: Springer Publishing; 2009.

25. De Vreese LP, Neri M, Fioravanti M, Belloi L, Zanetti O. Memory rehabilitation in Alzheimer's disease: A review of progress. *International Journal of Geriatric Psychiatry*. 2001 Aug;16(8):794–809.

26. Fuller A. Advice to caregivers: Reassure and Do Not Argue. Winston-Salem Journal. December 30, 2010. www.journalnow.com/. Accessed August 20, 2011.

27. Ibid.

28. Butcher J. Mind games: Do they work? *British Medical Journal*. 2008 Feb 2;336(7638):246–48; Karp A, Paillard-Borg S, Wang HX, Silverstein M, Winblad B, Fratiglioni L. Mental, physical and social components in leisure activities equally contribute to decreased dementia risk. *Dementia and Geriatric Cognitive Disorders*. 2006;21(2):65–73.

29. Cotrell V, Schulz R. The perspective of the patient with Alzheimer's disease: A neglected dimension of dementia research. *Gerontologist*. 1993 Apr;33(2):205–11.

30. Snyder L, Jenkins C, Joosten L. Effectiveness of support groups for people with mild to moderate Alzheimer's disease: An evaluative survey. *American Journal of Alzheimer's Disease and Other Dementias*. 2007 Feb–Mar;22(1):14–19.

31. Gonyea JG. Alzheimer's disease support groups: An analysis of their structure, format and perceived benefits. *Social Work in Health Care*. 1989;14(1):61–72.

32. Snyder, Jenkins, Joosten, Effectiveness of support groups.

33. Kaufer DI, Borson S, Kershaw P, Sadik K. Reduction of caregiver burden in Alzheimer's disease by treatment with galantamine. *CNS Spectrums*. 2005 Jun;10(6):481–88.

CHAPTER 19

1. Cleveland Clinic. Living with Early-Onset Alzheimer's Disease. www.cchs.net/. Accessed August 14, 2011.

2. Ibid.

3. Safe Kids (UK). The Terrible Twos Explained. www.safekids.co.uk/. Accessed August 14, 2011; Reebye P. Aggression during early years: Infancy and preschool. *Canadian Child and Adolescent Psychiatry Review*. 2005 Feb;14(1):16–20.

4. University of Iowa *portal*. Identity vs. Role Confusion. www.uiowa.edu/. Accessed August 26, 2011.

5. PRweb.com. Troubled Teen Son and His Mother Launch Website for Parents of Troubled Teens. March 27, 2009. www.prweb.com/. Accessed August 14, 2011.

6. Rabins PV, Blacker D, Rovner BW, Rummans T, Schneider LS, Tariot PN, Blass DM; Steering Committee on Practice Guidelines, McIntyre JS, Charles SC, Anzia DJ, Cook IA, Finnerty MT, Johnson BR, Nininger JE, Schneidman B, Summergrad P, Woods SM, Berger J, Cross CD, Brandt HA, Margolis PM, Shemo JP, Blinder BJ, Duncan DL, Barnovitz MA, Carino AJ, Freyberg ZZ, Gray SH, Tonnu T, Kunkle R, Albert AB, Craig TJ, Regier DA, Fochtmann LJ. American Psychiatric Association practice guideline for the treatment of patients with Alzheimer's disease and other dementias. 2nd ed. *American Journal of Psychiatry*. 2007 Dec;164(12 Suppl):5–56.

7. Doody RS, Stevens JC, Beck C, Dubinsky RM, Kaye JA, Gwyther L, Mohs RC, Thal LJ, Whitehouse PJ, DeKosky ST, Cummings JL. Practice parameter: Management of

dementia (an evidence-based review). Report of the quality standards subcommittee of the American Academy of Neurology. *Neurology.* 2001;56(9):1154–66.
8. Alzheimer's Society. Keeping Active and Staying Involved. 2011. www.alzheimers.org .uk/. Accessed August 26, 2011.
9. Snowdon D. *Aging with Grace: What the Nun Study Teaches Us About Leading Longer, Healthier, and More Meaningful Lives.* New York: Bantam Books; 2001.
10. Ohgi S, Loo KK, Mizuike C. Frontal brain activation in young children during picture book reading with their mothers. *Acta Paediatrica.* 2010 Feb;99(2):225–29.
11. Friedland RP, Fritsch T, Smyth KA, Koss E, Lerner AJ, Chen CH, Petot GJ, Debanne SM. Patients with Alzheimer's disease have reduced activities in midlife compared with healthy control-group members. *Proceedings of the National Academy of Sciences USA.* 2001;98(6):3440–45.
12. Alzheimer's Society, Keeping Active and Staying Involved.
13. Ibid.
14. Delaune S, Ladner P. *Fundamentals of Nursing: Standards and Practice.* 2nd ed. Farmington Hills, MI: Thompson; 2002.
15. Ibid.
16. Zarit S. *The Hidden Victims of Alzheimer's Disease: Families under Stress.* New York: New York University Press; 1985.
17. Mayo Clinic. Alzheimer's: Dealing with Family Conflict. www.mayoclinic.com/. Accessed August 14, 2011; Yaari R, Fleisher AS, Burke AD, Brand H, Dougherty J, Seward JD, Tariot PN. Why does mommy forget? *Primary Care Companion for CNS Disorders.* 2011;13(2).pii.
18. Mayo Clinic, Alzheimer's.
19. Arai Y, Washio M. Burden felt by the family caring for the elderly members needing care in southern Japan. *Aging and Mental Health.* 1999;3(2):158–64.
20. Mayo Clinic, Alzheimer's.
21. O'Rourke N, Tuokko HA. Psychometric properties of an abridged version of the Zarit burden interview within a representative Canadian caregiver sample. *Gerontologist.* 2003 Feb;43(1):121–27.
22. Boutoleau-Bretonnière C, Vercelletto M, Volteau C, Renou P, Lamy E. Zarit burden inventory and activities of daily living in the behavioral variant of frontotemporal dementia. *Dementia and Geriatric Cognitive Disorders.* 2008;25(3):272–77.
23. Hérbert R, Bravo G, Préville M. Reliability, validity, and reference values of the Zarit burden interview for assessing informal caregivers of community-dwelling older persons with dementia. *Canadian Journal on Aging.* 2000;19:494–507.
24. Dozeman E, van Schaik DJ, van Marwijk HW, Stek ML, van der Horst HE, Beekman AT. The Center for Epidemiological Studies Depression Scale (CES-D) is an adequate screening instrument for depressive and anxiety disorders in a very old population living in residential homes. *International Journal of Geriatric Psychiatry.* 2011 Mar;26(3):239–46.

CHAPTER 20

1. Li LW, Conwell Y. Pain and self-injury ideation in elderly men and women receiving home care. *Journal of the American Geriatric Society.* 2010 Nov;58(11):2160–65; Wilson RS, Boyle PA, Buchman AS, Yu L, Arnold SE, Bennett DA. Harm avoidance and risk of Alzheimer's disease. *Psychosomatic Medicine.* 2011 Oct;73(8):690–96.
2. Stanton SS. Alzheimer's Disease: A Family Affair and a Growing Social Problem. April 2001. www.csa.com/. Accessed December 30, 2011.

3. Erde EL, Nadal EC, Scholl TO. On truth telling and the diagnosis of Alzheimer's disease. *Journal of Family Practice*. 1988 Apr;26(4):401–6.

4. Skrastins R, Merry GM, Rosenberg GM, Schuman JE. Clinical assessment of the elderly patient. *Canadian Medical Association Journal*. 1982 Aug 1;127(3):203–6; Erlen JA. The frail elderly: A matter of caring. *Orthopedic Nursing*. 2007 Nov–Dec;26(6):379–82.

5. Zarit S. *The Hidden Victims of Alzheimer's Disease: Families Under Stress*. New York: New York University Press; 1985; Alzheimer's Society. Fact Sheets: Unusual Behaviour. www.alzheimers.org.uk/. Accessed December 31, 2011.

6. Zarit, *Hidden Victims*.

7. Scarmeas N, Luchsinger JA, Brickman AM, Cosentino S, Schupf N, Xin-Tang M, Gu Y, Stern Y. Physical activity and Alzheimer disease course. *American Journal of Geriatric Psychiatry*. 2011 May;19(5):471–81.

8. Giasson M, Leroux G, Tardif H, Bouchard L. Therapeutic touch [French]. *L'Infirmière du Québec (Order of Nurses of Quebec)*. 1999 Jul–Aug;6(6):38–47.

9. Sandell-Delaloye P, Guex P, Fivaz-Depeursinge E. The role of body language in physician-patient relations: A key for improved communication [French]. *Revue Médicale de la Suisse Romande (Medical Journal of Western Switzerland)*. 2003 Feb;123(2):121–23.

10. Patterns of discourse cohesion and coherence in Alzheimer's disease. *Journal of Speech and Hearing Disorders*. 1988 Feb;53(1):8–15; Orange JB, Molloy DW, Lever JA, Darzins P, Ganesan CR. Alzheimer's disease. Physician-patient communication. *Canadian Family Physician*. 1994 Jun;40:1160–68.

11. Caring, Inc. How to Sidestep Power Struggles with Elderly Parents. www.caring.com. Accessed December 30, 2011.

12. Sullivan K, Finch S, O'Conor F. A confidence interval analysis of three studies using the Alzheimer's disease knowledge test. *Aging and Mental Health*. 2003 May;7(3):176–81.

13. Ibid.

Glossary

acetylcholinesterase test. Specific blood tests performed in order to detect abnormalities for acetylcholine levels. Acetylcholine levels have been, in many cases, noticed to be irregular for Alzheimer's patients.

ADRDA. Alzheimer's Disease and Related Disorders Association.

Alzheimer's disease. A fatal disease that, in most severe cases, can take away one's ability to think, remember, and behave properly. Known in medical literature as Alzheimer disease or AD.

Ammon's horn. One of the two major interlocking gyri that exist beneath the surface of cortex. Also called hippocampus proper, Ammon's horn is known in medical literature as *Cornu ammonis*.

amygdala. Almond-shaped part of the brain and limbic system. The amygdala is situated in the temporal lobes of the cerebrum and controls emotional responses such as anger and fear.

amyloid beta (Aβ). A biomarker evidencing the plaques characteristic of Alzheimer's.

amyloid plaques. Structures consisting of amyloid protein tangles, amyloid plaques are one of the major pathological hallmarks of Alzheimer's disease. They generally accumulate in the nerve cells of the brain.

anterograde amnesia. Inability to generate new memories after an event of amnesia. Generally, this type of memory loss happens after serious brain damage.

apolipoprotein E4 gene (APOE-4). One of the major variations of the APO-E gene. Increases the occurrence of Alzheimer's disease. The presence of this risk gene can develop into the late onset, sporadic type of Alzheimer's disease.

apraxia. Physical symptom of Alzheimer's disease. Patients lose the ability to perform daily basic activities such as bathing, brushing teeth, or feeding themselves.

argyrophilic grain disease. A sporadic ailment that comes with old age and is typified by argyrophilic grains. Other names used include Braak's dementia and Braak's disease.

aseptic meningoencephalitis. Inflammation of the outer lining of the brain that does not involve bacteria.

association cortex. Cerebral cortex found in the outer edge of the primary areas. It strengthens sensory stimulation and smooths out complex mental functions.

astrocyte. A large, star-shaped cell of the nervous system.

autism spectrum disorder. Autism spectrum disorder is a group of developmental disorders characterized by social impairments and disabilities.

basal ganglia. A group of nuclei or interconnected subcortical mass in the gray matter. It is comprised of mesencephalic, claustrum, and diencephalic elements.

Binswanger's disease. A vascular dementia generally caused by damage to the white matter of the brain, due to the narrowing and thickening of arteries leading to the brain.

biomarker. A biochemical substance or physical trait used to track the progression of a disease.

carbamazepine A. Medication that used for epilepsy. Presently, carbamazepine A is a treatment method for Alzheimer's disease.

cerebellum. Highly important part of the brain. The term stems from a Latin lexicon meaning "little brain." The cerebellum is located just beneath the occipital lobe and is shaped like a cauliflower.

Chimaera monstrosa. A species of fish with smooth skin and a tail that looks similar to a string of thread. It is also known as the rat fish.

cholinesterase inhibitors. Structures that enhance the activities of acetylcholine. At times, cholinesterase inhibitors improve the condition of Alzheimer's patients.

computed tomography. A medical imaging method; CT scan.

condyloma latum. Secondary-stage manifestation of syphilis. It usually takes place in the surrounding areas of genitalia and anus.

corpus callosum. Neural fibers located under the cortex of the mammal brain. It helps in interhemispheric communications by linking cerebral hemispheres.

Creutzfeldt-Jakob disease. A fatal neurological disorder, sometimes ascribed as mad cow disease in humans, in which holes are created in brain tissues.

CSF (cerebrospinal fluid) Aβ42. A watery fluid, produced and absorbed in the ventricles of the brain. Flows around spinal cord and various parts of the brain. It is considered a cutoff value that may predict the development of MCI to Alzheimer's dementia.

cytopathology. Use of cytology to go over loose cells on microscope slides.

dementia. Latin-originated term that means a very serious loss of cognitive abilities in a person. Different types of dementia include cortical, subcortical, vascular, dementia with Lewy bodies, and frontotemporal.

dentate gyrus. One of two major interlocking gyri in the brain. It is contained in the hippocampus.

donepezil. The generic name for Aricept, this medication is thought to be the most popular of all the medications used for Alzheimer's disease.

dysthymic disorder. A kind of depression in which a person experiences depressed mood for most of the time, for at least two years. The symptoms are chronic but not as severe as in major depression. In this case, the person can execute his or her normal activities.

enzyme-linked immunoabsorbent assay (ELISA). Specific tests that are generally performed to find antibodies.

galantamine. One of the top prescription cholinesterase inhibitors currently. Galantamine is also known in the brand name Razadyne. It performs the important function of preventing the breakdown of the acetylcholine neurotransmitter and creates a balance among the neurotransmitters present in the brain.

ghost tangles. Tangles occurring outside the perimeter of a dead neuron.

Ginkgo biloba. A living tree species and a major traditional medicine of ancient China. It is highly effective on different kinds of ailments ranging from circulatory disorders, tinnitus, multiple sclerosis, and vitiligo. It is said that the herb can work miraculously in sharpening and enhancing a person's memory functions.

haematoxylin. A colored mixture that is applied to color a cell's nucleus before a microscopic examination. The haematoxylin mixture is rich in metal ions.

hippocampus. Part of the brain that regenerates the nerve cells that lose their capacity during Alzheimer's disease. It is situated on both sides of the brain and helps in retaining long-term memory. The hippocampus is affected first by Alzheimer's disease.

histology. The anatomical study of the microscopic observation of specific structures of plant tissues and animal tissues.

histopathological. Associated with the microscopic observation of the diseased tissue structure.

Huperzia serrata. A Chinese herb that is rich in antioxidant and neuroprotective properties. It may be beneficial for patients suffering from Alzheimer's disease and the early stages of dementia.

hypothalamus. A gland located in the middle base portion of the brain, serving as the temperature control of the body.

immunocytochemistry. Specific procedure of microscopic observation with the use of fluorescent dyes.

lobes. Areas of the brain distinguished by function, including causes, emotions, analysis, reasoning, and sensory functions. The right and left hemispheres of the cerebrum are both subdivided into four major lobes: frontal, parietal, temporal, and occipital.

logopenic progressive aphasia. Ailment in which a patient suffers from impaired naming capacity, slowed speech, and reduced syntactic understanding.

medulla. Latin-originated term for "marrow." Examples of medulla include medulla spinalis, medulla of ovary, medulla of thymus, adrenal medulla, renal medulla, medulla oddea, and medulla oblongata.

microtubuli. Small tunnel or empty fibrous rod that helps in shaping the cells of the human body. Found in eukaryotic cells, microtubuli are also referred to as microtubules.

mild cognitive impairment (MCI). Specific diagnosis adopted for individuals who have reportedly suffered from cognitive impairments. Amnestic MCI (memory loss) is considered a high risk factor in the cases of Alzheimer's.

mini-mental state exam (MMSE). A standard test that includes questions designed to determine a patient's mental state. This exam is also informally called mini-mental *status* exam.

neocortex. The layer that covers the outskirts of cerebral hemispheres. The original Latin term for neocortex means "new rind or bark."

neurodegeneration. Significant loss of neuron functions. Neurodegenerative ailments include Huntington's, Alzheimer's, and Parkinson's.

neurofibrillary tangles. Structures popularly known as the preliminary markers of Alzheimer's disease and generally characterized by tau protein.

neurotransmitters. Endogenous chemicals that send out signals from neurons to target cells. Neurotransmitters are connected via structures called synaptic vesicles.

Nissl method. A new procedure of staining cells to examine them under the microscope.

NMDA receptors. Structures that allow the transfer of brain signals from the brain to the spinal cord and to the rest of the body. NMDA receptors play a crucial role in specific and significant brain functions such as memory, cognition, and learning.

normal-pressure hydrocephalus. Abnormal expansion that takes place in ventricles of the brain. It is generally caused when cerebrospinal fluid accumulates. There are two major variants, acquired and congenital.

opioids. Synthetic narcotic drugs that create opiate-like impact and relieve pain. Opioids are usually prescribed by medical practitioners to relieve respiratory depression and for sedation.

paranoia. An inflated, baseless, and serious mental outcome of Alzheimer's disease in which the patients keep suspecting the motives of people around them. Delusions, introvertedness, depression, jealousy, and bitterness are among the related symptoms.

PET amyloid imaging. One of the major pathological tests for Alzheimer's disease. It helps in the early diagnosis of Alzheimer's and is also helpful in deciding treatment.

phosphatidylserine. An indispensable element produced by the human body. Phosphatidylserine plays an important role in keeping cells undamaged and whole as well as transporting nutrients into cells and driving out waste.

prana biotechnology 2 (PBT2). A therapeutic strategy that deals with pathological devices related to amyloid beta protein and can prevent the rapid growth of Alzheimer's.

progressive supranuclear palsy (PSP). A very rare kind of a degenerative ailment that causes destruction of nerve cells in the brain. The condition ultimately affects coordination in muscles, breathing, and eye movements. Due to slowed reaction time and malfunction of motor skills caused by damage in the subcortical regions of the brain. Also known as Steele-Richardson-Olszewski syndrome.

retrograde amnesia. Failure of the brain to record or remember the events that have taken place.

rivastigmine. Type of prescription cholinesterase inhibitor drug. Generally, it is given to patients suffering from mild to moderate dementia associated with Alzheimer's disease as well as Parkinson's disease.

single-photon emission computed tomography (SPECT). A specific imaging technique that is performed with gamma rays and tomographic nuclear medicine.

Steele-Richardson-Olszewski syndrome. *See progressive supranuclear palsy.*

substantia nigra. A Latin term that stands for black substance; refers to a structure in the brain that plays an important role in movement.

thalamus. Gray mass located in the center of the brain, below the corpus callosum. The thalamus supports the motor activities as well as the sensory functions of the brain.

thiamine deficiency. A severe form of deficiency that is caused by regular as well as excessive alcohol intake. Thiamine deficiency is the reduction of a vital nutrient called thiamine.

tramiprosate. An amyloid-beta antagonist that averts the buildup of a toxic protein called amyloid plaques that trigger a brain abnormality now largely recognized and held responsible for the development of Alzheimer's disease.

vermis. A structure that connects the left and the right hemisphere of the cerebellum.

Resources

Alzheimer's Disease
www.nlm.nih.gov/medlineplus/alzheimersdisease.html

Alzheimer's Disease Care
www.alzheimers-disease-care.com/

Alzheimer's Disease Fact Sheet
www.nia.nih.gov/Alzheimers/Publications/adfact.htm

Alzheimer's Disease: The Basics
http://www.alz.org/national/documents/brochure_basicsofalz_low.pdf

Alzheimer's Early Stages: First Steps for Families, Friends, and Caregivers
Daniel Kuhn, MD, and David A. Bennett
Hunter House, 2003
ISBN: 0897933974

Alzheimer's: Few Clues on the Mysteries of Memory
www.healingwell.com/library/alzheimers/hingley1.asp

Alzheimer's Patients and the Adjustment to Assisted Living
www.healingwell.com/alzheimers

Best Alzheimer's Products
www.store.best-alzheimers-products.com/merchant2

Care for the Caregiver: Managing Stress
www.ahaf.org/docs/pdf-publications/caringcaregiver_stress.pdf

Caring for the Alzheimer Patient
J. Thomas Hutton, MD, and R. L. Dippel
Prometheus Books, 1996
ISBN: 9781573921084

Holistic Approaches to Alzheimer's Disease
www.alzheimers.about.com/lw/Health-Medicine/Alternative-treatments/Taking-a-Holistic-Approach-to-Alzheimers-Disease.htm

Learning to Speak Alzheimer's: A Groundbreaking Approach for Everyone Dealing with the Disease
Robert M. Butler, MD, and Joanne Koenig Coste
Houghton Mifflin Harcourt, 2004
ISBN: 0618485171

Living with Alzheimer's Disease
www.ahaf.org/docs/pdf-publications/livingwithalzheimers.pdf

Maintaining Selfhood and Dignity in Alzheimer's Patients
www.healingwell.com/library/alzheimers/bryce1.asp

Memory Clinics for Alzheimer's Disease
www.alzheimers.about.com/od/helpyoumayneed/a/memory_clinics.htm

Safety and the Old Driver
www.ahaf.org/docs/pdf-publications/safety_olderdriver_adr.pdf

Staying Safe: Wandering and the Alzheimer's Patient
Alzheimer's Disease Research
www.ahaf.org/docs/pdf-publications/stayingsafe_wandering.pdf

10 Warning Signs of Alzheimer's Disease
www.alz.org/national/documents/brochure_10warnsigns.pdf

The 36-Hour Day
N. L. Mace and Peter Rabins, MD
Johns Hopkins University Press, 2011
ISBN: 9781421402796

Tips on Wandering in Alzheimer's Patients
www.healingwell.com/library/alzheimers/knox1.asp

Treatments for Alzheimer's Disease
www.alz.org/national/documents/topicsheet_treatments.pdf

TV Series Solution to Parents with Alzheimer's
www.healingwell.com/alzheimers

Understanding Alzheimer's Disease
www.nia.nih.gov/alzheimers/publication/understanding-alzheimers-disease

Bibliography

CHAPTER 1

[No author listed]. Alois Alzheimer (1864–1915), neurohistopathologist. *Journal of the American Medical Association.* 1969 May 12;208(6):1017–18.

Biegert C, Wagner I, Lüdtke R, Kötter I, Lohmüller C, Günaydin I, Taxis K, Heide L. Efficacy and safety of willow bark extract in the treatment of osteoarthritis and rheumatoid arthritis: Results of 2 randomized double-blind controlled trials. *Journal of Rheumatology.* 2004 Nov;31(11):2121–30.

Fabrega H. Mental health and illness in traditional India and China. *Psychiatric Clinics of North America.* 2001 Sep;24(3):555–67, ix.

Purse M. Mental illness in the past and future. www.pipolar.about.com. Updated October 4, 2011. Accessed November 6, 2011.

Sedivec V. [Mental disorders in the writings of Hippocrates]. *Ceskoslovenská Psychiatrie.* 1989 Aug;85(4):270–73.

Yapijakis C. Hippocrates of Kos, the father of clinical medicine, and Asclepiades of Bithynia, the father of molecular medicine [Review]. *In Vivo.* 2009 Jul–Aug;23(4):507–14.

CHAPTER 2

Akiguchi I, Tomimoto H, Suenaga T, Wakita H, Budka H. Alterations in glia and axons in the brains of Binswanger's disease patients. *Stroke.* 1997 Jul;28(7):1423–29.

Bech-Azeddine R, Waldemar G, Knudsen GM, Høgh P, Bruhn P, Wildschiødtz G, Gjerris F, Paulson OB, Juhler M. Idiopathic normal-pressure hydrocephalus: Evaluation and findings in a multidisciplinary memory clinic. *European Journal of Neurology.* 2001 Nov;8(6):601–11.

Davachi L, Mitchell JP, Wagner AD. Multiple routes to memory: Distinct medial temporal lobe processes build item and source memories. *Proceedings of the National Academy of Science.* 2003 Feb 18;100(4):2157–62.

de Jong LW, van der Hiele K, Veer IM, Houwing JJ, Westendorp RG, Bollen EL, de Bruin PW, Middelkoop HA, van Buchem MA, van der Grond J. Strongly reduced volumes of putamen and thalamus in Alzheimer's disease: An MRI study. *Brain.* 2008 Dec;131(Pt 12): 3277–85.

Derntl B, Windischberger C, Robinson S, Kryspin-Exner I, Gur RC, Moser E, Habel U. Amygdala activity to fear and anger in healthy young males is associated with testosterone. *Psychoneuroendocrinology.* 2009 Jun;34(5):687–93.

Merriam Webster. Ecophysiology. www.merriam-webster.com/dictionary. Accessed November 6, 2011.

Zentner J, Neumüller H. Modified impulse diminishes discomfort of transcranial electrical stimulation of the motor cortex. *Electromyography and Clinical Neurophysiology.* 1989 Mar;29(2):93–97.

CHAPTER 3

Adams A. Genetics of Alzheimer's Disease. Genetic Health online. http://www.genetichealth .com/alz_genetics_of_alzheimers_disease.shtml. Accessed May 31, 2011.

Alzheimer's disease. Alzheimer Society of Canada. http://www.alzheimer.ca/english/disease/ causes-riskfac.htm. Accessed May 22, 2011.

Alzheimer's disease. MedicineNet.com. http://www.medicinenet.com/alzheimers_disease_ causes_stages_and_symptoms/page4.htm#tocg. Accessed May 23, 2011.

Amen D, Shankle WR. *Preventing Alzheimer's.* New York: Penguin; 2004.

Arias HR, Tuppo EE. The role of inflammation and Alzheimer's disease. *International Journal of Biochemistry and Cell Biology.* 2004;37:289–305.

Causes and risk factors of Alzheimer's disease. WebMD. www.webmd.com/alzheimers/guide/ causes-risk-factors. Accessed May 22, 2011.

Forman LJ, Tuppo EE. Free radical oxidative damage and Alzheimer's disease. *Journal of the American Osteopathic Association.* 2001;101:11–15.

Mayo Clinic. Alzheimer's disease: Causes. Mayo Clinic. http://www.mayoclinic.com/health/ alzheimers-disease/DS00161/DSECTION=causes. Accessed May 23, 2011.

Mayo Clinic. Alzheimer's disease: Risk factors. http://www.mayoclinic.com. Accessed May 23, 2011.

Mayo Clinic. Amyloidosis. www.mayoclinic.com. Accessed May 31, 2011.

Mitchell D, Turkington C. *The Encyclopedia of Alzheimer's Disease.* 2nd ed. New York: Infobase Publishing; 2010.

Mulnard RA, Cotman CW, Kawas C, van Dyck CH, Sano M, Doody R, Koss E, Pfeiffer E, Jin S, Gamst A, Grundman M, Thomas R, Thal LJ. Estrogen replacement therapy for treatment of mild to moderate Alzheimer disease: A randomized controlled trial. Alzheimer's Disease Cooperative Study. *Journal of the American Medical Association.* 2000 Feb 23;283(8):1007–15.

Sadowski M, Wisniewski TM. *100 Questions and Answers about Alzheimer's Disease.* Sudbury, MA: Jones and Bartlett Publishers; 2004.

Strock M. Alzheimer's disease. National Institute of Mental Health;1996:1–5.

CHAPTER 4

Baker LD, Frank LL, Foster-Schubert K, Green PS, Wilkinson CW, McTiernan A, Cholerton BA, Plymate SR, Fishel MA, Watson GS, Duncan GE, Mehta PD, Craft S. Aerobic exercise improves cognition for older adults with glucose intolerance, a risk factor for Alzheimer's disease. *Journal of Alzheimer's Disease.* 2010;22(2):569–79.

Clark RE, Broadbent NJ, Zola SM, Squire LR. Anterograde amnesia and temporally graded retrograde amnesia for a nonspatial memory task after lesions of hippocampus and subiculum. *Journal of Neuroscience.* 2002 Jun 1;22(11):4663–69.

Cleveland Clinic. Types of Dementia. www.my.clevelandclinic.org. Accessed November 14, 2011.

Escandon A, Al-Hammadi N, Galvin JE. Effect of cognitive fluctuation on neuropsychological performance in aging and dementia. *Neurology.* 2010 Jan 19;74(3):210–17.

Fujiwara E, Brand M, Kracht L, Kessler J, Diebel A, Netz J, Markowitsch HJ. Functional retrograde amnesia: A multiple case study. *Cortex.* 2008 Jan;44(1):29–45.

Hoch DB, Zieve D, reviewers. Multi-infarct Dementia. www.ncbi.nlm.nih.gov. Last reviewed March 22, 2010. Accessed November 14, 2011.

Kennard C. Urinary Tract Infection and Alzheimer's Disease. www.alzheimers.about.com. Updated November 8, 2006. Accessed November 6, 2011.

Pendlebury ST. Stroke-related dementia: Rates, risk factors and implications for future research. *Maturitas.* 2009 Nov 20;64(3):165–71.

CHAPTER 5

Arnold SR, Ford-Jones EL. Congenital syphilis: A guide to diagnosis and management. *Pediatric Child Health.* 2000 Nov;5(8):463–69.

Copeland JR, Davidson IA, Dewey ME, Gilmore C, Larkin BA, McWilliam C, Saunders PA, Scott A, Sharma V, Sullivan C. Alzheimer's disease, other dementias, depression and pseudodementia: Prevalence, incidence and three-year outcome in Liverpool. *British Journal of Psychiatry.* 1992 Aug;161:230–39.

Donix M, Ercoli LM, Siddarth P, Brown JA, Martin-Harris L, Burggren AC, Miller KJ, Small GW, Bookheimer SY. Influence of Alzheimer disease family history and genetic risk on cognitive performance in healthy middle-aged and older people. *American Journal of Geriatric Psychiatry.* 2011 Feb 24.

Harciarek M, Jodzio K. Neuropsychological differences between frontotemporal dementia and Alzheimer's disease: A review. *Neuropsychology Review.* 2005 Sep;15(3):131–45.

Iliadou V, Kaprinis S. Clinical psychoacoustics in Alzheimer's disease central auditory processing disorders and speech deterioration. *Annals of General Hospital Psychiatry.* 2003 Dec 22;2(1):12.

Medical University of South Carolina. Acetylcholinesterase, Red Blood Cell Measurement. www.muschealth.com. Accessed August 19, 2011.

Otsuka M, Yamaguchi K, Ueki A. Similarities and differences between Alzheimer's disease and vascular dementia from the viewpoint of nutrition. *Annals of the New York Academy of Science.* 2002 Nov;977:155–61.

Pasquier F. Telling the difference between frontotemporal dementia and Alzheimer's disease. *Current Opinions in Psychiatry.* 2005 Nov;18(6):628–32.

Sunderland T, Hampel H, Takeda M, Putnam KT, Cohen RM. Biomarkers in the diagnosis of Alzheimer's disease: Are we ready? *Journal of Geriatric Psychiatry and Neurology.* 2006 Sep;19(3):172–79.

Swainson R, Hodges JR, Galton CJ, Semple J, Michael A, Dunn BD, Iddon JL, Robbins TW, Sahakian BJ. Early detection and differential diagnosis of Alzheimer's disease and depression with neuropsychological tasks. *Dementia and Geriatric Cognitive Disorders.* 2001 Jul–Aug;12(4):265–80.

CHAPTER 6

Bordji K, Becerril-Ortega J, Buisson A. Synapses, NMDA receptor activity and neuronal Aβ production in Alzheimer's disease. *Reviews in the Neurosciences.* 2011;22(3):285–94.

Crouch PJ, Savva MS, Hung LW, Donnelly PS, Mot AI, Parker SJ, Greenough MA, Volitakis I, Adlard PA, Cherny RA, Masters CL, Bush AI, Barnham KJ, White AR. The Alzheimer's therapeutic PBT2 promotes amyloid-β degradation and GSK3 phosphorylation via a metal chaperone activity. *Journal of Neurochemistry.* 2011 Oct;119(1):220–30.

Howland RH. Drug therapies for cognitive impairment and dementia. *Journal of Psychosocial Nursing & Mental Health Services.* 2010 Apr;48(4):11–14.

Massoud F, Léger GC. Pharmacological treatment of Alzheimer disease. *Canadian Journal of Psychiatry.* 2011 Oct;56(10):579–88.

Miller CA. How much of a breakthrough is Cognex for Alzheimer's disease? *Geriatric Nursing.* 1994 Jan-Feb;15(1):53–54.

Salomone S, Caraci F, Leggio GM, Fedotova J, Drago F. New pharmacological strategies for treatment of Alzheimer's disease: Focus on disease-modifying drugs. *British Journal of Clinical Pharmacology.* 2011 Oct 28.

Sparks DL. Alzheimer disease: Statins in the treatment of Alzheimer disease. *Nature Reviews Neurology.* 2011 Oct 18;7(12):662–63.

Venkataramani V, Rossner C, Iffland L, Schweyer S, Tamboli IY, Walter J, Wirths O, Bayer TA. Histone deacetylase inhibitor valproic acid inhibits cancer cell proliferation via down-regulation of the Alzheimer amyloid precursor protein. *Journal of Biological Chemistry.* 2010 Apr 2;285(14):10678–89.

CHAPTER 7

Amaducci L, Crook TH, Lippi A, Bracco L, Baldereschi M, Latorraca S, Piersanti P, Tesco G, Sorbi S. Use of phosphatidylserine in Alzheimer's disease. *Annals of the New York Academy of Sciences.* 1991;640:245–49.

Guan JZ, Guan WP, Maeda T, Makino N. Effect of Vitamin E administration on the elevated oxygen stress and the telomeric and subtelomeric status in Alzheimer's disease. Gerontology. 2011 Sep 7. Published online ahead of print.

Ha GT, Wong RK, Zhang Y. Huperzine A as potential treatment of Alzheimer's disease: An assessment on chemistry, pharmacology, and clinical studies. *Chemistry and Biodiversity.* 2011 Jul;8(7):1189–204.

Hashimoto M, Hossain S. Neuroprotective and ameliorative actions of polyunsaturated fatty acids against neuronal diseases: Beneficial effect of docosahexaenoic acid on cognitive decline in Alzheimer's disease. *Journal of Pharmacological Sciences.* 2011;116(2):150–62.

Ihl R, Tribanek M, Bachinskaya N. Efficacy and Tolerability of a Once Daily Formulation of Ginkgo biloba Extract EGb 761 in Alzheimer's Disease and Vascular Dementia: Results from a Randomised Controlled Trial. *Pharmacopsychiatry.* 2011 Nov 15. Published online ahead of print.

Martineau E, de Guzman JM, Rodionova L, Kong X, Mayer PM, Aman AM. Investigation of the noncovalent interactions between anti-amyloid agents and amyloid beta peptides by ESI-MS. *Journal of the American Society for Mass Spectrometry.* 2010 Sep;21(9):1506–14.

Omura Y, O'Young B, Jones M, Pallos A, Duvvi H, Shimotsuura Y. Caprylic acid in the effective treatment of intractable medical problems of frequent urination, incontinence, chronic upper respiratory infection, root canalled tooth infection, ALS, etc., caused by asbestos & mixed infections of Candida albicans, Helicobacter pylori & cytomegalovirus with or without other microorganisms & mercury. *Acupuncture & Electro-therapeutics Research.* 2011;36(1–2):19–64.

Spindler M, Beal MF, Henchcliffe C. Coenzyme Q10 effects in neurodegenerative disease. *Journal of Neuropsychiatric Disease and Treatment.* 2009;5:597–610.

CHAPTER 8

Beach TG, Sue LI, Walker DG, Sabbagh MN, Serrano G, Dugger B, Mariner M, Yantos K, Henry-Watson J, Chiarolanza G, Hidalgo J, Souders L. Striatal amyloid plaque density predicts Braak neurofibrillary stage and clinicopathological Alzheimer's disease: Implications for amyloid imaging. *Journal of Alzheimer's Disease.* 2011 Nov 23. Published online ahead of print.

Ewers M, Mielke MM, Hampel H. Blood-based biomarkers of microvascular pathology in Alzheimer's disease. *Experimental Gerontology.* 2010 Jan;45(1):75–79.

Keeney JT, Swomley AM, Harris JL, Fiorini A, Mitov MI, Perluigi M, Sultana R, Butterfield DA. Cell cycle proteins in brain in mild cognitive impairment: Insights into progression to Alzheimer disease. *Neurotoxicity Research.* 2011 Nov 15.

Leoni V. The effect of apolipoprotein E (ApoE) genotype on biomarkers of amyloidogenesis, tau pathology and neurodegeneration in Alzheimer's disease. *Clinical Chemistry and Laboratory Medicine.* 2011 Mar;49(3):375–83.

Weigand SD, Vemuri P, Wiste HJ, Senjem ML, Pankratz VS, Aisen PS, Weiner MW, Petersen RC, Shaw LM, Trojanowski JQ, Knopman DS, Jack CR Jr. Transforming cerebrospinal fluid Aβ42 measures into calculated Pittsburgh Compound B units of brain Aβ amyloid. *Alzheimer's & Dementia.* 2011 Mar;7(2):133–41.

CHAPTER 9

Arima K, Nakamura M, Sunohara N, Nishio T, Ogawa M, Hirai S, Kawai M, Ikeda K. Immunohistochemical and ultrastructural characterization of neuritic clusters around ghost tangles in the hippocampal formation in progressive supranuclear palsy brains. *Acta Neuropathologica.* 1999 Jun;97(6):565–76.

Braak H, Braak E. Frequency of stages of Alzheimer-related lesions in different age categories. *Neurobiology of Aging.* 1997 Jul–Aug;18(4):351–57.

Ikeda K, Haga C, Oyanagi S, Iritani S, Kosaka K. Ultrastructural and immunohistochemical study of degenerate neurite-bearing ghost tangles. *Journal of Neurology.* 1992 Apr;239(4):191–94.

MacDonald AB. Alzheimer's disease Braak stage progressions: Reexamined and redefined as Borrelia infection transmission through neural circuits. *Medical Hypotheses.* 2007;68(5):1059–64.

Zhan J, Brys M, Glodzik L, Tsui W, Javier E, Wegiel J, Kuchna I, Pirraglia E, Li Y, Mosconi L, Saint Louis LA, Switalski R, De Santi S, Kim BC, Wisniewski T, Reisberg B, Bobinski M, de Leon MJ. An entorhinal cortex sulcal pattern is associated with Alzheimer's disease. *Human Brain Mapping.* 2009 Mar;30(3):874–82.

CHAPTER 10

Abe N, Fujii T, Nishio Y, Iizuka O, Kanno S, Kikuchi H, Takagi M, Hiraoka K, Yamasaki H, Choi H, Hirayama K, Shinohara M, Mori E. False item recognition in patients with Alzheimer's disease. *Neuropsychologia.* 2011 Jun;49(7):1897–902.

Correia Sde M, Morillo LS, Jacob Filho W, Mansur LL. Swallowing in moderate and severe phases of Alzheimer's disease. *Arquivos de Neuro-psiquiatria.* 2010 Dec;68(6):855–61.

Friedlander AH, Norman DC, Mahler ME, Norman KM, Yagiela JA. Alzheimer's disease: Psychopathology, medical management and dental implications. *Journal of the American Dental Association.* 2006 Sep;137(9):1240–51.

Ripich DN, Terrell BY. Patterns of discourse cohesion and coherence in Alzheimer's disease. *Journal of Speech and Hearing Disorders.* 1988 Feb;53(1):8–15.

CHAPTER 11

Agitation. Wrongdiagnosis.com. www.wrongdiagnosis.com/sym/agitation.htm. Accessed May 31, 2011.

Aggression. Wrongdiagnosis.com. www.wrongdiagnosis.com. Accessed May 31, 2011.

Dementia. Medicinenet.com. www.medicinenet.com/dementia/article.htm. Accessed June 3, 2011.

Dementia: Hope through Research. Office of Communications and Public Liaison: National Institute of Neurological Disorders and Stroke. www.ninds.nih.gov. Updated March 23, 2011. Accessed May 29, 2011.

Depression. Familydoctor.org. January 1996. www.familydoctor.org. Updated May 2010. Accessed May 30, 2011.

Mental Health: Depression. World Health Organization. www.who.int/mental_health. Accessed May 31, 2011.

Mental Health: A Report from the Surgeon General. www.surgeongeneral.gov/library/mental-health. Accessed May 28, 2011.

A Report of the World Health Organization. Department of Mental Health and Substance Abuse in collaboration with the Prevention Research Centre of the Universities of Nijmegen and Maastricht. 2004. www.who.int. Accessed June 2, 2011.

CHAPTER 12

Adler CH. Premotor symptoms and early diagnosis of Parkinson's disease. *International Journal of Neuroscience.* 2011;121 Suppl 2:3–8.

Chitravas N, Jung RS, Kofskey DM, Blevins JE, Gambetti P, Leigh RJ, Cohen ML. Treatable neurological disorders misdiagnosed as Creutzfeldt-Jakob disease. *Annals of Neurology.* 2011 Sep;70(3):437–44.

Côté M, Misasi J, Ren T, Bruchez A, Lee K, Filone CM, Hensley L, Li Q, Ory D, Chandran K, Cunningham J. Small molecule inhibitors reveal Niemann-Pick C1 is essential for Ebola virus infection. *Nature.* 2011 Aug 24;477(7364):344–48.

Czosnyka M, Czosnyka Z, Whitehouse H, Pickard JD. Hydrodynamic properties of hydrocephalus shunts: United Kingdom shunt evaluation laboratory. *Journal of Neurology, Neurosurgery, & Psychiatry.* 1997 Jan;62(1):43–50.

Devenny DA, Wegiel J, Schupf N, Jenkins E, Zigman W, Krinsky-McHale SJ, Silverman WP. Dementia of the Alzheimer's type and accelerated aging in Down syndrome. *Science of Aging Knowledge Environment.* 2005 Apr 6;2005(14).

Hasosah M, Satti M. Hepatobiliary and pancreatic: Niemann-Pick disease. *Journal of Gastroenterology and Hepatology.* 2011 Dec;26(12):1813.

Kertesz A. Frontotemporal dementia, Pick's disease. *Ideggyógyászati Szemle (Neurological Review).* 2010 Jan 30;63(1–2):4–12.

Kwok JB. Role of epigenetics in Alzheimer's and Parkinson's disease. *Epigenomics.* 2010 Oct;2(5):671–82.

Nath A, Schiess N, Venkatesan A, Rumbaugh J, Sacktor N, McArthur J. Evolution of HIV dementia with HIV infection. *International Review of Psychiatry.* 2008 Feb;20(1):25–31.

Panegyres PK, Beilby J, Bulsara M, Toufexis K, Wong C. A study of potential interactive genetic factors in Huntington's disease. *European Neurology.* 2006;55(4):189–92.

Winogrodzka A, Wagenaar RC, Booij J, Wolters EC. Rigidity and bradykinesia reduce interlimb coordination in Parkinsonian gait. *Archives of Physical Medicine and Rehabilitation.* 2005 Feb;86(2):183–89.

Zigman WB, Lott IT. Alzheimer's disease in Down syndrome: Neurobiology and risk. *Mental Retardation and Developmental Disabilities Research Reviews.* 2007;13(3):237–46.

CHAPTER 13

Fisher-Morris M, Gellatly A. The experience and expression of pain in Alzheimer patients. *Age and Ageing.* 1997 Nov;26(6):497–500.

Giamberardino MA, Affaitati G, Costantini R. Chapter 24: Referred pain from internal organs. *Handbook of Clinical Neurology.* 2006;(81):343–61.

Gibson SJ, Voukelatos X, Ames D, Flicker L, Helme RD. An examination of pain perception and cerebral event-related potentials following carbon dioxide laser stimulation in patients with Alzheimer's disease and age-matched control volunteers. *Pain Research & Management.* 2001 Fall;6(3):126–32.

Jolivalt CG, Mizisin LM, Nelson A, Cunha JM, Ramos KM, Bonke D, Calcutt NA. B vitamins alleviate indices of neuropathic pain in diabetic rats. *European Journal of Pharmacology.* 2009 Jun 10;612(1–3):41–47.

Lopez-Garcia E, Schulze MB, Fung TT, Meigs JB, Rifai N, Manson JE, Hu FB. Major dietary patterns are related to plasma concentrations of markers of inflammation and endothelial dysfunction. *American Journal of Clinical Nutrition.* 2004 Oct;80(4):1029–35.

Phantom limb pain: Mechanisms and treatment approaches. *Pain Research and Treatment.* 2011. Published online ahead of print.

Pollatos O, Dietel A, Herbert BM, Wankner S, Wachsmuth C, Henningsen P, Sack M. Blunted autonomic reactivity and increased pain tolerance in somatoform patients. *Pain.* 2011 Sep;152(9):2157–64.

Russell WJ. The impact of Alzheimer's disease medication on muscle relaxants. *Anaesthesia and Intensive Care.* 2009 Jan;37(1):134–35.

Scherder E, Oosterman J, Swaab D, Herr K, Ooms M, Ribbe M, Sergeant J, Pickering G, Benedetti F. Recent developments in pain in dementia. *British Medical Journal.* 2005 Feb 26;330(7489):461–64.

Shereen J. Anti-Inflammatory Foods. www.nutrition.about.com. Updated March 18, 2012. Accessed April 4, 2012.

Straube S, Derry S, Moore RA, McQuay HJ. Vitamin D for the treatment of chronic painful conditions in adults. *Cochrane Database of Systematic Reviews*. 2010 Jan 20;(1).

CHAPTER 14

Barnes L, Perry D, Woodcock J. Alzheimer's Disease/Effects on Federal Spending and Industry Innovation [Presented at Audio Conference]. Avalere Health: Washington, DC; July 25, 2007:2–13.

Bloom BS, de Pouvourville N, Straus WL. Cost of illness of Alzheimer's disease: How useful are current estimates? *Gerontologist*. 2003 Apr;43(2):158–64.

Kingsbury K. Tallying Mental Illness' Costs. Time. May 9, 2008. www.time.com. Accessed December 13, 2011.

Jönsson L. Economic evidence in dementia: A review. *European Journal of Health Economics*. 2004 Oct;5 Suppl 1:S30–35.

McKenzie J. Rising Cost of Caring for Alzheimer's. ABC News. March 24, 2009. www.abcnews.go.com. Accessed December 13, 2011.

Plunkett JW. Plunkett's Health Care Industry Almanac 2011: Health Care Industry Market Research, Statistics, Trends & Leading Companies. Houston; Plunkett Research. 2010: 722.

Wimo A, Jönsson L, Gustavsson A, McDaid D, Ersek K, Georges J, Gulácsi L, Karpati K, Kenigsberg P, Valtonen H. The economic impact of dementia in Europe in 2008: Cost estimates from the Eurocode project. *International Journal of Geriatric Psychiatry*. 2011 Aug;26(8):825–32.

CHAPTER 15

Atamna H, Kumar R. Protective role of methylene blue in Alzheimer's disease via mitochondria and cytochrome c oxidase. *Journal of Alzheimer's Disease*. 2010;20 Suppl 2:S439–52.

Chen M, Maleski JJ, Sawmiller DR. Scientific truth or false hope? Understanding Alzheimer's disease from an aging perspective. *Journal of Alzheimer's Disease*. 2011;24(1):3–10.

Hollingworth P, Sweet R, Sims R, Harold D, Russo G, Abraham R, Stretton A, Jones N, Gerrish A, Chapman J, Ivanov D, Moskvina V, Lovestone S, Priotsi P, Lupton M, Brayne C, Gill M, Lawlor B, Lynch A, Craig D, McGuinness B, Johnston J, Holmes C, Livingston G, Bass NJ, Gurling H, McQuillin A, GERAD Consortium, National Institute on Aging Late-Onset Alzheimer's Disease Family Study Group, Holmans P, Jones L, Devlin B, Klei L, Barmada MM, Demirci FY, Dekosky ST, Lopez OL, Passmore P, Owen MJ, O'Donovan MC, Mayeux R, Kamboh MI, Williams J. Genome-wide association study of Alzheimer's disease with psychotic symptoms. *Molecular Psychiatry*. 2011 Oct 18. Published online ahead of print.

Holtzman DM. CSF biomarkers for Alzheimer's disease: Current utility and potential future use. *Neurobiology of Aging*. 2011 Dec;32 Suppl 1:S4–9.

Hock C, Nitsch RM. Clinical observations with AN-1792 using TAPIR analyses. *Neurodegenerative Diseases*. 2005;2(5):273–76.

Kawas CH, Clark CM, Farlow MR, Knopman DS, Marson D, Morris JC, Thal LJ, Whitehouse PJ. Clinical trials in Alzheimer disease: Debate on the use of placebo controls. *Alzheimer Disease & Associated Disorders*. 1999 Jul–Sep;13(3):124–29.

Liddell BJ, Paul RH, Arns M, Gordon N, Kukla M, Rowe D, Cooper N, Moyle J, Williams LM. Rates of decline distinguish Alzheimer's disease and mild cognitive impairment relative to normal aging: Integrating cognition and brain function. *Journal of Integrative Neuroscience.* 2007 Mar;6(1):141–74.

Liu ZP, Wang Y, Zhang XS, Xia W, Chen L. Detecting and analyzing differentially activated pathways in brain regions of Alzheimer's disease patients. *Molecular BioSystems.* 2011 May;7(5):1441–52.

Pietrzak M, Rempala G, Nelson PT, Zheng JJ, Hetman M. Epigenetic silencing of nucleolar rRNA genes in Alzheimer's disease. *PLoS One (Public Library of Science).* 2011;6(7):e22585.

Rafii MS, Aisen PS. Recent developments in Alzheimer's disease therapeutics. *BioMed Central Medicine.* 2009 Feb 19;7:7.

Schneider LS, Sano M. Current Alzheimer's disease clinical trials: Methods and placebo outcomes. *Alzheimer's & Dementia.* 2009 Sep;5(5):388–97.

Schoonenboom NS, Reesink FE, Verwey NA, Kester MI, Teunissen CE, van de Ven PM, Pijnenburg YA, Blankenstein MA, Rozemuller AJ, Scheltens P, van der Flier WM. Cerebrospinal fluid markers for differential dementia diagnosis in a large memory clinic cohort. *Neurology.* 2011 Dec 14. Published online ahead of print.

CHAPTER 16

Dorgeret B, Khemtémourian L, Correia I, Soulier JL, Lequin O, Ongeri S. Sugar-based peptidomimetics inhibit amyloid β-peptide aggregation. *European Journal of Medicinal Chemistry.* 2011 Dec;46(12):5959–69.

Drew B, Leeuwenburgh C. Aging and the role of reactive nitrogen species. *Annals of the New York Academy of Sciences.* 2002 Apr;959:66–81.

Harding A. Diabetes Doubles Alzheimer's Risk. CNN. September 19, 2011. www.cnn.com. Accessed December 23, 2011.

Morris MC. Diet and Alzheimer's disease: What the evidence shows. *Medscape General Medicine.* 2004 Jan 15;6(1):48.

Morris MC, Evans DA, Bienias JL, Tangney CC, Bennett DA, Aggarwal N, Schneider J, Wilson RS. Dietary fats and the risk of incident Alzheimer disease. *Archives of Neurology.* 2003 Feb;60(2):194–200.

Phivilay A, Julien C, Tremblay C, Berthiaume L, Julien P, Giguère Y, Calon F. High dietary consumption of trans fatty acids decreases brain docosahexaenoic acid but does not alter amyloid-beta and tau pathologies in the 3xTg-AD model of Alzheimer's disease. *Neuroscience.* 2009 Mar 3;159(1):296–307.

Ringman JM, Frautschy SA, Cole GM, Masterman DL, Cummings JL. A potential role of the curry spice curcumin in Alzheimer's disease. *Current Alzheimer Research.* 2005 Apr;2(2):131–36.

Viña J, Lloret A, Giraldo E, Badia MC, Alonso MD. Antioxidant pathways in Alzheimer's disease: Possibilities of intervention. *Current Pharmaceutical Design.* 2011 Sep 20. Published online ahead of print.

CHAPTER 17

Andel R, Crowe M, Pedersen NL, Fratiglioni L, Johansson B, Gatz M. Physical exercise at midlife and risk of dementia three decades later: A population-based study of Swedish twins. *Journals of Gerontology Series A: Biological Sciences and Medical Sciences.* 2008 Jan;63(1):62–66.

Logan D, Kiemel T, Dominici N, Cappellini G, Ivanenko Y, Lacquaniti F, Jeka JJ. The many roles of vision during walking. *Experimental Brain Research*. 2010 Oct;206(3):337–50.

Rogers ME, Fernandez JE, Bohlken RM. Training to reduce postural sway and increase functional reach in the elderly. *Journal of Occupational Rehabilitation*. 2001 Dec;11(4):291–98.

Tak E CP, van Uffelen J GZ, Chin A Paw MJ, van Mechelen W, Hopman-Rock M. Adherence to exercise programs and determinants of maintenance in older adults with mild cognitive impairment. *Journal of Aging and Physical Activity*. 2012 Jan;20(1):32–46.

Winward C, Sackley C, Meek C, Freebody J, Esser P, Soundy A, Barker K, Hilton Jones D, Minns Lowe C, Elsworth C, Paget S, Tims M, Parnell R, Patel S, Wade D, Dawes H. Supporting community-based exercise in long-term neurological conditions: Experience from the Long-term Individual Fitness Enablement (LIFE) project. *Clinical Rehabilitation*. 2011 Jul;25(7):579–87.

Zhou R, Deng J, Zhang M, Zhou HD, Wang YJ. Association between bone mineral density and the risk of Alzheimer's disease. *Journal of Alzheimer's Disease*. 2011;24(1):101–8.

CHAPTER 18

Alzheimer's disease. MedicineNet.com. www.medicinenet.com. Accessed June 9, 2011.

Bartolini M, Coccia M, Luzzi S, Provinciali L, Ceravolo MG. Motivational symptoms of depression mask preclinical Alzheimer's disease in elderly subjects. *Dementia and Geriatric Cognitive Disorders*. 2005;19(1):31–36.

Birchenall JM, Streight ME, Streight E. *Mosby's Textbook for Home Care Aide*. 2nd ed. St. Louis, MI: Mosby Publishing; 2003.

Brawley EC. *Designing for Alzheimer's Disease*. New York: Wiley; 1997.

Callone P, Vasiloff B, Brumback R, Manternach J, Kudlacek C, Callone PR. *Alzheimer's Disease: A Handbook for Caregivers, Family and Friends*. Sydney, Australia: Accessible Publishing Systems; 2008.

Caring for an Alzheimer's Patient. Alzheimer's Disease. www.alzheimersdisease.com. Accessed June 7, 2011.

Cohen GD, Firth KM, Biddle S, Lloyd Lewis MJ, Simmens S. The first therapeutic game specifically designed and evaluated for Alzheimer's disease. *American Journal of Alzheimer's Disease and other Dementias*. 2008 Dec–2009 Jan;23(6):540–51.

Douglas S, James I, Ballard C. Non-pharmacological interventions in dementia. *Advances in Psychiatric Treatment*. 2004;10:171–77.

Forstmeier S, Maercker A, Maier W, van den Bussche H, Riedel-Heller S, Kaduszkiewicz H, Pentzek M, Weyerer S, Bickel H, Tebarth F, Luppa M, Wollny A, Wiese B, Wagner M. Motivational reserve: Motivation-related occupational abilities and risk of mild cognitive impairment and Alzheimer disease. *Psychology and Aging*. 2011 Aug 29. Published online ahead of print.

Kong EH, Evans LK, Guevara JP. Nonpharmacological intervention for agitation in dementia: A systematic review and meta-analysis. *Aging & Mental Health*. 2009 Jul;13 (4):512–20.

Living with Alzheimer's. Alzheimer's Association. www.alz.org. Accessed June 8, 2011.

Lunde, A. Dementia Journey Affects Family relationships. Mayo Clinic. www.mayoclinic.com. Accessed June 7, 2011.

O'Neil ME, Freeman M, Christensen V, Telerant R, Addleman A, Kansagara D. A Systematic Evidence Review of Non-pharmacological Interventions for Behavioral Symptoms of Dementia [Internet]. *VA Evidence-based Synthesis Program Reports.* 2011 Mar.

Ritchter R, Ritcher BZ. *Alzheimer's Disease: A Physician's Guide to Practical Management.* Totowa, NJ: Humana Press; 2004.

Snyder L. Living Your Best with Early Stage Alzheimer's. North Branch, MN: Sunrise River Press; 2010.

Stevenson JP. Family stress related to home care of Alzheimer's disease patients and implications for support. *Journal of Neuroscience Nursing.* 1990 Jun;22(3):179–88.

Thomas P, Clément JP, Hazif-Thomas C, Léger JM. Family, Alzheimer's disease and negative symptoms. *International Journal of Geriatric Psychiatry.* 2001 Feb;16(2):192–202.

Tornatore JB, Grant LA. Family caregiver satisfaction with the nursing home after placement of a relative with dementia. *Journals of Gerontology Series B: Psychological Sciences and Social Sciences.* 2004 Mar;59(2):S80–88.

Villaume WA, Berger BA, Barker BN. Learning motivational interviewing: Scripting a virtual patient. *American Journal of Pharmaceutical Education.* 2006 Apr 15;70(2):33.

Williams AK. Motivation and dementia. *Topics in Geriatric Rehabilitation.* April/June 2005; 21(2):123–26.

CHAPTER 19

Albert SM, Marks J, Barrett V, Gurland B. Home health care and quality of life of patients with Alzheimer's disease. *American Journal of Preventative Medicine.* 1997 Nov–Dec;13(6 Suppl):63–68.

Gay CL, Lee KA, Lee SY. Sleep patterns and fatigue in new mothers and fathers. *Biological Research for Nursing.* 2004 Apr;5(4):311–18.

Gershon RRM, Pogorzelska M, Qureshi KA, Stone PW, Canton AN, Samar SM, Westra LJ, Damsky MR, Sherman M. Home health care patients and safety hazards in the home: Preliminary findings. *Advances in Patient Safety.* 2008 Aug.

Goodlin-Jones BL, Burnham MM, Gaylor EE, Anders TF. *Journal of Developmental & Behavioral Pediatrics.* 2001 Aug;22(4):226–33.

Grant LA, Kane RA, Stark AJ. Beyond labels: Nursing home care for Alzheimer's disease in and out of special care units. *Journal of the American Geriatric Society.* 1995 May;43(5):569–76.

Holstein M, Parks JA, Waymack MH. *Ethics, Aging, and Society: The Critical Turn.* New York: Springer; 2011.

Kadushin G. Home health care utilization: A review of the research for social work. *Health & Social Work.* 2004 Aug;29(3):219–44.

Pelluck P. Giving Alzheimer's Patients Their Way, Even Chocolate. New York Times. January 1, 2011:A1.

Rodiek S, Benyamin S, eds. *Outdoor Environments for People with Dementia.* Binghampton, NY: Haworth Press; 2007.

Varela G, Varona L, Anderson K, Sansoni J. Alzheimer's care at home: A focus on caregivers strain. *Professioni Infermieristiche (Nursing Professions).* 2011 Apr–Jun;64(2):113–17.

Zhu CW, Torgan R, Scarmeas N, Albert M, Brandt J, Blacker D, Sano M, Stern Y. Home health and informal care utilization and costs over time in Alzheimer's disease. *Home Health Care Services Quarterly.* 2008;27(1):1–20.

CHAPTER 20

[No authors listed]. The patient's confidence. *British Medical Journal*. 1971 Nov 6;4(5783):316.

Cummings JL, Frank JC, Cherry D, Kohatsu ND, Kemp B, Hewett L, Mittman B. Guidelines for managing Alzheimer's disease: Part II. Treatment. *American Family Physician*. 2002 Jun 15;65(12):2525–34.

Davies M. When Do You Break a Patient's Confidence? BBC. www.bbc.co.uk. Updated April 7, 2010. Accessed December 31, 2011.

de Fijter JW. Counselling the elderly between hope and reality. *Nephrology Dialysis Transplantation*. 2011 Jul;26(7):2079–81.

DeJong R, Osterlund OW, Roy GW. Measurement of quality-of-life changes in patients with Alzheimer's disease. *Clinical Therapeutics*. 1989 Jul–Aug;11(4):545–54.

Glazier RH, Dalby DM, Badley EM, Hawker GA, Bell MJ, Buchbinder R. Determinants of physician confidence in the primary care management of musculoskeletal disorders. *Journal of Rheumatology*. 1996 Feb;23(2):351–56.

Kylmä J, Isola A. [Nursing research on the dynamics of hope in the elderly: A review]. *Sairaanhoitajien Koulutussäätiö (Finland)*. 1997;9(2):66–75.

Index

About the Author

Naheed Ali, MD, is the author of *Diabetes and You: A Comprehensive, Holistic Approach* and *The Obesity Reality: A Comprehensive Approach to a Growing Problem*. He began writing professionally while still an undergraduate. Since then, he has appeared as a special guest on numerous talk shows and has been quoted in many national print magazines and TV websites across the United States. Additional information is available online at NaheedAli.com.